LINCOLN CHRISTIAN UNIVE   P9-DEO-918

Crisis Intervention Case Book

ALAN A. CAVAIOLA
Monmouth University

JOSEPH E. COLFORD
Georgian Court University

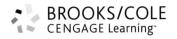

BROOKS/COLE
CENGAGE Learning™

Australia • Brazil • Japan • Korea • Mexico • Singapore • Spain • United Kingdom • United States

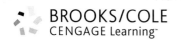
BROOKS/COLE
CENGAGE Learning™

Crisis Intervention Case Book
Alan A. Cavaiola and Joseph E. Colford

Acquisitions Editor: Seth Dobrin

Editorial Assistant: Rachel McDonald

Marketing Manager: Trent Whatcott

Marketing Assistant: Darlene Macanan

Marketing Communications Manager: Tami Strang

Project Management: Pre-Press PMG

Creative Director: Rob Hugel

Art Director: Caryl Gorska

Print Buyer: Paula Vang

Rights Acquisitions Account Manager, Text: Roberta Broyer

Production Service: Pre-Press PMG

Cover Designer: Cheryl Carrington

Cover Image: © Whit Richardson/Aurora/Getty Images

Compositor: Pre-Press PMG

© 2011, Brooks/Cole, Cengage Learning

ALL RIGHTS RESERVED. No part of this work covered by the copyright herein may be reproduced, transmitted, stored, or used in any form or by any means graphic, electronic, or mechanical, including but not limited to photocopying, recording, scanning, digitizing, taping, Web distribution, information networks, or information storage and retrieval systems, except as permitted under Section 107 or 108 of the 1976 United States Copyright Act, without the prior written permission of the publisher.

For product information and technology assistance, contact us at **Cengage Learning Customer & Sales Support, 1-800-354-9706**.

For permission to use material from this text or product, submit all requests online at **www.cengage.com/permissions**. Further permissions questions can be e-mailed to **permissionrequest@cengage.com**.

Library of Congress Control Number: 2009940810

ISBN-13: 978-0-618-94631-0

ISBN-10: 0-618-94631-4

Brooks/Cole
20 Davis Drive
Belmont, CA 94002-3098
USA

Cengage Learning is a leading provider of customized learning solutions with office locations around the globe, including Singapore, the United Kingdom, Australia, Mexico, Brazil, and Japan. Locate your local office at **www.cengage.com/global.**

Cengage Learning products are represented in Canada by Nelson Education, Ltd.

To learn more about Brooks/Cole, visit **www.cengage.com/brookscole**

Purchase any of our products at your local college store or at our preferred online store **www.CengageBrain.com.**

Printed in the United States of America
1 2 3 4 5 6 7 8 13 12 11 10

Brief Contents

123873

Contents

Preface

Our interest in writing this casebook began almost immediately after the completion of our earlier work, *A Practical Guide to Crisis Intervention*, in 2006. We still strongly believe that training in crisis intervention is an important component in any undergraduate or graduate program in psychology, counseling, social work, nursing, and other human services specialty areas. Our first book, however, provided a model of crisis intervention without enough case study material to bring crisis intervention to life, thus our interest in this casebook.

The purpose of this book was to serve as a supplement to our earlier work and to provide more extensive case examples in order to illustrate various types of personal and community crises as well as intervention strategies for them. This book, however, can also stand alone as a text for those interested in understanding crisis types and crisis intervention.

Our casebook includes other crisis types not included in the original book: crises found at adolescence, at midlife, in the workplace, and those due to health-related issues. We thought that the addition of these four chapters would broaden the field of study for those students seeking more information for their particular areas of professional interest.

Another driving force in writing this book was to make it not only instructor-friendly, but student-friendly as well. Instructors will find great utility in this book. Each chapter begins with discussion questions designed to get students thinking and talking about the chapter's crisis type. Then, after some introductory background information, the chapters present crisis case examples followed by actual intervention strategies, general guidelines for intervention, and suggestions for follow-up ("homework") activities for students. It is as if the format of each chapter presents to the instructor a built-in lesson plan for each class. Additionally, the 14 chapters lend themselves to a 14-week school semester.

Students will also find this book is clearly written and designed for the practitioner rather than the theoretician. The introductory material for each chapter provides more hard data than theory, and the cases themselves will resonate with students, having been taken from the lives of real people. We designed this book as more of a workbook than a textbook so that readers will find it to be informative, engaging, and very student-friendly.

Biographical Information

Alan A. Cavaiola, Ph.D. is a Professor in the Department of Psychological Counseling at Monmouth University. He began doing crisis intervention in 1975 while working in the outpatient mental health services at Monmouth Medical Center. He later went on to become Clinical Director of the substance abuse treatment programs at Monmouth Medical Center.

Dr. Cavaiola has published extensively in the field of addictions and has presented at many national and international conferences. Dr. Cavaiola has co-authored three books: *Toxic Co-workers* (which has been translated into six languages), *Assessment and Treatment of the DWI Offender,* and *A Practical Guide to Crisis Intervention.*

In addition to his teaching, Dr. Cavaiola is a Practicing Clinician, a Licensed Psychologist, a Licensed Clinical Alcohol/Drug Counselor, a Licensed Professional Counselor, and a New Jersey certified Disaster Response Crisis Counselor.

Joseph E. Colford, Ph.D. is an Associate Professor in the Psychology Department at Georgian Court University and is the Director of the Graduate Program in School Psychology. He has had extensive experience in public education as a School Psychologist, in private practice as a Licensed Psychologist, and in higher education as an Associate Professor. His experiences in working with school-age children in the aftermath of a variety of crisis types lead to his collaboration with Dr. Cavaiola in this casebook and in their earlier work *A Practical Guide to Crisis Intervention.*

Dr. Colford also created a graduate-level course, *School Crisis Prevention and Intervention,* for his program incorporating sound practices for crisis prevention and for crisis intervention with children, adolescents, and their schools and families. The political and social landscape of the 21st century convinced him that such a casebook was important for mental health professionals who work in a variety of settings.

Acknowledgments

We are grateful to so many people who have assisted us in bringing this case book to completion. First of all, we salute our wives, Jeanne and Carolann, and our sons Matthew, Michael, Jay, and Chris for their support and encouragement and for letting us take up more than our fair share of computer time in our home offices. We also want to acknowledge the reviewers of our initial manuscript for their insightful and helpful suggestions and Seth Dobrin, our editor at Cengage, who stayed with this project and moved it along after its transition from Houghton-Mifflin. Our thanks also go to our copy editor, Shannon Walsh, and to our project manager at Pre-Press, Timothy Vitagliano, for his critical role in getting this case book ready to be handed over to the folks who run the presses.

To our graduate students for sharing their insights and experiences pertaining to crisis intervention, we extend our gratitude. To those who shared stories of their own personal crisis experiences with us for this book—particularly Danielle, Courtney, and Kristin—we thank you. A special thanks also goes to those other professionals and caring individuals who provided us with invaluable assistance in completing these chapters, specifically Eileen Allen and Linda Altieri who work tirelessly for victims of sexual assault, and our Middletown friends, Detective Joe Capriotti, Janet Dluhi, and Eileen Theall, who told us of the tragedy and the resiliency of a community devastated after 9/11.

Crisis Intervention Case Book Reviewer List

Casey Ann Barrio	University of North Texas
Alfred Carlozzi	Oklahoma State University
Mimi daSilva	Georgian Court University
Noreen Glover	University of Texas-Pan American
Elizabeth Stroot	Lakeland College

Crisis Intervention

An Introduction

DISCUSSION QUESTIONS

When was the last time a friend called on you to help work through a crisis event in his or her life? What was that experience like for you? What did you do to assist with the resolution of the crisis?

Close your eyes for a moment and think back to a particular crisis you had in your own life. Who was most helpful to you in dealing with it? What did they do that was so helpful?

Discuss what you think are some of the typical types of crises that an individual faces in the 21st century. What crises do larger organizations face (such as schools or communities)?

INTRODUCTION

Evening news programs and morning newspapers are replete with high-profile, attention-grabbing headlines, stories of local tragedies that often override larger stories of more international significance: a neighborhood fire kills multiple members of a single family; the reckless driver kills a woman and her baby in the carriage she pushed; and the high school star football player hangs himself at home, much to the numbed disbelief of all who knew him.

Most individuals who experience a crisis event in their lives are able to re-cover sufficiently after a few weeks without the intervention of the mental health system; the presence of a personal support system consisting of family, friends, neighbors, clergy, and other members of their social network is quite curative and therapeutic, making the psychologist in private practice superfluous in most cases. Caplan (1964) thought that a typical crisis state lasted from four to six weeks and that one's own support network helped one through it. Even those exposed to severe trauma see their symptoms subside within three months, with only 25% developing stress disorders. The psychologist who labored long and hard assisting the rescue workers at Ground Zero, the site of the collapsed Twin Towers after the terrorist attacks of 9/11, replied, "I call my mother," when asked what she did to help herself after being immersed in the tragedy day after day.

Other victims of a crisis may talk to a friend, a family member, or the clergy, or a favorite teacher or sports coach; they may attend a service at their church or temple, carry on the normal activities that keep them in contact with familiar faces, or they may anonymously call a hotline for support. In recounting a similar feeling of loss and depression that she felt after a personal tragedy as a teenager, the widow of a 9/11 victim told her neighbor that what helped her through that earlier event was the fact she went to church. "I always felt safe in church," she said; "I remembered that, whenever I was in church, there was nothing to fear."

The passage of time and their own support system is often all that is needed for crisis victims to return to some sense of equilibrium. However, there are times when they require more than just the passage of time to resolve the emotional aftermath of the event.

For example, resilient individuals recover more quickly than those who had difficulties with transition or with change before the crisis, whereas others possess additional vulnerability factors that put them at risk for a more severe crisis reaction. These factors include an avoidant coping style, preexisting mental illness, poor regulation of emotion, poor problem-solving skills, history of other trauma, low self-esteem, social isolation, and poverty or financial stress (Brock, 2002). Ascetic loners with little family or social support will be left to fend for themselves after a crisis, whereas victims who typically are surrounded by large, extended families will have those resources to help them through it.

CRISIS DEFINED

The word *crisis* itself is rich with meaning. The two symbols that combine to create the character *crisis* in Chinese writing mean *danger* and *opportunity*. Although seemingly mutually exclusive terms, they actually are quite compatible in the field of crisis intervention. *Danger* is inherent in any precipitating crisis event; it is those physical, emotional, and psychological challenges that strain the resources of individuals in coping with crisis successfully, something that propels them into a state of disequilibrium and disorder. Crises of all types (see page 5) can contribute to this *danger*.

Opportunity, on the other hand, refers to the crisis outcome that provides victims with the chance to emerge from the event successfully, perhaps even stronger than before. For example, crisis victims who recover with the understanding that they were "survivors," that they had considerable inner resources to draw upon, and that they truly had a strong support group behind them

realize that the crisis was indeed an *opportunity* for personal growth. These survivors become better able to cope with future crises and change their lives in a positive direction by becoming helpers or advocates for others (Brock, Nickerson, Reeves, Jimerson, Lieberman, & Feinberg, 2009).

Stories abound of parents who, after suffering the deaths of their children through random violence or a drunk driver's collision, recover to form support groups to assist other parents who experience a similar crisis, lobby Congress for changes in the laws pertaining to these events, and speak with other groups and individuals about overcoming tragedy. Few examples of this kind of outcome are more profound than that of the family of Melissa Aptman, a young college student who was murdered just two weeks before her graduation. To honor her memory, prevent violence, and assist victims of violence, Melissa's family and friends established the Melissa Institute for Violence Prevention and Treatment in her hometown of Miami, Florida. This nonprofit organization is committed to the prevention of violence through education, and it sponsors research specific to this topic. This crisis response is a terrific example of the *opportunity* inherent in the word *crisis*.

The word *crisis* also is derived from the Greek word, *krinein*, meaning *to decide*. The connotation of this word suggests that individuals in the midst of crisis have a choice to make, whether to meet the demands of the crisis (i.e., address and cope with the emotional aftermath in a productive way) or to avoid them altogether. These decisions have a profound impact on the ultimate outcome for the person after the crisis has ended. Does the victim of a sexual assault, for example, decide to pursue her attacker through law enforcement and rape advocacy resources to keep him from assaulting other women, or do shame and guilt lead her to stay silent about her assault, telling no one about it?

Crises can be random and unpredictable or predictable. There is a consensus among many mental health professionals regarding what constitutes a crisis. Elements of crisis include the following:

- perception of an event, either expected or unexpected, as being extremely negative, significant, and threatening
- realization that traditional coping methods are not sufficient to lessen the impact of the event
- sense of hopelessness, powerlessness, and loss of control
- creation of increased fear, tension, and/or confusion
- creation of a high level of subjective discomfort
- creation of a state of disequilibrium

Crisis generally disrupts people's routines, those reassuring and predictable things people do day-by-day to help them manage their lives; it forces people from their typical comfort zones, keeping them, at least temporarily, from getting their off-balance world back into balance. Crisis events typically occur suddenly, unexpectedly, and without warning, leaving the individual with relatively little time to adjust and to prepare (Carlson, 1997). Those gradual and predictable events, like the death of a loved one after a lengthy illness, generate less traumatic stress than those that are sudden and unpredictable, like a school shooting or an accidental death (Brock et al., 2009). These latter events leave the survivors with little time to make cognitive and emotional adjustments (Saylor, Belter, & Stokes, 1997).

COMMON CRISIS REACTIONS

Many of the crisis reactions listed below are normal reactions to traumatic events. These reactions subside over time for most people, but those who experience a crisis vary in their reactions to it. Those crisis reactions that are normal and that are to be expected in the aftermath of crisis include the following:

Physical	Cognitive
■ sleep disturbances	■ flashbacks to the event
■ fatigue and exhaustion	■ inattention
■ stomachache	■ poor concentration
■ headache	■ memory loss
■ problems breathing	■ indecision
■ rapid heartbeat	■ thoughts of "going crazy"
■ startle reactions	■ poor problem-solving
Emotional	**Behavioral**
■ grief or depression	■ social withdrawal
■ fear or anxiety	■ need to cling to others
■ anger	■ increase in drug or alcohol use
■ survivor guilt	■ suspiciousness
■ shock or denial	■ aggressiveness
■ confusion	■ behavioral regression
■ emotional liability	■ self-destructive acts
■ helplessness	■ temper tantrums

Despite the commonality of these reactions, not all individuals will be affected equally by crisis. For the reasons discussed above, the need for crisis intervention varies from person to person. Some will require considerable assistance, and others will need very little, if any. The "one size fits all" approach does not work in crisis intervention. In fact, providing it for those who do not need it may do more harm than good by convincing individuals that they were unable to help themselves and that the crisis event was too overwhelming for them. Similarly, the typical reactions of shock and denial also serve as protective mechanisms for individuals after crisis. These reactions allow people temporarily to avoid the crisis, to "dull the pain" of the event, providing them with time while they begin, slowly but surely, to come to terms with it and to develop more effective coping strategies. To challenge this denial in crisis victims might force them to confront a trauma before they are ready to do so, eliminating the protective value of these crisis reactions.

CRISIS TYPES

Crisis can be considered to be any one of three different types (Brammer, 1985): *developmental crises, traumatic event crises,* and *existential crises.* This book also has included a fourth type, *psychiatric crises.*

Developmental Crises   Erikson (1963) was a developmental theorist who conceptualized development as occurring in eight different stages, each one providing its own crisis or challenge. A primary theme of his theory involves the ongoing issue of identity formation and the challenge of individuals to redefine themselves continually as they encounter new experiences and life changes.

Individuals go through Erikson's stages from the infants' initial development of a trusting and reassuring bond with a caregiver through subsequent stages in which they consolidate a sense of autonomy and independence, mastery of social and academic skills, and ultimately form a sense of identity in adolescence. Crises, he proposed, could develop in any one of these school-age stages:

- The crisis of the "terrible twos" when, after ambulation allowed them to be quite adventurous and independent for some time, toddlers realize that this new-found independence put them "out there" into a world that turned out to be a lonely and frightening place.
- The crisis of the children who realize that they cannot compete successfully with their peers in an academic or social setting.
- The adolescents who experience a sense of isolation and despair after being unable to decide who they are or where they are going.

The crises of adulthood also are varied, according to Erikson. Issues related to the development of intimate relationships, dealing with increasingly difficult adolescent children and their own aging parents, retirement from one's professional career, and adjusting to aging and increasing physical limitations were some of the challenges inherent in these later developmental stages. Crises specific to these later stages include:

- separation or divorce
- career problems
- rebellious children
- death of parents or spouse
- menopause
- "empty nest" realization

- health problems
- loneliness and despair

Traumatic Event Crises   This crisis typically involves a clear precipitating event which one cannot predict or control. Unlike some of the more predictable crises inherent in the above developmental stages, the crisis event is more random and unpredictable, something that individuals have no forewarning of and, as a result, it forces them to rely on familiar coping strategies to deal with it effectively. Development and crisis events are inextricably linked, however, because the developmental stage in which the event occurs has a profound impact on the individual's ability to manage crisis, which ultimately impacts the victim's outcome.

Crisis events can affect the lives of individuals or they can have a profound impact on entire communities. They can be human-made crises or natural or environmental disasters. Terrorists' attacks on the Twin Towers on 9/11 or the Murrah Federal Building bombing in Oklahoma City are extreme examples of human-made crises, as are school shootings that claim the lives of students and staff alike. Fatal car accidents, sexual assault, and other random acts of violence devastate not only individual victims, but their families and friends as well.

Natural disasters include any adverse weather condition that lays waste to entire communities and claims thousands of victims in an instant: hurricanes, tornados, drought, and tsunamis. Other environmental disasters include the spillage of toxic chemicals in a highway truck accident and the spread of a deadly flu virus without sufficient inoculation capabilities to combat it.

Existential Crises   An existential crisis takes place when the individual begins to question the meaning of life or the meaninglessness of one's existence, the lack of connectedness to other people, or the futility of one's work or profession (Cavaiola & Colford, 2006). Probably the most difficult of all the crisis types to identify, the person experiencing an existential crisis may experience other symptoms like physical ailments, lethargy, or other depressive problems. A traumatic event may serve as a precipitant to an existential crisis; for example, the middle-aged mother who loses her only child in an auto accident begins to question the meaning of her own life, or the highly publicized suicide of a popular high school student leads other adolescents to question the worth of their own lives.

Psychiatric Crises   People who meet the criteria for any of the disorders found in the *Diagnostic and Statistical Manual of Mental Disorders (DSM-IV)* of the American Psychiatric Association can find themselves in crisis if they pay insufficient attention to their symptoms. The individual with panic disorder who experiences another panic attack while on the subway going to work, the individual with bipolar disorder who enters a manic state and starts calling the president with a plan for world peace, and the person with major depressive disorder who contemplates suicide are all examples of people in psychiatric crisis. Not all individuals with a psychiatric diagnosis, however, find themselves in crisis, but the existence of such a condition can significantly compromise their ability to cope with a crisis when it occurs.

ELEMENTS OF CRISIS INTERVENTION

Crisis intervention is short-term and crisis-specific. That is, its goal is to help the crisis victim recover from it and return to a previous level of functioning. It is not psychotherapy. The purpose of crisis intervention is not to "rescue" the victim of crisis. People in the crisis field who harbor these "rescue fantasies" encourage dependency in the victim and make the mistake of maintaining control of a situation when this control should be placed in the hands of the individual in crisis. The notion of *opportunity* in the definition of crisis can be considered the chance for the victim to acquire more effective problem-solving skills, greater self-awareness and fulfillment, and more positive feelings of competence and self-efficacy.

Crisis intervention should empower individuals to rise from the ashes and to resume control of their lives with a regained sense of hopefulness. To be effective, therefore, crisis intervention must be both empowering and flexible. Young (2001) suggested that the primary goal of crisis intervention was to help victims restore control over their lives. Fraser (1998) maintained that intervening in a crisis should assist the victim in striving for something more than just returning to a pre-crisis level of functioning, maintaining that crisis should be an opportunity to get people to grow to even a higher, more competent level. Recognizing the inner resourcefulness and resilience of crisis victims is a first step in helping them accomplish this goal.

Resourceful individuals have a variety of strategies that have served them well in past times of stress. The crisis counselor's belief in the victim's resourcefulness is essential, since it recognizes that the road toward crisis resolution lies in the hands of the crisis victim. Since the individual's response to crisis depends upon a myriad of different factors that are distinctly different from one person to the next, effective crisis intervention also must be flexible. The crisis counselor must be able to make a quick evaluation of many factors that contribute to the crisis reaction of the victim. Some of these factors include:

- The victim's cognitive appraisal of the crisis event —that is, what they think of it, how they evaluate it and answer questions such as: How or why did it happen? Am I to blame or am I responsible? Have I done something wrong to deserve it? How can I go on? Will I ever feel better? Can I really survive in such a tragic world?

- The context in which it occurred —context is defined by the type of crisis it was; whether the individual was the sole victim or one of many; their age and developmental level; cultural, religious, and ethnic practices or beliefs about why crisis happens; the reactions of and support from family and friends.

Crisis intervention cannot be effective without appreciating these factors as well as the manner in which the individual interacts with them. To be cognizant of these influences is to create a template that will guide the crisis counselor's response to the crisis victim in a meaningful way.

EFFECTIVE CRISIS COUNSELORS

The core conditions of sound counseling are universal: empathy, genuineness, acceptance, and positive regard (Carkhuff, 1969; Rogers, 1951). Each is essential to the establishment of a sound therapeutic alliance. Empathy allows the therapist to communicate to the client their understanding of their pain, whereas genuineness is the openness and honesty of therapists who are comfortable with themselves as well as with their clients. Acceptance and positive regard are the therapist's acceptance of all clients, regardless of differences, and their consistent and unwavering caring for them.

Besides these core counseling values, however, crisis intervention requires additional traits. Some of these important traits include (Cavaiola & Colford, 2006):

- **Tolerance for Ambiguity** — The ability to enter a high stress environment without at first fully understanding the event itself or the victim's involvement in it is a critical trait for the crisis counselor.

- **A Calm, Neutral Demeanor** — The counselor must be able to maintain a calm, reassuring demeanor to manage the waves of emotion expressed by the victim. Remaining neutral and not being shocked by the strong feelings expressed by the client also are critical. This demeanor will show the client that it is safe to communicate strong emotions without overpowering or frightening the counselor. Additionally, the counselor can serve as a role model of strength and serenity for the client to emulate in the face of the crisis.

- **Tenacity** — It may only be the determination and tenacity of the counselor that will allow them to "hang in there" with the client and to persist through the crisis until a resolution is reached.

- **Optimism** — The counselor's belief that people are resilient and resourceful creatures, capable of recovering from horrific circumstances and emerging (perhaps) stronger than before is a core value in crisis intervention. Without this belief, the counselor would have difficulty developing an action plan for the client.

- **Adventurousness** — The unpredictable nature of crisis, the sense of never knowing what to expect, and its frenetic pace all cry out for adventurousness in any individual seeking this kind of work.

- **Flexibility** — As the counselor observes client needs and as crisis demands shift and change over time, they must also have the ability to adapt to these changes and to be flexible enough to adjust the course of the intervention.

- **Confidence** — The counselor's self-knowledge and a strong belief in one's self-efficacy in helping others are critical ingredients for success in crisis work.
- **Little Need to Rescue** — As mentioned above, the counselor's "rescue fantasy" invites over involvement with a client, tends to assume ownership of the problem, and obscures objectivity in crisis work.
- **Capacity for Listening** — The crisis counselor must be able to demonstrate effective listening skills and all that listening implies. The counselor with a capacity for listening knows when to let the victim lead the way, when to be active in gathering information, and how to avoid being too intrusive with a distressed victim wishing to talk.
- **Awareness of Trauma Indicators** — The counselor must be prepared to make decisions based upon observations of the client's response to crisis. Are there more critical safety issues that should be addressed? Medical concerns? Need to move to a more secure environment?
- **Openness to Individual Crisis Reactions** — Because crisis victims bring to the experience their own unique contexts consisting of family relationships, learning histories, unmet and satisfied needs, and their own unique modes of perceiving and responding to the world around them, the effective crisis counselor will not enter this encounter with any preconceived notions about how the client *should* react to crisis. Rather, the counselor will understand the client by listening to their expression of the crisis experience.
- **Capacity for Information Management** — When information floods the counselor, they must be able to sort it out and make an assessment of the client pertinent to the action plan.

CRISIS INTERVENTION TECHNIQUES

A rule of thumb offered by the National Organization for Victim Assistance (NOVA), the nation's oldest victim advocacy group founded in 1975, is that the sooner the crisis intervention services are offered, the better. Even though there is no way for anyone to predict when crisis will strike, who will be affected, or the scope and nature of the crisis, NOVA reports that early response to victims of a crisis may prevent or greatly reduce crisis symptoms and their impact.

In training for its Crisis Response Teams which respond to communities affected by crisis, NOVA (Young, 2001) emphasized certain core crisis intervention techniques and some hints for helping crisis victims in the aftermath of trauma. These techniques are listed below:

1. **Safety and security**
   - Ensure the physical safety of the individual.
   - If they are not safe, keep them informed about the extent of the threat (if a rapist is still at large, gather information about his likely whereabouts).

- Assess need for emergency medical aid.
- If responding to a telephone crisis call, ask, "Are you safe now?"
- Make sure that the victim *feels* safe. (Is the victim removed from the scene of the crisis? Is he or she cold and uncomfortable? Has the assailant been apprehended?)
- Assure victims of confidentiality (or clearly explain limits of confidentiality to them).
- Promote opportunities for them to regain control of events.

2. **Hints for helping**
   - Sit down to talk.
   - Ask the victims where they would feel safest talking to you and move to that location.
   - Identify yourself (and your agency) clearly.
   - If possible, keep the media away from the victims or help them in responding to media questions.
   - Find out about any loved ones they are concerned about and try to ease these concerns through some action. (For example, the mother who has been a victim on the way home from work may be worried about her children at home; help her contact a neighbor or relative to go to the home to provide childcare.)
   - Give them permission to express any reactions and respond nonjudgmentally. Say: "You have a right to be upset over this tragedy, so don't be afraid to tell me what you are thinking."

3. **Respond to the need for nurturing**
   - Be wary of being a "rescuer" whom the victim will become dependent.
   - Take care of practical things that need to be done but are beyond the victim's ability to accomplish at this time. (For example, arrange to have a rape victim's friend bring a change of clothes to her, provided the forensic examination is completed and permission is given to do so.) However, do not assume that you know what the victims need; take their lead in determining these things.
   - Offer to provide childcare, transportation, make telephone calls, and so on.

4. **Help victims to re-establish a sense of control over the small things, then the larger ones, in their lives**
   - It is important to allow them to make decisions for themselves and to take an active role in planning their future.
   - Offer a sense of control by asking them simple questions involving choices that are easily made, such as:
   - "What name would you like me to use in talking to you?"

- "Where would you like to sit while we talk?"
- "Would you like a glass of water?"

5. **Allow for *ventilation* and *validation***

   a. ***ventilation*** – The process of allowing the victims to "tell their story."

      - They may need to tell it over and over again, as they try to put the pieces together and to cognitively organize the event to make sense of it.

      - They may need help in finding the right words to express their feelings ("outrage" may be more expressive of their feelings than "anger," just as "crash" describes a drunk driving death more accurately than "accident" by suggesting the criminal element of the act).

   b. ***validation*** – The process through which the counselor makes it clear that most reactions to horrific events are "normal."

      - Validation should be content-specific; rather than saying, "I can't imagine how upset you are," it is preferable to say, "I can't imagine how upset you are about your son's death in the car crash."

      - Validate their experience as unique, telling them that their reactions are "not uncommon."

      - Repeat victims' actual phrases that they use to describe the experience; if they claim that they cannot sleep at night because they are afraid, an appropriate response would be, "It's not unusual for you to be afraid after such a terrifying experience. If you can't sleep at night, that only shows how afraid you are."

      - Assure them that they are not "crazy," it is just that their lives have been thrown into chaos.

In talking with victims, NOVA first suggests that the counselors encourage them to talk about the event, including all details about whom they were with and what they saw, heard, said, or did. Keeping the interview focused on specific, concrete details of the event will assist victims in creating some order in their minds about it. Second, victims should be encouraged to describe their own reactions and responses, with the counselor validating these reactions as they are expressed.

Asking victims about the events that followed the crisis is also important, because this information will reveal whether victims have gained additional support and compassion from their support network or simply suffered other indignities from a rejecting or absent family and friends network. Since victims' reactions to crisis can take many different forms over a period of time, counselors should not assume anything; the controlled calm at the present time may change into periods of tearfulness or rage in a few weeks.

Other NOVA suggestions:

Don't Say Things Like	Do Say Things Like
Your feelings ...	Your reactions ...
I understand	You are safe now (if true).
It sounds like ...	I'm glad you're here with me now.
I'm glad you can share those feelings.	I'm glad you're talking with me now.
You're lucky that ...	I am sorry it happened.
It'll take some time, but you'll get over it.	It wasn't your fault.
I can imagine how you feel.	Your reaction is not an uncommon response to such a terrible thing.
Don't worry; it's going to be all right.	
Try to be strong for your children.	It must have been really upsetting to see that.
Calm down and try to relax.	
	I can't imagine how terrible you are feeling.
	You are not going crazy.
	Things may never be the same, but they can get better.

Finally, to help crisis victims regain control of their lives, providing them with information about the crisis and what will come next is critical. Practical information regarding subsequent legal issues in the event an assailant is prosecuted, the possible relocation of a victim in the aftermath of a flood or house fire, and information about medical issues and their treatment are just some of these areas in which information would be helpful. Equally important, counselors should provide victims with information regarding possible longer-term crisis reactions which they might experience over the course of weeks, months, or even years. These reactions might include difficulties with sleep or appetite, recurring feelings of anger or anxiety, unavoidable reminders of the event, and the ongoing reactions of significant others (overprotectiveness, revulsion, blame for the event, or avoidance of it altogether).

CULTURAL CONSIDERATIONS IN CRISIS INTERVENTION

"Traumatic events do not exist in a vacuum. Like other social phenomena, they should be understood within the social and cultural context in which they occur." (Young, 1998, p. 42)

Culture influences how a crisis event is perceived and what meaning is assigned to it. Particularly when the event involves death, crisis responders must be prepared to understand the survivor's cultural and religious attitudes toward death in order to be able to assist them in the grieving process (Athey & Moody-Williams, 2003). Young (1998) offered a protocol to be followed in crisis work across cultures; she suggested that crisis workers:

- Understand the meaning of death, life, and suffering and pain in that culture.

- Ask the survivors what they would like you to do.

- Be aware of the appropriateness of specific communication techniques such as eye contact, integrating food and drink in discussions, body language, and so on.

- Understand access rituals and participate in them as allowed or requested (such as those involving ceremony, food, and expressions of good will).

- Explain the purpose of the intervention and the need for reciprocal questions. Even though many cultures find questions intrusive, they are the only way to clarify differences in language and customs.

- Express an appreciation and respect for the culture's strengths in coping with trauma.

- Express a willingness to learn about the ethnic group involved.

- Acknowledge your limitations and differences regarding the inability to speak their language and the lack of understanding of their customs and rituals.

- Dress appropriately; men wear suits and women wear dresses in most cultures, so the attire must be appropriate and congruent with the culture's expectations.

Crisis workers should take great care in being able to identify the culture-related needs of the community; they should know how to gain access to interpreters, religious figures, or other "culture brokers" — those individuals identified as representing that particular group. Different cultural groups also have different values, beliefs and certain preferences for accessing social support (Brock et al., 2009). Understanding these preferences prior to making an intervention is critical, lest the intervention appear intrusive and inappropriate to the survivor. Racial and ethnic minorities who turn to extended family members for support in times of need may prefer the presence of an aunt, an uncle, or a grandparent to that of a trained professional in order to heal. Understanding this preference should guide the nature and extent of the crisis responder's work.

THE LAPC MODEL: PUTTING IT ALL TOGETHER

Cavaiola and Colford's LAPC model (2006) provides a comprehensive model of crisis intervention that incorporates each of the components of crisis management described above. Their model involves four simple steps: **L**isten, **A**ssess, **P**lan, **C**ommit.

Listen   This first step should communicate three important messages to the crisis victim: they are safe, they are heard, and they are in control. Allowing victims to talk about their emotional experiences during and after the crisis without reacting in a judgmental way is perhaps the most important of all four steps in this model. Putting all the core counseling skills of empathy, genuineness, and unconditional acceptance of the victim into practice is critical. Using active listening techniques reassures victims that the counselor understands and is empathic to their own unique responses to the event; these techniques also facilitate communication from victims and encourage them to expand on the issues they raise.

Listening is an active process that involves the counselor's attention to both verbal and nonverbal messages communicated by the crisis victim. Listening skills — including clarifying, paraphrasing, and summarizing the client's verbal messages to depict accurately the victims' experience of the crisis — are invaluable tools in crisis intervention.

Assess   Being able to make an assessment of all the verbal and nonverbal communications received from the victim is important in directing the course of the intervention. The counselor must be attuned to information regarding the emotional health and welfare of victims and must be able to assess the depth of their emotional reactions (inconsolable? hopeless? angry? terrified?), their behavior (agitated? lethargic? clingy and dependent?), their thoughts (their perceptions of the event? the meaning it has for them? their perceptions of their ability to cope?), and the level of their support system (Are there family members or friends to support them after the crisis? Are they alone and solitary? Do they have people to call upon when in need?).

Answers to the above questions will assist the counselor in determining the course of the crisis intervention. These assessment considerations apply to crisis work with individuals as well as with larger systems such as schools and entire communities. For example, people involved with crisis intervention must also be able to determine the emotional health of a school staff after a school crisis, an important step in planning a school-wide intervention. (See school crisis and community response chapters later in this book.)

Plan   The outcome of crisis intervention actually is twofold: First, help the individuals recover from the emotional impact of the event. Second, communicate to the victims a sense of hope and empowerment by assisting them in developing a plan for the future, both immediate and longer-term. Planning, however, cannot be accomplished without the first two steps being implemented effectively: That is, listening and assessing the individual and their post-crisis situation provide the counselor with information specific to that individual and then bring them to the planning stage. The assumption of individuals' resourcefulness and resilience also contributes to the counselor's ability to develop a plan of action with the victim. It is the responsibility of the crisis counselor to assist victims in tapping into their inner resources in order to help them move forward with some kind of articulated plan, keeping in mind that the plan should not be imposed by the counselor, but rather developed along with the victim by using their strengths and problem-solving ability to determine the plan.

Those with a rich spiritual life might develop a post-crisis plan that involves contacting a familiar member of the clergy, whereas those with a large and supportive extended family might plan to contact them for specific needs or for general support. Still others without such a support system might plan to seek out the services of a mental health professional or simply to call a local hotline for solace. Finally, there are those victims who simply might plan to return to the familiar routine of work as a response and still others who prefer a support group at the local community health center for ventilation of their feelings related to the crisis. Several different plans, however, might be discussed with the victim along with the advantages and disadvantages of each one before a plan is chosen.

Commit   In this final step of the LAPC model, the victim agrees to commit to the plan developed above. This commitment empowers crisis victims and helps them regain some sense of equilibrium. The advantage of this step is that it allows the individual the opportunity to follow up with the counselor or with another member of the support system to choose another plan if the present one did not lead to a successful outcome.

SOME FINAL THOUGHTS

Crisis intervention is different from more typical approaches to psychotherapy. It requires the skills of a counselor as well as the knowledge of how crisis affects individuals and how they, in turn, respond to the crisis. Those involved in the field have to be a special breed; they have to possess qualities that are not necessarily found in other traditional therapists. They must be calm in the face of chaos, in control without taking control, and committed to a short-term, rather than long-term relationship with the people with whom they work. The provision of effective crisis intervention after an event ultimately can go a long way to precluding the need for longer-term psychotherapy.

This book has been written for graduate students as well as for community college and four-year college students in psychology, sociology, social work, counseling, education, nursing, and human services programs. Completing the readings and the assignments included in each chapter will not suffice to completely train students in the field of crisis intervention, but will expose students to many different crisis events and the most efficacious manner of responding to them. This book at least will provide a knowledge base regarding the process of crisis intervention for those entering the mental health field.

RECOMMENDATIONS FOR CHAPTER ENRICHMENT

SUGGESTED ACTIVITIES

1. Contact a local hotline and arrange to speak with one of the volunteers. Inquire about the kinds of calls volunteers receive and the specific techniques they use in assessing the emotional health of their callers. Ask if he or she would permit you to sit with them during a shift to observe calls and responses.

2. Survey the course offerings for various counseling programs in universities and colleges (this can be done online). How many of them provide courses in crisis intervention? Are separate courses offered in this area, or do the course descriptions address crisis intervention within the content of more generic counseling courses?

3. Select a group of your friends (or your current classmates) and discuss with them their own experiences with developmental crises. That is, find out what life stages were particularly problematic, vis-à-vis typical developmental (not event-related) crises? Were they crises related to adolescence? to the beginning of school as a youngster? to dating? to working?

4. Pay a visit to several funeral home directors in culturally and racially diverse communities. Ask them about the differences they see in the grieving rituals and practices among members of different groups. Do they approach families differently when discussing funeral arrangements? Do the arrangements themselves vary significantly from group to group?

2

Child Maltreatment

DISCUSSION QUESTIONS

What are some common disciplinary practices currently used by parents? Which practices are promoted by the popular press? by visiting child psychologists on your local talk shows?

Did you ever suspect that any friends or schoolmates were being maltreated by their parents? by someone else (clergy, teacher, coach)? What was your response?

What do you consider to be some of the typical stresses and strains in family life today that might influence how parents discipline their children?

INTRODUCTION

Child maltreatment is a tragedy of human error and human consequences. At its most basic level, child maltreatment denotes parenting failure—failure to protect the child from harm and to provide the positive aspects of a parent–child relationship that can foster development. The responsibility for this failure is shared not only by the individual parents for not adequately providing for their child, but also by society, for not adequately providing the parents with supports and safety nets (Wekerle & Wolfe, 2003).

Child maltreatment—the term used to include physical abuse, neglect, emotional abuse, and sexual abuse—is a significant problem, not only for America's youth but also for society in general.

In *Child Maltreatment, 2005*, the 16th and most recent annual report from the Department of Human Services' (DHHS) National Center on Child Abuse and Neglect Data System (NCANDS), 1,460 children were reported to have died as a result of child maltreatment that year, a rate of four children every day. Another 3.6 million children were accepted by state and local Child Protective Services (CPS) agencies for investigation or assessment of possible maltreatment; investigators substantiated 899,000 of these reported cases of maltreatment as true cases of abuse or neglect. Most of these children, approximately 564,572 of them, were victims of neglect, whereas another 150,000 child victims suffered physical abuse and 84,000 were victims of sexual abuse. According to this report, however, these data reflect only a small part of the problem, since many cases of abuse and neglect are never reported to the police or to social service agencies.

Maltreatment that occurs at an early age also can damage children in ways that extend well beyond the present day. Abuse and neglect contribute to a legacy of chronic problems for children that last well into adolescence and adulthood, including poor school performance, an increased need for special education services, juvenile delinquency, relationship difficulties, and adult criminality.

There are those children, however, who possess a sense of resiliency that protects them from these lifelong problems. A relatively new term in the psychological lexicon, *resilience* refers to the tendency for some children to develop psychological and behavioral competence, even in the face of other multiple risk factors (Weis, 2008). Those protective factors which make up resilience occur spontaneously and are rarely planned. Mash and Dosois (2003) list several such factors:

- an "easy" temperament that makes the child good-natured and easy to deal with
- high intelligence and scholastic competence
- effective problem-solving skills
- positive self-esteem
- the will to be or do something

Still others (Weis, 2008) described the protective value of a child who has a supportive relationship with a significant adult outside the family (a teacher, coach, or neighbor who values them and serves as a positive role model), the importance of adequate educational opportunities, or the possession of a special skill that is valued by others. These factors as well as others serve as buffers between some children and the possible toxic aftereffects of a legacy of maltreatment.

However, for those children who do not have a high level of resilience, abuse can have a high cost. Prevent Child Abuse America's Annual Report (2006) documented the following long-term effects of maltreatment:

- 90% of imprisoned male felons were abused as children
- 70% of teenage drug abusers reported abuse in childhood
- more than 50% of female criminals were sexually or physically abused as children
- 95% of teenage prostitutes have child abuse histories
- abused children often become adults who repeat these violent, abusive acts

HUMAN COSTS OF MALTREATMENT

The costs to society of child maltreatment are incalculable. Prevent Child Abuse America (2001) attempted to approximate its financial costs by looking at confirmed cases of abuse and neglect as well as the many unreported cases of maltreatment, those children simply considered to be "accident prone" and those other silent victims of maltreatment whose cries are never heard outside the family's walls. Its estimate of $94 billion per year was considered a conservative amount, at least.

Just some of the broad range of physical, psychological, cognitive, and social effects caused by this social ill includes:

Physical   Victims of physical abuse often suffer broken bones, bruising, burns, and a host of other perpetrator-inflicted wounds. Head trauma in particular can lead to neurological damage, and as many as 35% of physically abused children suffer injuries serious enough to require medical or psychiatric treatment to prevent long-term problems (Sedlak & Broadhurst, 1996). Approximately 25%–30% of infants who are victims of Shaken Baby Syndrome (SBS), the violent shaking of an infant back and forth, die from their injuries. Those infants who do not die from SBS, however, often suffer varying degrees of visual, motor, and cognitive impairments (National Center on Shaken Baby Syndrome, 2005).

Psychological   Children who suffer maltreatment experience an elevated risk of developing adverse health conditions and behaviors, including smoking, alcoholism, drug abuse, eating disorders, depression, suicide, and sexual promiscuity (Runyan, Wattam, Ikeda, Hassan, & Ramiro, 2002). Maltreated children also are more likely than non-abused peers to develop anxiety disorders, particularly Posttraumatic Stress Disorder (PTSD), a condition whose symptoms can last years beyond the abuse itself (Weis, 2008).

Other psychological conditions which often result from child maltreatment include a number of disruptive behavior disorders; Oppositional Defiant Disorder (ODD), a condition characterized by argumentativeness toward caregivers and teachers, poor self-control, and open defiance of established rules, is one such condition. Older children and adolescents also may develop Conduct Disorder (CD), a condition which involves serious antisocial behaviors such as stealing, cheating, animal cruelty, and physical assault (Weis, 2008).

Cognitive   Maltreated children also show more cognitive delays than their non-abused peers. These problems include difficulties with executive functioning (planning, organizing, and problem-solving), working memory (the ability to hold information temporarily in memory while performing some operation with it), and language (Eigsti & Cicchetti, 2004). Cognitive problems such as these are long-lasting and have a significant impact on a child's performance, both outside school and within it. Academic achievement of abused children also suffers significantly across all areas of functioning. The combination of the aforementioned behavioral difficulties associated with maltreatment as well as the cognitive sequelae of abuse contributes to the academic woes of abused children (Kolko, 2002).

Social   A history of troubled relationships with others, even into adulthood, often characterizes the life of the maltreated child. These children may experience a life-long pattern of absent or troubled relationships as they find it difficult to trust others and participate in interpersonal relationships (Prevent Child Abuse America, 2006). Infants and young children who suffer severe neglect also are at risk for a specific psychological condition known as Reactive Attachment Disorder (RAD). In the Inhibited Type of RAD, children do not initiate or respond, even to care-givers, when physical comfort is offered; because they avoid close contact with caregivers, they are difficult to soothe. The Disinhibited Type of RAD is marked by the child's indiscriminate sociability; that is, these children seek comfort and attention from anyone, including strangers, and are often described as "needy" and as requiring constant reassurance from others (Weis, 2008).

DEFINITIONAL ISSUES IN MALTREATMENT

The key piece of federal legislation that addressed child abuse and neglect was the Child Abuse Prevention and Treatment Act (CAPTA), originally enacted in 1974. The Act underwent several changes over the years, with the most re-cent changes taking place in 2003 when CAPTA was reauthorized by the Keep-ing Children and Families Safe Act of 2003.

In addition to providing federal funding to the states in support of preven-tion, assessment, and treatment of child abuse and neglect, CAPTA also set forth a minimum definition of abuse and neglect and identified the federal govern-ment's role in supporting research, technical assistance, and data collection activ-ities. It also established the Office on Child Abuse and Neglect and mandated Child Welfare Information Gateway, a service that provides access to print and electronic resources in many areas, including child abuse and neglect, for indivi-duals concerned for the welfare of children and families.

Within CAPTA's minimum definitional standards, each state must provide its own definitions of child abuse and neglect. CAPTA's definition of child abuse and neglect refers to:

> Any recent act or failure to act on the part of a parent or caretaker
> which results in death, serious physical or emotional harm, sexual abuse,
> or exploitation, or an act or failure to act which presents an imminent
> risk of serious harm.

Most states recognize four major types of child maltreatment:

- physical abuse
- neglect
- sexual abuse
- emotional abuse

Physical Abuse   Generally defined as "any accidental physical injury to the child," the definition can include striking (with a hand, stick, strap, or other object), kick-ing, burning, shaking, throwing, stabbing, choking, or any action that results in a physical impairment of the child. The definitions in approximately 36 states also include acts or circumstances that threaten the child with harm or create a substantial risk of harm to the child's health or welfare.

Neglect   Frequently defined in terms of deprivation to the child of adequate food, clothing, shelter, medical care, or supervision, neglect also may include the failure to provide for educational needs (failure to educate or to attend to special education needs) and emotional needs (failure to provide psychological care or permitting a child to use drugs or alcohol). Approximately 21 states actually include failure to educate in their definitions of neglect, and seven states define as medical neglect the withholding of medical or mental health care needed by the child.

Sexual Abuse   All states include sexual abuse in their definitions of child abuse. States vary in how it is defined, however; some states refer to it in general terms, whereas others specify various acts as sexual abuse. This form of abuse typically includes activities by a parent or caretaker such as fondling a child's genitals, penetration, incest, rape, sodomy, indecent exposure, and exploitation of children through prostitution or the production of pornographic materials.

Emotional Abuse   All states except two include emotional maltreatment as part of their definitions of child abuse and neglect. Approximately 22 states provide specific definitions of emotional abuse or mental injury to the child. The language usually used in these definitions includes "injury to the psychological capacity or emotional stability of the child as evidenced by an observable or substantial change in behavior, emotional response, or cognition" or by "anxiety, depression, withdrawal, or aggressive behavior."

It is generally agreed, however, that the definition of emotional abuse involves those behaviors which impair a child's emotional development or sense of self-worth such as constant criticism, threats, or rejection, as well as withholding love, support, or guidance.

The problem with this type of abuse lies in the fact that it is difficult to prove, thereby preventing the local CPS personnel from intervening; without evidence of harm to the child, CPS help is not likely. However, emotional abuse is considered to be almost always present when other forms of abuse are identified and documented.

PREVALENCE OF CHILD ABUSE AND NEGLECT

Among the many amendments to CAPTA in 1988 was the mandate for the DHHS to establish a national data and analysis program for child abuse and neglect reporting information. As a result of this mandate, the DHHS created NCANDS (see Introduction section for recent maltreatment data) as a voluntary national reporting system. Other NCANDS data included in its report were statistics on types of maltreatment, victim characteristics, and perpetrator characteristics.

Types of Maltreatment

- 63% of the confirmed child victims experienced neglect
- 17% were physically abused
- 9% were sexually abused
- 7% were psychologically maltreated
- 2% were medically neglected

Victim Characteristics

- 51% of the victims were girls; 47% of victims were boys.

- The youngest children were the most victimized of all age groups, with the highest rate of victimization occurring among infants and children from birth through three years of age (16.5 per 1,000 same-age children); this group accounted for 77% of the 1,460 child maltreatment fatalities; SBS alone, the violent shaking of an infant or child, affects 1,200–1,600 children each year (National Center on Shaken Baby Syndrome).

- The rate of victimization was inversely related to the age of the child, with ages 4–7 being the second most victimized group (13.5 per 1,000) followed by ages 8–11 (10.9 per 1,000), ages 12–15 (10.2 per 1,000), and ages 16–17 (6.2 per 1,000).

- About one-half of all victims were white, one-quarter were African American, and 17% were Hispanic; highest rates of victimization by race were found among African American children (19.5 per 1,000) followed by American Indian/Alaska Native children (16.5) and Pacific Islander children (16.1); white children and Hispanic children had similar rates of victimization (10.8 and 10.7 per 1,000, respectively).

- Although living arrangements of victims were not reported by many states, more than 20% of victims were living with a single parent in those states that did report.

- Children with a disability requiring more care and attention than is typically required of children without a disability accounted for nearly 8% of the victims of abuse and neglect.

Perpetrator Characteristics

- Most victims (83%) were abused by parents acting alone or with another person.
- 40% of victims were maltreated by their mothers acting alone; 18% by fathers acting alone, and 17% by both parents.
- Women abusers typically were younger than men (31 years versus 34 years, respectively); almost half of these women (45%) were younger than 30 years.
- 55% of abusers were White, 21% African American, and 18% Hispanic.
- Most abusers (61%) neglected children, whereas 11% physically abused them and approximately 8% sexually abused them.

Although there is no single profile of the child abuser, multiple risk factors that contribute to child maltreatment include mental health problems and substance abuse in the parent or caregiver, the use of ineffective and coercive discipline practices, domestic violence, and single parenthood, which often means high stress, low income, and poverty.

POSSIBLE INDICATORS OF CHILD
ABUSE AND NEGLECT

There is no single indicator of child maltreatment, nor is there a "profile" of a maltreated child. Physical signs or behavioral problems are only unreliable indicators of abuse. A child's direct verbal report is far more reliable (McConaughy, 2005). Nevertheless, those who work with children should be aware of some of the more common signs of child maltreatment. The Child Welfare Information Gateway and the National Children's Advocacy Center provide information on these signs and symptoms.

Type of Abuse	Physical Indicators	Behavioral Indicators
Physical Abuse	**Child-Related**	**Child-Related**
	■ unexplained bruises in various stages of healing ■ unexplained burns, especially cigarette burns or immersion burns ■ unexplained fractures, lacerations, or abrasions ■ swollen areas ■ evidence of delayed or inappropriate treatment for injuries	■ self-destructive ■ behavioral extremes: withdrawn and/or aggressive ■ arrives at school early or stays late as if afraid to be at home ■ seems frightened of the parents and protests or cries when it is time to go home ■ shrinks at the approach of adults ■ reports injury by a parent or another adult caregiver ■ chronic runaway (adolescents) ■ complains of soreness or moves uncomfortably ■ wears clothing inappropriate to the weather in order to cover body ■ bizarre explanation of injuries **Parent-Related** ■ offers conflicting, unconvincing, or no explanation for the child's injury ■ describes the child as "evil" or in some other very negative way ■ uses harsh physical punishment with the child ■ has a history of abuse as a child

Physical Neglect	Child-Related	Child-Related
	■ **abandonment** ■ unattended medical or dental needs, immunizations, or eyeglasses ■ consistent lack of supervision ■ consistent hunger, inappropriate dress, poor hygiene ■ lice, distended stomach, emaciated ■ inadequate nutrition	■ states that there is no one at home to provide care ■ frequent absences from school; tardy often ■ begs or steals food or money ■ regularly displays fatigue or listlessness, falls asleep in class ■ self-destructive ■ school dropout (adolescents) ■ extreme loneliness and need for affection **Parent-Related** ■ appears to be indifferent to the child ■ seems apathetic or depressed ■ behaves irrationally or in a bizarre manner ■ is abusing drugs or alcohol
Sexual Abuse	**Child-Related**	**Child-Related**
	■ torn, stained, or bloody underclothing ■ pain, swelling, or itching in genital area ■ difficulty walking or sitting ■ bruising or bleeding in genital area ■ contracts venereal disease or becomes pregnant, particularly if under age 14 ■ frequent urinary or yeast infections ■ massive weight change	■ suddenly refuses to change for gym or to participate in physical activities ■ reports nightmares or bedwetting ■ sudden change in appetite ■ demonstrates bizarre, sophisticated, or unusual sexual knowledge or behavior ■ runs away ■ reports sexual abuse by a parent or other adult caregiver ■ excessive seductiveness ■ role reversal, overly concerned for siblings ■ suicide attempts (especially adolescents) ■ threatened by physical contact, closeness

Parent-Related

- is unduly protective of the child
- severely limits the child's contact with other children, especially those of the opposite sex
- is secretive and isolated
- is jealous or controlling with family members

Emotional Abuse	Child-Related	Child-Related
	▪ delayed physical or emotional development	▪ habit disorder (sucking, rocking, biting)
	▪ substance abuse	▪ antisocial, destructive
	▪ ulcers, asthma, severe allergies	▪ neurotic traits (sleep disorders, inhibition of play)
		▪ delinquent behavior (especially adolescents)
		▪ shows extremes in behavior, such as overly compliant or demanding behavior, extreme passivity, or aggression
		▪ is either inappropriately adult (parenting other children) or inappropriately infantile (frequently rocking or head banging, for example)
		▪ has attempted suicide
		▪ reports a lack of attachment to the parent
		Parent-Related
		▪ constantly blames, belittles, or berates the child
		▪ appears unconcerned about the child
		▪ refuses to consider offers of help for the child's problems
		▪ overtly rejects the child

The following four cases are varied; the first two involve the events surrounding the reporting of child abuse by responsible adults, and the second two concern intervention directly with an abused child.

C A S E   P R E S E N T A T I O N : Physical Neglect and the Neighbor

---

Billy was a seven-year-old boy who frequently played with his neighbor's five-year-old son, David, in an assortment of games and activities in a neighborhood that was short of school-age children and long on older, mature families. As a result of this demographic, the two boys were locked into a friendship due to mutual need rather than to a true friendship bond. Billy had Fetal Alcohol Syndrome (FAS), a condition caused by his mother's excessive use of alcohol during her pregnancy with him. He was undersized for his age, very thin and frail, and his facial features were distinctive and were characteristic of others with FAS. Billy's mother had not been employed in some time, and she had recently been widowed, leaving her as the sole caregiver for Billy. After repeated suspicions among the neighbors that Billy had been unsupervised for extended periods of time, these suspicions became acute when Billy was invited to have dinner with his friend's family. The manner in which he ate ravenously, as if he hadn't eaten in a while, prompted his friend's father to inquire about his eating habits at home.

Intervention:

FATHER: Billy, you seemed very hungry tonight.

BILLY: I was!

FATHER: Did you have any lunch today?

BILLY: No, my mom was asleep.

FATHER: Does she sleep a lot?

BILLY: She usually sleeps in the daytime and I sleep in the nighttime.

FATHER: Who feeds you during the daytime?

BILLY: I usually get food myself.

FATHER: What did you have for dinner last night?

BILLY: I made myself some cereal (naming his two favorite breakfast cereals).

FATHER: Do you have cereal for dinner a lot?

BILLY: Yeah.

FATHER: Do you get hungry sometimes for other kinds of food?

BILLY: Yeah, but sometimes my mom tells me that she can't go to the store to buy stuff, and sometimes she just tells me to have cereal.

FATHER: What are some of your favorite foods?

BILLY: Well, when my daddy was here, he used to take us to the diner where I used to get different things. I don't know what it was called, but it was good. My mom says she doesn't have enough money now to take me there anymore.

FATHER: It sounds like you would like to have other kinds of food for dinner besides cereal. I know that there are ways that I can help you and your mom have enough other kinds of food to eat. I know that there are people I can call whose job it is to help families who need help with things like food and money.

BILLY: Really?

FATHER: Yes. First, let's go over to see your mom so that I can tell her about my plan to call these people. They are social workers who will come to visit you and your mom.

BILLY: O.K.

Case Discussion/Crisis Resolution

When David's father escorted Billy home later that evening, there was no answer to a knock on the door. Left unlocked, Billy and David's father entered the house to find his mother, Helen, slumped across the kitchen table, oblivious to their presence until Billy nudged her awake. Seeing that it was clear that she was unable to provide for Billy's needs that night, David's father walked Billy back to his own home in order to spend the night with David. Meanwhile, David's father called the local CPS office to report his concerns over the apparent physical neglect of Billy and then returned to Billy's home to make sure that his mother was not in any danger herself. When he told her that he had called CPS to report his observations, she was neither angry nor upset; rather, she told him that she already had a caseworker, having been reported to CPS once before when pulled over by the local police for driving under the influence of alcohol with Billy in the car.

David's father took care to express his concerns to Helen that his call to CPS was not a vindictive one, but rather one borne out of his concerns for Billy's safety as well as for her needs for assistance from other agencies, given her single-parent status and other life stresses. Helen nodded in agreement with this assessment and awaited the next phone call and home visit from the CPS worker assigned to the family.

In applying Cavaiola and Colford's LAPC model of crisis intervention, it was important to follow the four steps:

Listen. Be attentive to Billy's description of his dietary habits at home. Questions posed to children, particularly someone like Billy, a seven-year-old developmentally challenged boy, must be short and simple and geared toward the understanding of the child. It is important not to be judgmental nor reactive to the content of his answers, lest one runs the risk of having him "shut down" as a result of one's reactions to him. One also must listen not only to the verbal responses to the questions asked, but also to those nonverbal messages that accompany the verbal (such as avoidance of eye contact, squirming in discomfort due to the questions, possible withholding of information out of shame, embarrassment, and so on).

Assess. What does all this information mean? The lingering suspicions of neglect, Billy's overall appearance, and his ravenous approach to the meal offered to him all suggested that the course of action chosen by the father was the appropriate one. Although seemingly not forlorn or depressed, his physical health continued to be compromised due to lack of proper nutrition and to a mother struggling with a probable alcohol addiction. The father's assessment of all these factors that he observed and heard from Billy guided him in deciding to call the local CPS office.

Plan. Of primary concern, based on his assessment, was for the physical well-being of Billy and his mother, thus the immediate plan to keep Billy for the night for a "sleepover" with David and to establish the safety of his mother as well. The plan for a longer-term intervention was for the father to contact CPS so that Billy's health and safety would be assured via the agency's monitoring of the family by providing it with appropriate financial and other resources.

Commit. In this step of the process, it is important to get the client to commit to following the plan as outlined in the previous step. In the case of Billy, however, it was preferable, but not required, that Billy and his mother make a commitment to the plan to call CPS. That is, whether they agreed to it or not, the father was still legally obligated to contact CPS, even if Billy's mother asked him not to do so; his strong suspicion of neglect bound him to be proactive to make sure that Billy's health and safety be monitored by CPS. Billy's mother's consent to the plan to call CPS was fortunate in this case, but not essential.

CASE PRESENTATION: Physical Abuse and the Third Grader

Ms. Spatzer, a third-grade teacher in one of the neighborhood public schools, came to see the school psychologist one day to ask his opinion about her concerns about one of her students. She reported that she had just observed for the second time in as many weeks suspicious bruising on the upper arms of her student, Lloyd. Thinking nothing of it at first, attributing it to a "boys will be boys" bit of horseplay with one of his friends, she asked him about the bruises several days later when she happened to have a quiet and private time with him. According to her, Lloyd's behaviors, both verbal and nonverbal, raised some suspicions in her when she questioned him about the source of the bruises. She said that he became noticeably agitated when questioned, averted eye contact when Ms. Spatzer raised the issue with him, and began to pull down on his sleeves as if to cover the bruising. His hesitation in presenting an explanation about the cause of the bruises, as if he were struggling to create a fictional account of what they were from, also alarmed her.

Lloyd's reticence in this encounter also convinced Ms. Spatzer that some of her previous observations of Lloyd may have been significant after all. She always thought that he tended to be more withdrawn and passive immediately after a weekend break from school, and there were times when he wore clothing that was not particularly seasonal, particularly long-sleeved shirts on hot, humid days. She also learned from conversation in the teachers' room that his parents had separated recently and that he stayed with his father on weekends. After consideration of these observations, Ms. Spatzer decided to seek out the school psychologist for a consultation.

Intervention:

TEACHER: I have a strong suspicion that one of my students, Lloyd, may be being abused by one of his parents, probably his father.

PSYCHOLOGIST: Tell me about your suspicions.

TEACHER: Well, it's just that I have noticed a second set of bruises in the last couple of weeks, and when I tried to talk with him about it, he became very secretive and uncomfortable and couldn't tell me clearly of any reason that might account for the bruises. I also recall some times when he wore oversized clothing that was not in keeping with the weather conditions. Could this also be a sign that he was hiding some other signs of physical abuse?

PSYCHOLOGIST: All of what you have just told me could be the result of several things, but one of them is possible child abuse. Since you have these suspicions, you are required to report it to the local Child Protective Services. It is up to them to investigate suspicions like yours and to make sure that Lloyd is safe. Have you ever made a call like this before?

TEACHER: No, I haven't. I've only been teaching for three years, and I have never had this experience before. One of my college professors warned us, though, that one day we would have an abused child in our classes. I don't even know what to do; couldn't you make the call for me with all that I told you? And what if I am wrong? Can I get in trouble? I mean, what if his bruises really are the result of his playing around with his friends? I just am not sure what to do.

PSYCHOLOGIST: I certainly can assist you with the call, but the CPS intake worker will have some specific questions about what you saw and what Lloyd told you, all things that only you can answer accurately. I will sit with you and make the call with you, but you are the best one to speak directly to the CPS worker. Just remember that you also can make the call anonymously and that anyone who makes a report of suspected abuse "in good faith" cannot be held liable, even if the suspected abuse was not corroborated by the investigation. Your observations seem to me to be sufficient reason for contacting CPS.

TEACHER: Is there anything else I need to do after I make this call?

PSYCHOLOGIST: That will be up to the CPS worker assigned to Lloyd. There is a good chance that they will come to school to interview him today; they also may want to see you as well. Afterward, they will visit Lloyd's parents and ascertain the ongoing danger to his health and safety and then decide on the best placement for him. Just be assured that your call will go a long way toward guaranteeing his protection from further abuse.

TEACHER: O.K., I'm new at this, unfortunately, but let's go make the call. Can we use your office?

PSYCHOLOGIST: Of course.

Case Discussion/Crisis Resolution

Within minutes Ms. Spatzer and the psychologist were in his office making the call to CPS. Although he initiated the contact with the intake worker, Ms. Spatzer handled the telephone interview and answered all the intake worker's questions related to her observations of Lloyd's suspected abuse. A subsequent CPS investigation of her suspicions corroborated them as factual, leading to several interventions for Lloyd and his family.

Despite that the largest percentage of calls to CPS offices regarding suspected child maltreatment come from educators (see page 36 for breakdown), making such a call is nevertheless unnerving for most professionals. Fears of being wrong in their suspicions, worries over lawsuits from angry parents, and a general uneasiness about being the one to call contribute to this sense of dread. All school districts are required to have in place an Emergency Response and Crisis Management Plan (see Chapter 12) that is designed to address all potential crises that might arise within the school or the community. Among the issues addressed are the school's organized responses to many potential crisis events, including school shootings, natural and human-made disasters, and teacher- or student-reported suspicions of suicidal talk or child abuse.

Ms. Spatzer followed the protocol for a reporting of child maltreatment as outlined in her district's crisis plan: contact the psychologist first with your suspicions and be prepared to be the one to contact CPS. Although Lloyd was the individual who was most in crisis and needful of CPS intervention, Ms Spatzer herself required some reassurances for her actions. According to the LAPC model:

Listen. The psychologist heard what Ms Spatzer said about this crisis: Lloyd definitely showed signs of possible abuse that seemed to peak after visits with his father. The case required a call to CPS on behalf of Lloyd, but despite the appropriateness of this response, the teacher also was in a high state of agitation over this course of action. Her reaction became quite clear to the psychologist after listening to her description of Lloyd's physical condition and observing her nonverbal messages such as hand wringing, voice shaking, and general level of anxiety over being in this situation.

Assess. The psychologist had to make a dual assessment in this case: whether or not CPS was to be contacted and the emotional state of the reporting teacher. He decided that it was clearly a case for CPS to make sure that Lloyd would be safe from further harm; he also concluded that Ms. Spatzer required a lot of support herself in making the CPS call.

Plan. After assuring Ms. Spatzer that her suspicions warranted CPS involvement and that her call was to be made "in good faith," thus precluding any legal actions against her, the psychologist explained the plan of how the call would be made and what the outcome would be.

Commit. Ms. Spatzer agreed with this plan and made the phone call along with the psychologist.

C A S E   P R E S E N T A T I O N : Self-Disclosure of Abuse

Brian visited the nurse's office in his middle school one morning several times. He was a frequent visitor, she reported, so his multiple visits this one particular morning did not raise any suspicions in her mind. It was during his fourth trip that morning, however, when he announced to her that his father had beaten him with a belt the night before.

Brian's family had a contentious relationship with the school district for a variety of reasons, so this self-disclosure of abuse was a delicate one. The school nurse reported Brian's statements to the school principal who was unclear as to how to proceed, considering the sensitive nature of the issue that was superimposed on a difficult home–school relationship. Fears of a lawsuit and of other repercussions from the family clouded her thinking for the moment.

The first person she consulted was the school counselor who had had most of the contact with the family ever since Brian's arrival in the middle school one year earlier. She asked the counselor to speak with Brian and to proceed with the appropriate CPS referral.

The school counselor asked Brian's classroom teacher to send him to the counselor's office after his lunch period ended. In sensitive matters such as this one, the counselor always tried to be as unobtrusive as possible in singling out students for a visit to her office, lest other classmates suspect that something was up with their friend. Confidentiality and privacy issues are paramount, particularly in cases of child maltreatment. Brian himself was considered somewhat of an oddity by his peers, since he lacked those social skills typical for his age group. Although not disliked by them, they viewed him as just a bit "different," and they were not inclined to invite him to many of the weekend birthday and holiday parties that included so many of the other classmates.

When Brian entered the counselor's office, he looked perplexed as to the purpose of his visit. He had been in the counselor's office many times before, but he usually was the one who initiated the visit, dropping in from time to time to talk about nothing of great consequence. This visit was different, he suspected.

Intervention:

SCHOOL COUNSELOR: Hello, Brian. Please take a seat.

BRIAN: Sure. Why did you want to see me? Am I in trouble?

SCHOOL COUNSELOR: No, of course not, Brian. I just wanted to talk with you about something, that's all.

BRIAN: Should I close the door (looking nervously at the entrance to the office)?

SCHOOL COUNSELOR: Yes, Brian. I would like to talk with you about what you told the school nurse this morning.

BRIAN: What do you mean?

SCHOOL COUNSELOR: She told me that you said that your father beat you with a belt last night.

BRIAN: Oh, that! No, I was only kidding! Nothing like that really happened. My father's a great guy; he would never do that to me! I was just kidding! (Brian averted eye contact with the counselor and started to stare at the floor while uttering his protest. He was noticeably agitated.)

SCHOOL COUNSELOR: Brian, one of my jobs here as counselor is to do what I can to make sure that all children in this school are safe and that no one hurts them.

BRIAN: You mean, like, other kids, bullies, people like that?

SCHOOL COUNSELOR: Yes, certainly, but I also mean parents; they also don't have the right to hurt their children, even though they love them and want them to behave.

BRIAN: So a father, I mean, a parent can hit their kids and still love them, right?

SCHOOL COUNSELOR: Yes. It's just that there are better ways for a parent to deal with their children's behavior without hitting or hurting them.

BRIAN: Oh.

SCHOOL COUNSELOR: I'm wondering if that might not be true for your father: you know, loving you and hitting you sometimes?

BRIAN: (Sitting silently with his eyes welling up with tears)

SCHOOL COUNSELOR: (Allowing for a period of silence first) Is it, Brian?

BRIAN: (Starting to cry) I just don't want to get him in trouble, and I don't want to be taken away. I'll just tell everyone that I made it up before! Can't we just keep this a secret?

SCHOOL COUNSELOR: Remember what I told you once before, Brian? There are many things that a counselor can keep secret or confidential, but when a counselor learns that children are thinking of hurting themselves or someone else or if they themselves are being hurt, then the counselor has to break confidentiality and tell other people to make sure that those children are safe. Do you understand?

BRIAN: Yes, but it's not his fault! He's used the belt before, but last night I talked back to him and made him mad, so he hit me more than he usually does. I just don't want to get him in trouble for something that I did.

SCHOOL COUNSELOR: Brian, when a child is hurt by a parent, it's never his fault. Parents are adults and have to learn ways of disciplining their children without hurting them or humiliating them. It sounds like your father has to learn other ways to deal with you when you talk back or do other things that children do.

BRIAN: Now what are you going to do?

SCHOOL COUNSELOR: Brian, the law says that I or anyone else who works in a school has to contact a group of people called Child Protective Services if they suspect that a child has been hurt. I will make the phone call now and tell them all that you have told me and the school nurse. Then they will either come to the school to meet with you first or make direct contact with your father. The way they proceed will be their decision. Their job is to help families by having them change the ways they deal with their children.

BRIAN: But I won't be in trouble, will I?

(continued)

C A S E   P R E S E N T A T I O N :   Self-Disclosure of Abuse (*continued*)

SCHOOL COUNSELOR: No, Brian. The caseworker who visits you or your family will try to make sure that you don't get in trouble for telling us what happened. In fact, what you did was a very hard thing to do; it took a lot of courage to come forward to tell us what happened. I also will be here when the caseworker comes and sit with you, if that's O.K. with you.

BRIAN: Sure.

Case Discussion/Crisis Resolution:

The counselor then made the phone call to the agency. Although inclined to make a visit to Brian's home within 24 hours, the agency instead dispatched a caseworker to see Brian in school before the end of the school day, since he let it be known that he was afraid to return home that afternoon.

Generally, the messages that should be communicated clearly to the child throughout this process include (Cavaiola & Colford, 2006):

- Children are entitled to be safe and not hurt.
- Children should not have to be afraid to go home.
- Adults, even parents, are not permitted to hurt children.
- Abuse is not the child's fault.
- A child will not get into trouble for telling someone about abuse.
- Hitting is not the right way for parents to punish bad behavior.
- There are ways that counselors and other people can help parents so that they will stop doing hurtful things.
- The goal of the involvement of Child Protective Services is to help the family.

The familiarity that Brian had with the school counselor made the counselor's role less problematic than it could have been, had they not known each other. There was undoubtedly a level of trust that facilitated the counselor's LAPC intervention.

Listen. The counselor listened to Brian's initial denial of the abuse admission, then heard him minimize it by accepting the blame for it. One of the protective factors for children experiencing physical abuse is whether or not they blame themselves for the abuse (Grych, Jouriles, Swank, McDonald, & Norwood, 2000). That is, children who blame the abusers rather than themselves for the abuse tend to have a better outcome than those who think that they were the ones who deserved the abuse. The counselor heard statements of self-blame from Brian, his wish to protect his father and to keep the family intact, and his eventual relief that something was going to be done about it.

Assess. The counselor's assessment was that abuse had taken place at the father's hands and that Brian continued to be at risk for future harm. Of great concern to the counselor was Brian's acceptance of blame for the abuse. It was clear that a call to CPS was essential at this point.

Plan. The counselor described his plan to Brian in order to let him know what the next step in the process was. Ideally, he hoped that Brian also agreed to the plan, even though he was obligated to make the call, with or without Brian's agreement.

Commit. With the counselor's support, Brian committed to the counselor's plan.

C A S E   P R E S E N T A T I O N : Self-Blame and Abuse

Cindy, an eight-year-old second grader in the local public school, presented as a very frail, undernourished young girl. Although the teachers who knew her never really suspected anything in the way of abuse at home, they always encouraged her to eat more. She was very affectionate, appearing at times to be very "clingy" with her teachers. She interacted well with her fellow classmates, although she tended to be quite passive and to take orders from others in her class. Her appearance, including the dark circles under her eyes, escaped her teachers' scrutiny for any abuse or neglect in the home. A neighbor of Cindy's, however, had many more opportunities to observe her home life. He decided to make a call to CPS, citing multiple instances of abuse and neglect that he observed around the neighborhood. He had witnessed her father and her mother strike her several times, and he voiced other concerns about the time she was left alone to take care of her younger brother, Jake. The social worker from CPS received the neighbor's phone call and went to see her in school that same day. The principal summoned Cindy from class when the social worker arrived.

SOCIAL WORKER: Hello, Cindy, my name is Jane.

CINDY: Hello. (Looking very confused and uncertain of why she was sitting with a stranger in the principal's office)

SOCIAL WORKER: I just wanted to ask you a few questions, if I might. You are not in trouble in any way. I am what they call a social worker. My job is to talk to parents, children, and families just to make sure that everything is going well. Do you mind if I ask you some questions?

CINDY: O.K.

SOCIAL WORKER: First of all, how old are you?

CINDY: I am eight.

SOCIAL WORKER: And you are in the second grade, right?

CINDY: Yes, I am in Ms. Fielder's class.

SOCIAL WORKER: Tell me what your favorite thing to do in school is.

CINDY: (Smiling, as if comfortable with this initial neutral line of questioning) My favorite part of school is the specials; I like Art, because we get to do lots of different things. We draw, play with clay, and look at pretty pictures that the teacher shows us.

SOCIAL WORKER: What other specials do you like?

CINDY: Gym, because we get to run around a lot and play different games. I get a little tired, though.

SOCIAL WORKER: Yes, I remember how I also liked to play gym when I was in school. Do you mind if I ask you some more questions?

CINDY: O.K.

SOCIAL WORKER: Tell me, Cindy, who else lives at home with you?

CINDY: My mom, my stepdad, and my brother, Jake.

SOCIAL WORKER: How old is Jake?

CINDY: Five, I think. Yeah, he's five, that's right. He's funny, but sometimes he bothers me, like he takes my stuff and cries a lot.

(continued)

CASE PRESENTATION: Self-Blame and Abuse (*continued*)

SOCIAL WORKER: And who takes care of Jake?

CINDY: Mostly I do, because my stepdad works, and my mom works sometimes and sleeps sometimes.

SOCIAL WORKER: What kinds of things do you do for Jake?

CINDY: Well, I wake him up and give him his breakfast, get his clothes out for him to wear—he goes to kindergarten here—and then I get dressed. Oh yeah, and then I wake my mom for her to drive us to school.

SOCIAL WORKER: And what do you do after school?

CINDY: Well, I wait for Jake and we sometimes walk home together, because sometimes my mom forgets to pick us up.

SOCIAL WORKER: Is your mom or stepdad home when you eat dinner?

CINDY: Sometimes, but if she isn't, she leaves us something to eat ourselves.

SOCIAL WORKER: You and Jake?

CINDY: Yes.

SOCIAL WORKER: Do you get punished sometimes, like if you didn't do your chores or something?

CINDY: (Looking more apprehensive) Yes.

SOCIAL WORKER: Tell me what your punishment is.

CINDY: Sometimes I have to kneel in the corner on the floor in my kitchen until my mom tells me I don't have to any more.

SOCIAL WORKER: Have your mom or stepdad used other kinds of punishment?

CINDY: (Clearly uncomfortable at this point and silent)

SOCIAL WORKER: Cindy, I know that these questions are hard questions to answer, but I really appreciate how you have been able to talk with me here today. I know that it is hard for lots of children your age to talk about these things. I really would like you to tell me the other kinds of punishment that is used at home.

CINDY: (Starting to cry) Sometimes, if I'm really bad, I get hit and I cry.

SOCIAL WORKER: Who hits you?

CINDY: Mostly my stepdad, but he hits my mom too, sometimes, and some-times my mom hits me, too, like if I forget to clean up or if I have a fight with Jake. But I'm older, I should know better.

SOCIAL WORKER: You should know better?

CINDY: Yeah, I'm older and I should know better. I should be more responsible. I should be better, too. Jake looks up to me, he needs me to be better.

General Guidelines for Reporting Suspected Child Abuse and Neglect

Once an individual observes signs of maltreatment in a child (see page 23), he/she must contact the local CPS office with these suspicions. All states have statutes identifying mandatory reporters of child maltreatment. Individuals

SOCIAL WORKER: Cindy, you are such a good, caring big sister, but maybe being an eight-year-old is too young to have to do so much at home. I don't think that you have to be better at all. One of the things that I do is to talk to parents about ways to help their children without hurting them or hitting them. Sometimes parents make mistakes and hurt their children, but nobody should hurt other people, especially children. I also want to make sure that your mom is safe and that your stepdad doesn't hurt her anymore. What I want to do is to go to see your mom and stepdad and talk to them about other ways of helping you and Jake. I can talk to them about lots of other things that they can do instead of hitting you and hurting you. There also are other people that they can see who can help. I also will tell them that I talked with you today.

CINDY: But I don't want to get into more trouble.

SOCIAL WORKER: I will tell your mom that you were very brave in answering some very hard questions and that you shouldn't get in trouble for it. I also will give her some help so that she is safe.

CINDY: O.K.

Case Discussion/Crisis Resolution

As with the case of Brian (see page 30), Cindy blamed herself for the maltreatment; if she were only "more responsible" it wouldn't have happened. In other words, she deserved it. The social worker who responded to the neighbor's call was aware of this belief of Cindy's and tried to reassure her that this was not the case. The social worker utilized the LAPC approach in her interview of Cindy.

Listen. She sensed Cindy's initial discomfort with the interview, talked first about more neutral school-related issues, and then gradually introduced the more emotionally laden topic of her home life. She also heard the blame for the abuse that Cindy heaped upon herself.

Assess. The assessment was clear to the social worker that Cindy was the victim of maltreatment within the confines of a home where there also was domestic violence. The blame she accepted for it made her numb to what was happening and undoubtedly required additional community and mental health services for Cindy and her family.

Plan. Making a visit to the home was critical in this case to assess the level of safety for the children and their mother.

Commit. As with the previous cases in this chapter, even a child's refusal to commit to the plan cannot be heeded, given the ethical and legal obligations to report abuse and to allow CPS to intervene on behalf of children. Nevertheless, Cindy did seem to be agreeable to the plan after the social worker's explanation of what she intended to do.

typically designated as mandatory reporters are those who have frequent contact with children, including social workers, school personnel, healthcare workers, mental health professionals, childcare providers, medical examiners or coroners, and law enforcement officers. Approximately 18 states (although these laws change regularly) require all citizens to report suspected abuse or neglect, regardless of profession. These reporters often are referred to as "permissive reporters."

Although the standards used to determine when a mandatory report should be made vary from state to state, a report must be made when the reporter suspects that a child has been abused or neglected. Reporters may make these reports anonymously, although states find it helpful to know the identity of the reporter. Most states have provisions to maintain the confidentiality of the reporters and to protect the disclosure of their identity to the alleged abuser. Failure to report suspected child maltreatment or filing a false report against someone in most states results in penalties ranging from fines to imprisonment. However, professionals are protected from civil and criminal liability in all states if reports are made in good faith, even if later the reports are deemed unfounded by the investigation.

The most recent NCANDS report claimed that 24% of reports of physical abuse were made by teachers, 23% by police officers or lawyers, and almost 12% by medical staff. Overall, professionals accounted for 75% of reports of physical abuse and nonprofessionals provided the other 25%. However, reports of neglect and sexual abuse were made primarily by police officers and lawyers.

Considering the high rate of reports made by teachers, it is incumbent upon them to familiarize themselves with the laws of the state in which they teach regarding the reporting of abuse and neglect, as well as of the school district's policy identifying procedures for reporting and those designated as reporters. Investigating reported allegations of maltreatment, however, is not within the purview of teachers, but rather the responsibility of the CPS staff or of other professionals who have received special training in interviewing children, particularly in the investigation of abuse claims. Nevertheless, school-based professionals often are the first ones to know if a child has been abused; children spend almost 40 hours per week in the schools, raising the likelihood that a teacher may observe evidence of possible abuse, that a child may self-disclose abuse at home, or that a friend will report on the abuse of a peer.

When disclosure of possible maltreatment of a child is made, the local CPS office will be contacted. Prior to this contact, however, the initial interviewer often will be another professional, perhaps a school teacher, counselor, psychologist, or social worker. McConaughy (2005) provided general guidelines for responding to all children who report maltreatment. These guidelines are not investigative in nature, since it is not the job of the interviewer to gather evidence or to establish guilt; rather, they are designed to provide a framework for reassurance and support for a maltreated child after a disclosure has been made. These guidelines suggest that the professional:

- conducts the interview in a private place
- maintains an atmosphere of informality and trust
- believes the child (or at least take the child's report at face value)
- reassures the child that he/she has done nothing wrong and will continue to have the professional's support
- does not display negative reactions such as horror, shock, or disapproval of the child or parents
- is sensitive to the child's nonverbal cues

- asks for clarification if what the child says is ambiguous
- uses language that the child understands
- uses the child's terms for body parts and sexual behaviors, but also obtains the child's definition of such terms
- does not suggest answers to the child and avoids probing and pressing for answers
- gives the child a clear and understandable reason that reporting to the local CPS agency is necessary
- does not suggest that the child conceals the interview from the parents
- keeps clear notes of the interview and the child's disclosure statements, as well as of any subsequent actions regarding reporting

Fears of retribution by the abuser, concerns about the break-up of the family after the disclosure has been made, and guilt over reporting an abuser, particularly if he or she is a parent are only some of the reasons that children are reluctant to self-disclose or to participate in an interview with a professional after being reported by a peer. Therefore, in age-appropriate terms and language, the interviewer must validate these fears for children, recognize their courage in coming forward, and provide other reassurances that the outcome of the process will result in keeping them safe. Discussing the limits of confidentiality with the child also is critical (the mandate to report whenever someone has been hurt or is intending to hurt themselves or someone else). CPS investigators of the report also should be portrayed to the child as being in a position to protect the child so that further abuse does not happen. The initial interviewer, however, should not make personal promises to protect the child.

All professionals who work with children should learn how to contact their local CPS or law enforcement agencies. Many states have toll-free numbers to call to report suspected child abuse or neglect. The National Child Abuse Hotline, however, is staffed 24 hours per day, seven days per week, by trained crisis counselors who have access to a database of over 50,000 emergency, social service, and support resources; all calls are anonymous. The phone number is: **1-800-4-A-CHILD.**

RECOMMENDATIONS FOR CHAPTER ENRICHMENT

SUGGESTED FILMS

This Boy's Life **(1993)** Leonardo DiCaprio portrays the stepson of a brutal and controlling stepfather played by Robert DeNiro. The emotional and physical abuse handed down by the stepfather culminates in a final confrontation between the two men. Even before the actual abuse begins, the film suggests a cold, detached emotional climate in the household. The movie is based upon a personal memoir by American novelist Tobias Wolfe.

Radio Flyer **(1992)** Two young brothers are the chronic victims of their violent, drunken stepfather's physical abuse. Resorting to fantasy to escape the abuse, they imagine that their Radio Flyer wagon can take them away and allow them to escape the torment they must endure.

Dolores Claiborne **(1995)** The title character in the film is a middle-aged woman who is a suspect in the mysterious death of the elderly woman she took care of for several years. There also were strong suspicions that she had a hand in her husband's death 15 years before. When her estranged daughter, a newspaper reporter, visits her to inquire about the case, the family secret of sexual abuse rises to the surface.

Suggested Activities

1. Contact the local Child Protective Services agency and interview one of the caseworkers about the caseloads, the kinds of cases CPS investigates, and examples of some of the most difficult cases.

2. Research how your particular state defines different forms of child maltreatment, mandatory versus permissive reporters, and the consequences of failing to report suspicions of abuse and neglect or of filing a knowingly false report.

3. Research the issue of corporal punishment and the roles that culture, ethnicity, and religion play in its acceptability as a parenting practice? What are your thoughts on the use of spanking as an appropriate discipline strategy?

Student Activity: What Would You Do?

You are a college student who befriends another student during the first semester of freshman year. You both begin a cordial relationship with each other, taking classes together when possible and socializing on weekends. You enjoy each other's company, and little by little, you begin to share personal stories. Your friend, Sasha, tells you laughingly one Monday morning about how drunk her stepfather was over the weekend. Although a commuter to campus, Sasha holds down a part-time job on the weekends, so she was out of the house and not around to witness firsthand the entire drunken episode. Much of what she reports to you came from the personal account of her 11-year-old brother, Ian.

Ian apparently told Sasha that his father "took the paddle to him" and gave him a good "whooping." According to Sasha, corporal punishment such as this was not new to her or to Ian. Sasha explained that it was just that her stepfather was more abusive than usual when he was drunk and that no one knew this more than Ian. When you questioned Sasha further about all this, she laughed and said that she was just waiting to afford an apartment so that she could get away from her stepfather entirely. When questioned about Ian, she told you that she didn't have time to worry about him and that "he would just have to deal with it like she did all those years."

Answer the following questions as if you were the friend to whom Sasha disclosed this information:

1. How would you respond to Sasha's stories of abuse, particularly the ongoing stories about Ian's abuse?

2. Would you take any proactive steps to stop it?

3. How would you respond to Sasha if she told you not to tell anyone about her story, lest it lead to additional repercussions at the hands of her stepfather?

4. Does her threat of her loss of friendship with you deter you from doing what you might have planned to do about this issue?

3

Adolescent Crises

DISCUSSION QUESTIONS

Talk to your parents or a few other adults who are the same age as your parents. Ask them about the major issues they faced as adolescents.

Then talk to your own peers about the issues that adolescents face today.

How would you compare the stresses and strains faced by your parents or their peers with those faced by the adolescents of today?

Watch a little television. Look for those stations that broadcast the popular shows from the 1960s to 1970s and watch them with an eye toward their depiction of the typical American family and the major obstacles they faced on a week-to-week basis. Compare those issues with the ones portrayed in a contemporary situation comedy today.

What impact on the today's adolescents have the attacks of 9/11 had on their development? Similarly, how have technological advances like the Internet, multipurpose cell phones, and access to personal Webpages like *MySpace* affected the lives of adolescents today?

INTRODUCTION

What exactly is adolescence? Who determines what it is? Is it synonymous with the teenage years? Is it a life stage determined by age alone, or by mastery of certain developmental tasks? Finally, is there really a discernable beginning and end to this period?

The word itself, *adolescence*, if from the Latin word, *adolescere,* meaning *to grow* or *to grow into maturity* (Rice & Dolgin, 2008). Although perhaps not a sufficient definition of the term to satisfy some of the questions raised above, it nevertheless suggests a period of transition, a bridge of sorts between an earlier time of child-hood and the eventual stage of adulthood. The World Health Organization takes a more simplified approach, defining it as the ages of 10 to 19, and the American Academy of Pediatrics define it as the interval between child and adult status, ac-knowledging also that the exact period of adolescence varies in length according to differences in certain historical periods, cultures, and societies.

In fact, deciding when adolescence begins and ends may be more a matter of opinion rather than of actual fact (Steinberg, 2005). Does one consider the phys-ically precocious fourth grader, all of nine years of age, to be an adolescent or a child? Is the 23-year-old graduate school student who still lives at home and de-pends on parents for support considered an adolescent or an adult?

Using puberty as an indicator of adolescence is misleading. From the Latin word, *pubescere,* meaning *to grow hairy or mossy,* the appearance of body hair varies consider-ably from person to person and from one racial or ethnic group to the next, thereby precluding it as a reliable and universal marker of adolescence. The signs of puberty also come years before a child becomes fertile, so the physical signs that accompany puberty are not, in themselves, sufficient to reveal the onset of adolescence.

What is clear, however, is that the period of adolescence has lengthened con-siderably in recent years. Physical maturation has begun earlier and earlier over the last century for young people due to advances in medical treatment and in nutrition, whereas individuals at the other end of this age-range delay entering the world of work due to longer stays in undergraduate and graduate education programs. They also put off marriage for longer periods. The median ages for marriages in 1970 were 23.2 for men and 20.8 for women; in 2004, these ages increased to 27 for men and 26 for women (Popenoe & Whitehead, 2005). These data suggest that the parameters that previously defined adolescence have been expanded significantly in recent decades. For these reasons, it may make more sense to think of adoles-cence as beginning around age 10 and ending in the early 20s (Steinberg, 2005).

HISTORICAL PERSPECTIVES ON ADOLESCENCE

Adolescence has been the focus of much debate among the psychological estab-lishment over the years. G. Stanley Hall was the first psychologist to use scientific methods to study adolescence. He described this life stage as a period of *sturm und drang* ("storm and stress"), a reflection of his views of adolescence as a time of great turbulence and unrest.

Sigmund Freud did not focus much of his time or attention on adolescence, other than to discuss it in terms of his stages of psychosexual development. His daughter Anna assigned much greater importance to adolescence than he did. She saw it as playing an important role in character development and characterized it as a time of great inner conflict and erratic, unpredictable, and contradictory behavior: An adolescent was submissive and rebellious, selfish and idealistic, enthusiastic and apathetic.

These theorists and others have long viewed adolescence as a stressful develop-mental time, complete with pitfalls that are unavoidable to the typical adolescent.

The media also tends to portray adolescents as being only a failed romantic relationship away from a mass killing or a suicide attempt. Still other portrayals suggest that they, as a group, are shiftless and aimless, caught in an existential void of meaninglessness and pessimism. And then there are those who view them as highly emotional and much more random and unpredictable in their behavior than they are as children or adults. Anecdotal records of individual adolescent's mental health problems and behavioral shortcomings tend to be generalized to include all members of this developmental stage.

More contemporary thinking (Rice & Dolgin, 2008), however, suggests that certain problems such as conflicts with parents, mood swings, and risk-taking behaviors are more common in adolescence than in childhood or adulthood but that their presence does not mean that these issues are universal throughout this stage. Rather, the majority of adolescents do not get into serious trouble and if they do, these troubles are very intermittent and are of short duration.

Steinberg (2005, p. 18) claimed that adolescents were one of the most stereotyped groups in contemporary society:

> If they are not cast as juvenile delinquents—the usual role in which they are cast—adolescents are depicted as sex-crazed idiots (if they are male), giggling school girls (if they are female), or tormented lost souls, searching for their place in a strange, cruel world (if they aren't delinquent, sex-crazed, or giggling). It's not only fictionalized portrayals of teenagers that are stereotyped—studies of local television newscasts find that the majority of stories on youth are about violence.

None of the theorists mentioned above had any scientific evidence that the adolescent period was anymore turbulent than that of other life stages, but the stereotype persists. The Carnegie Foundation of New York, in its *Great transitions: Preparing adolescents for a new century*, concluded:

> Most American adolescents navigate the critical transition years from 10 to 18 with relative success. With good schools, supportive families, and caring community institutions, they grow up to meet the requirements of family life, friendship, the workplace, and citizenship in a technically advanced, democratic society. Even under difficult conditions, most young people grow into responsible, ethical, problem-solving adults.

A more balanced view on the influences on the adolescent journey appears to consider an interactive effect between the social and cultural influences of contemporary society and the inner biological/cognitive influences promulgated by many of the earlier researchers in the field. This provides a clearer picture of today's adolescent.

WHAT THE DATA SAY

Data on the behavior of American adolescents and their involvement with drugs and with other risky pursuits, often considered typical for this age group, are equivocal. That is, they are encouraging on the one hand, yet not altogether promising on the other hand. The data below will provide a look at three areas of concern in the study of the adolescent of today: drug and alcohol use, high-risk behaviors, and sexuality practices.

Alcohol and Drug Use   In its comprehensive survey of approximately 50,000 high school adolescents, the University of Michigan's Monitoring the Future (MTF), a long-term study of adolescents, college students, and adults through age 45, found the following among eighth, tenth, and twelfth graders:

- Gradual decline in the reported use of any illicit drug across all three grade levels between 1996 and 2006: down by more than a third of eighth graders, a quarter of tenth graders, and about 14% of twelfth graders during these same years.

- Marijuana, the most prevalent of the illicit drugs, is the most common drug responsible for this decline, as are amphetamines, Ritalin, and methamphetamine.

- Among the drugs showing practically no change during this time, however, were LSD, powder cocaine, crystal methamphetamine, heroin, tranquilizers, "club drugs" (Ketamine, Tohypnol, and GHB), and anabolic steroids. Prevalence rates for these drugs are low, however.

- Cigarette use is by far the adolescent problem behavior that is the most resistant to change.

- Alcohol use remains widespread. Almost three-quarters of students have consumed alcohol by the end of high school. 56% of twelfth graders and 20% of eighth graders in 2006 reported having been drunk at least once in their lives.

High-Risk Behaviors   These behaviors also appear to be part of the adolescent experience. Perhaps due to Elkind's (1967) idea of the *personal fable,* the typical adolescent believes that "nothing can happen to me, despite the risks presented by my behavior," thus putting them at risk of death or injury. It's as if adolescents usually perceive themselves as invulnerable and immune to the laws that apply to others. Yet again, contemporary neuroscience research suggests that the rational, organized, problem-solving part of the brain, the frontal lobe, is not fully developed until later in adolescence, thus the behavior of many adolescents is not governed by rational thought.

In its Youth Risk Behavior Surveillance Survey (YRBSS, 2005), the Centers for Disease Control and Prevention reported on the findings of its survey of those health-risk behaviors which contribute to the leading causes of morbidity and mortality among youth and adults. The reporting period of the survey was October 2004 to January 2006.

The YBRSS found:

- 71% of all deaths among persons 10-24 years of age result from four causes: motor vehicle crashes, other unintentional injuries, homicide, and suicide.

- During the 30 days preceding the survey, many high school students increased their risk of death by engaging in any one of four behaviors: driving a car while under the influence of alcohol (9.9%), carrying a weapon (18.5%), drinking alcohol (43.3%), and using marijuana (20.2%).

- 37.2% of sexually active high school students had not used a condom during their last sexual intercourse, thus exposing themselves to pregnancy and to a sexually transmitted disease (STD).

- 8.4% had attempted suicide in the previous 12-month period.

- 67% did not attend daily physical education classes.

- 13.1% were overweight.

- 10.2% of students had rarely or never worn a seatbelt when riding in a car driven by someone else.

- 28.5% had ridden in a car or other vehicle driven by someone else who had been drinking alcohol.

Sexuality Practices   The YBRSS also surveyed the sexual practices of adolescents, and the Kaiser Family Foundation (KFF), a nonprofit organization that researches healthcare issues, completed a *National survey of adolescents and young adults: Sexual health knowledge, attitudes, and experiences* (2003). Below are some of their findings:

YBRSS

- 9.2% of students had been hit, slapped, or physically hurt by their boyfriend or girlfriend in the year preceding the survey.
- 10.8% of high school females were forced to have sexual intercourse.
- 46.8% of students have had sexual intercourse.
- 14.3% reported having had sexual intercourse with four or more partners.

KFF

- One in four sexually active young people contract a STD every year.
- Young people feel a great pressure to have sex.
- 75% of sexually active adolescents engage in oral sex.
- 20% of adolescents are unaware that STDs can be transmitted through oral sex.
- 20% of sexually active teens reported having unprotected sex after drinking or taking drugs.
- 75% of adolescents expressed a need for more information about sexual health topics.

Although surveys such as the ones discussed above are far from perfect in the information they gather, their data suggest that many of today's adolescents place themselves at risk of a number of physical, psychological, and sexual dilemmas.

The facts and figures provided do not necessarily imply that the individuals surveyed possess chronic and persistent problems in these areas, but they do portray a trend in the behaviors of many adolescents of today. Even if many of these behaviors do not reach crisis proportions for most adolescents, they reveal patterns of behavioral choices for some members of this age group that reflect the uncertainties of this developmental period and the adolescent's search for identity, for independence from parents, and for acceptance by peer group members.

ADOLESCENT CRISES

This next section will address those crises in adolescence that are more chronic and aberrant than is typical for the average adolescent. Adolescents who experience a crisis which requires mental health treatment do not constitute the norm; rather, they are in the minority. A discussion of all the potential problems of nonclinical significance that might befall a typical adolescent is beyond the scope of this chapter; issues related to school underachievement, family conflict, and other challenges to the mastery of adolescent developmental tasks are left to chapters on adolescent development rather than to those devoted to adolescent crises. Instead, the following narrative and case examples will focus on three crises which often are associated with the adolescent stage: eating disorders, suicide, and self-injurious behavior (also known as cutting). Another case regarding identity development is included here as well, not because it is a crisis in the magnitude of the aforementioned three, but because it represents a challenge common to many adolescents.

EATING DISORDERS

An eating disorder is a psychological disorder that is characterized by an excessive desire to be thin as well as an intense fear of gaining weight. Individuals with the disorder limit their food intake to health-threateningly small amounts or use other techniques (excessive exercising, laxatives, diuretics, and vomiting) as weight control strategies. Eating disorders tend to be placed into two categories: anorexia nervosa and bulimia nervosa. Those with anorexia are known for their refusal to maintain a minimal body weight, defined as 85% of the body weight considered normative for their age and height. Those with the restricting type of anorexia limit their intake of food to the point that they experience starvation, whereas the binge-eating and purging types use various inappropriate compensatory behaviors like self-induced vomiting after they eat. The emaciated appearance of individuals with anorexia is an external indicator of the disorder.

Individuals with bulimia, however, maintain a fairly typical body weight, thus making it difficult to determine who has the disorder based on appearance alone. Their behaviors are marked by recurring episodes of binge-eating followed by various attempts to purge themselves of what they consumed by the misuse of laxatives, diuretics, various medications, or by exercising excessively.

> **C A S E   P R E S E N T A T I O N :** Danielle, A Story of Anorexia

For Danielle, it all started when she was a 12-year-old seventh grader who had just entered the middle school in her local district. A sensitive girl conscious of her appearance and of her body shape, she began what was to be years of food restricting in an attempt to get to and maintain a weight that seemed reasonable to her, one that was more comparable to the tall, thin young girls with whom she took dance lessons. However, to her friends and to her teachers, there was nothing reasonable about her weight status; they brought it to her attention and explained this thing called anorexia nervosa, but Danielle didn't think that problem applied to her at all. Changes in her life over the years of her disorder were stressful for her and made it difficult for her to maintain a normal weight: her family's move in the eighth grade to a different town, the death of a close grandfather two years later, and finally the diagnosis of terminal brain cancer in her own mother the following year.

When she entered the tenth grade, her thin frame didn't escape the notice of her friend's mother who promptly called Danielle's mother to express her concerns. Her first appointment with a psychologist who specialized in the treatment of eating disorders followed after her father's confronting her about her food restricting. Danielle saw the psychologist only once, preferring not to return to him after he attributed her eating disorder to anger at her parents for the forced middle school relocation, a conceptualization with which she strongly disagreed. However, she did see another therapist on a regular basis along with a nutritionist who developed a meal plan for her and supervised her adherence to it.

Although she continued in therapy, she got better at lying about her dietary habits, even to her therapist. She even went so far as to put things in her pockets so that she would be heavier at her regular weigh-ins. Her charade was over, however, when, later that tenth grade year, she passed out on the way to her first period class. Helped up by her friends and escorted to the class, Danielle recalled not remembering much for the next few minutes until the school nurse arrived with a wheelchair and took her to her office. A call to Danielle's parents summoned them to school where they took her to the first of many hospitals she was to visit in the next few years.

At the end of her 11th grade after her mother's diagnosis of brain cancer, she completely fell apart, eating no solid food for 18 straight days; all that sustained her was water and coffee with a little milk. This event began years of visits to inpatient units, outpatient units, day treatment programs, and partial hospitalization programs that became part of her routine through the rest of her high school and beyond.

Case Discussion/Crisis Resolution

Now several years into recovery, Danielle is able to reflect on her journey through her anorexia. She is able to speak of it publicly and has, in fact, become a leader of a support group at a local eating disorder treatment center. She also is nearing completion of a graduate program in social work with further plans to obtain her license as a clinical social worker so that she can become a therapist for others with eating disorders. "I want to raise awareness; it helps keep me in recovery."

In the following interview, she provides insight and advice for those who treat eating disorders and for adolescents themselves. Unlike other cases in this book, the following exchange between Danielle and her counselor provides a retrospective, rather than an interventionist look, on the early stages of her anorexia.

COUNSELOR: We all know what the research says about the personality type of the individual who develops an eating disorder. Tell me what you were like as a young person.

DANIELLE: I was just a typical kid. I was teased by the proverbial school bullies just like everyone else my age was, but I took it more personally than the others. It always bothered me more.

COUNSELOR: Tell me when things started to change for you.

DANIELLE: In grade seven when I was 12 years old, things were important; looks became important, clothes were important, all those shallow things. I didn't want to wear glasses, and my shoes and everything had to be a brand name.

COUNSELOR: Middle school can be a significant transition for young adolescents. Was that transition a smooth one for you or a difficult one?

DANIELLE: It was around that time that things started to change for me. I started gaining weight but not growing tall; I was a little pudgy, maybe at most, 10 pounds overweight.

COUNSELOR: Was that a problem for you?

DANIELLE: It wasn't only that. I had been a dancer from ages 3 through 15 or 16, and I started to compare my body to other dancers' bodies, those tall, lean bodies. My stomach was a sore issue, then my thighs. I could never have a flat enough stomach.

COUNSELOR: What did you do about these thoughts and feelings?

DANIELLE: Well, I decided that perhaps a diet was in order, so I cut back drastically on my food intake. I stopped eating breakfast and lunch completely. I was unable to avoid having dinner with my family, so I had to eat at that time in order to keep from arousing suspicion in my parents.

COUNSELOR: Was there a change in your eating habits after you moved with your family to a new town? I know that you were angry over having to leave your friends behind, and you were now an eighth grader.

DANIELLE: I just added new tricks to my dieting. I still refused to eat any breakfast or lunch, and I avoided dinners whenever possible, telling my parents that I ate dinner at a friend's house or that I had something to eat on the way home from school. I would make food, and then either throw it out in the outside garbage so my family wouldn't notice or feed it to the dogs. Sometimes I would put the food in my mouth and then spit it into a napkin, but I tried not to do this too often, because I was afraid of absorbing any of the calories.

COUNSELOR: Weren't your parents suspicious?

DANIELLE: They said nothing to me at the time, but they told me years later that they had their suspicions of my problem.

COUNSELOR: How did the rest of your eighth grade go?

DANIELLE: I had a growth spurt in the eighth grade that added a few more inches in height and accentuated my thinness all the more. However, I was into my "grunge-look phase"; all that large, oversized, and ill-fitting clothing let me be fashionable while using it to conceal my shrinking frame from my parents. The only one to notice was my Health teacher who took me aside one day and told me about eating disorders, but I was convinced that the problem didn't apply to me.

(continued)

CASE PRESENTATION: Danielle, A Story of Anorexia
(continued)

COUNSELOR: So things began to peak in the eighth grade. What was your high school experience like?

DANIELLE: In high school I met another girl my age who also thought that she was overweight, so we began to compare notes with each other about our food restricting, and we learned tricks to get over. I would leave dirty knives and forks around the kitchen to suggest that I had eaten, and I'd pack a picnic lunch at home, only to throw it all in the dumpster once away from my parents. Eventually two high school teachers approached me and talked to me about not eating lunch in the school cafeteria. I dreaded the cafeteria with the conflict between the smell of good food and the desire not to eat anything. I only put food in my mouth if somebody was watching me; otherwise I just pushed the food around the plate.

COUNSELOR: When did you make your first visit to the hospital?

DANIELLE: I was 15 years old and in the tenth grade. I passed out in school; I hadn't eaten in days. The hospital didn't admit me, though. I know now that it was because of some insurance issue, but I was convinced at that time that the hospital was telling me that I was not sick, that I didn't have an eating disorder. But I was still too weak to attend school, so I stayed home from school for two weeks.

COUNSELOR: Any other hospital visits?

DANIELLE: Anymore! I had many more hospital visits and all sorts of other treatment program stays. I was in and out of them for the next few years.

COUNSELOR: And now how are you?

DANIELLE: My last stay in an eating disorders treatment program was when I was 23 years old. I knew that it was my last resort. I am in recovery now, but I will always struggle. For me, it was always an issue of control. I couldn't control my family moving, I couldn't control my mother dying, but I could control eating or not eating. I will never be happy with my body, but it doesn't control me anymore.

Bulimia is diagnosed twice as often as anorexia, and bulimia sufferers are more likely to seek treatment.

There are more estimates of the prevalence of eating disorders than there are actual statistics, particularly among adolescents, since most individuals who suffer with eating disorders keep them secret and fail to acknowledge their symptoms. Therefore, survey data may reveal only a minimal estimate of the disorder, considering the large number of unreported cases. Another confounding problem in determining the prevalence of eating disorders is the number of adolescents, primarily female, who do not exhibit all the diagnostic indicators of the disorders as determined by the *Diagnostic and Statistical Manual of Mental Disorders* (*DSM-IV*), published by the American Psychiatric Association, yet who exhibit disordered eating habits and other excessive dieting regimens.

Estimates of the number of those adolescents actually diagnosed with an eating disorder are approximately 1% for anorexia and 4% for bulimia among college-age women (Anorexia Nervosa and Related Eating Disorders Inc., 2004). Others (Polivy & Herman, 2002), however, placed the estimate at between 3% and 10% of women between the ages of 15-29. Despite these seemingly low prevalence rates for diagnosed eating disorders, there is a far greater number of adolescent females who experience eating problems that fall just below a *DSM-IV* diagnosis.

Documenting this larger number was the YRBSS, which, in tracking all health-risk behaviors of adolescents, also surveyed the dieting practices of this age group. Some of its findings among adolescent females and their attempts to lose weight are listed below:

- 38.1% described themselves as overweight

- 61.7% reported that they were trying to lose weight

- 60% had exercised to lose weight

- 17% had gone for 24 hours or more without eating

- 8.1% had taken diet pills, powders, or liquids without a doctor's advice within 30 days of the survey

- 6.2% had vomited or taken laxatives in the last 30 days

Guidelines for Intervening with Eating Disorders

One of Havighurst's (1972) developmental tasks of adolescence had to do with "accepting one's physique," and it is precisely this task that many adolescents, particularly females, find difficult. The causes of eating disorders are varied, and it is the interplay among multiple factors than determines the course the disorder follows in individuals who suffer with them. Both internal and external factors share responsibility in the occurrence of the disorder.

Among some of the internal factors is the personality trait of perfectionism that is central to eating disorders. Individuals with the disorder also tend to be overachievers, popular, and academically successful (Weis, 2008). Rigidity and over control also mark individuals with eating disorders, and they are eager to please and are overly concerned with their appearance and the way they present themselves to others. Low self-esteem also haunts them (Tozzi, Thornton, Klump, Fichter, Halmi, & Kaplan, 2005).

Other external or environmental factors that play a causative role in the disorder are the media-driven ideal of the perfect body and the glorification of a standard of beauty that is more the ideal than the real. The demands on young girls in particular to lose weight and to be attractive are powerful. Seligman (1998) referred to "the pursuit of thinness" in describing these contemporary pressures on young women, a notion echoed by other researchers (Smolak, 2006) who address the "idealization of thinness" that contributes to body dissatisfaction and, as a result, various dietary restrictions to get to the ideal body size and shape.

Individuals with anorexia in particular are convinced that they need to lose weight. Their sense of body distortion leads them to overestimate their weight and the size of their bodies. Denial about the disorder keeps them from addressing this health-threatening condition. What causes them psychological and emotional distress is not the emaciated appearance of their bodies, but rather the chronic fear that they will continue to remain overweight.

Danielle's case illustrates much of what is true for others with the disorder: denial that her extreme weight loss was a problem, an inability to view her frame as far too thin, and a sense of perfectionism and a need for control. She illustrated these issues in her description of one of her hospitalizations, this one for six weeks. She spent most of this time being fed through a feeding tube, a practice which accounted for a four-pound weight gain in the first week. Her only thought, however, was that the staff was trying to make her fat.

AN IDENTITY CRISIS IN ADOLESCENCE

Erik Erikson modified many of Freud's views on development of the individual, particularly Freud's views on adolescence. He deemphasized Freud's notion of the strength of sexual and biological drives as primary forces in personality development. What he proposed instead was a *psychosocial* rather than a *psychosexual* theory of development, placing greater emphasis on social and cultural influences on development.

Stage five of his eight-stage theory, *identity vs role confusion*, is the most germane to a discussion of adolescent development. He believed that acquiring a strong identity was dependent upon the consistent and positive recognition of the child's achievements throughout the earlier stages. As the individual develops, interactions with peers, other significant adults outside the family, and the community in general help to shape the adolescent's identity.

The adolescent "tries on" different identities, just as one might try on a suit of clothes to see how it fits before deciding to purchase the right one. The feedback received from these other sources (peers, nonfamilial adults, community) influences the adoption of the one true identity that just seems to "fit." Thus, Erikson explained, the adolescent life stage is filled with experimentation and exploration as a means toward the development of a firm identity. To master the challenge posed by the question, *Who am I?* is the goal of this developmental stage.

Guidelines for Addressing Issues of Identity Development

As Erikson (see above) suggested, the major crisis for the adolescent is the development of an identity, answering the question, "Who am I?" Toward this end, experimentation with different looks, different attitudes and beliefs, and different lifestyles is not only typical for the adolescent, but healthy as well. Without having this range of other experiences to choose from in order to establish one's

---

C A S E   P R E S E N T A T I O N : David: A Case of Identity

---

David, a 17-year-old high school junior, always appeared to be wandering through his adolescence searching for an identity that fit him just right. Like any other adolescent who was trying on different identities in an attempt to find the most comfortable one, much in the same way one tries of different suits of clothes before settling on the right one, David had a hard time finding the right "fit."

From all accounts, his middle school years, the early stage of his adolescence, was marked by a delayed onset of puberty and his slightly overweight body type was characterized by some of his peers as "girly": a reference to his soft, chubby appearance and breasts considered oversized for boys of his age group. His teachers reported at the time that he never seemed to have settled into a regular group of friends, preferring instead to wander from group to group, as if looking for one that would accept him. He also spent many afternoons after the school day ended hanging around with any one of several teachers he professed to like. Whereas other students his age were at home socializing with friends, David chose instead to spend this time with trusted adults.

Although David was a bright young man, his grades always tended to hover around the "C" range. A self-described avoider of homework and of out-of-classroom assignments, he was content with just getting by with his grades. By the time he entered high school, his teachers, almost to a person, began their descriptions of him with the statement, "He's so bright, but …." The latter part of this statement typically ended with observations of his lack of effort, his failure to complete important assignments, or some other achievement-related shortcoming. But never did teachers ever complain about his classroom behavior; David remained respectful of teachers and compliant with school rules despite that he completed little, if any, work. Although he cut classes from time to time and reported smoking marijuana with some regularity, his discipline record was unremarkable. Despite grades that kept him on the brink of academic failure and with the threat of being a five- or six-year high school student, he presented the outward demeanor of a satisfied, happy-go-lucky individual, always greeting passers-by in the school corridors with a big smile.

A number of positive things happened for David when he entered high school, the most important of which was his discovery of, and acceptance by, a new group of friends. This group of approximately ten students was just like David: disenfranchised from the typical school experience, particularly its emphasis on academic achievement, and largely ignored by other more "mainstream" social groups. Nevertheless, David felt very much at home with this newfound group of friends, regardless of the identity it provided for him. His membership in this "fringe" group helped him define himself by giving him an identity that, for him, seemed to "fit." Researchers may refer to such a group as part of a resistance culture (Woolfolk, 2007), but David would describe it as being home among friends.

David's identifiable "trademark" was a full-length, trench-coat-like black leather duster that he wore consistently every day, regardless of the weather; days of low temperatures and days of high humidity did not dissuade David from this attire. The trench coat became his "calling card," the one thing that set him apart from others, even the other members of his own social group. Whereas some adolescents sport purple hair and others, multiple facial piercings to make a statement of their identity, David chose this coat as his statement.

The trench coat, however, also served another purpose for David. Still a slightly overweight, chubby individual, there was an air of body-consciousness to David, an explanation of his cutting gym class more often than other classes and of his refusal to change for gym on those days when he did attend. Exposing his body to others in the locker room was something he preferred not to do at all costs. Therefore, his trench coat allowed him to cover his body and to keep it from the judgmental eyes of fellow students.

(continued)

C A S E P R E S E N T A T I O N : David: A Case of Identity (continued)

Then on April 20, 1999, two students named Eric Harris and Dylan Klebold entered the halls of Columbine High School in Colorado armed with several guns, killed 12 fellow students and a teacher, wounded 24 others, and then committed suicide. The shooters had been members of a fringe group not unlike David's group, a counterculture, resistance culture group that had been informally labeled the Trench Coat Mafia because of the black leather dusters worn by the shooters. Like David's group, the Columbine group had banded together for much the same reason: to form a haven for those not accepted by the mainstream students. The Trench Coat Mafia had been in existence long before the shooters had joined it, and none of the other members were implicated in the shooting.

In a knee-jerk reaction to the media-saturated images of Harris and Klebold dressed in their trench coats before the killings, many school districts, including David's, banned the wearing of trench coats in school, fearing that those who wore them could easily conceal firearms and bring them into school. And so it was with David: within days of the news of the Columbine killings, the school principal called David, the lone wearer of a trench coat in his school, into his office and told him to remove it. David reluctantly complied and then found his way to the school psychologist's office; as well as he knew David, the psychologist also had never seen him without him wearing his trademark trench coat.

Intervention:

DAVID: (Pushing open the door to the office with such force that the psychologist had never before seen in him) I can't believe it, I'm gonna kill him!

PSYCHOLOGIST: I've never seen you angry like this before. Let's sit down together so that you can tell me about it.

DAVID: It's Clement (the principal)—He says I can't wear my coat!

PSYCHOLOGIST: You can't wear your coat?

DAVID: Yeah, he says that it's a new rule because of what happened in Columbine. What does he think, that I'm going to go out there and shoot somebody? I haven't hurt anybody in my entire life!

PSYCHOLOGIST: It sounds as if that coat is very important to you.

DAVID: Yeah, I've been wearing it since middle school and nobody told me I couldn't wear it until now.

PSYCHOLOGIST: Is there anyone else in the high school, a friend of yours maybe, who also has been wearing a similar coat?

DAVID: None of my friends do, and I don't know of anyone else who might. But that doesn't really matter to me, anyway. I just want to wear my coat. I just feel too weird without it. Like I said, I've been wearing it since the seventh grade.

PSYCHOLOGIST: Was there anything special about seventh grade that made you decide to start wearing it then?

DAVID: No, but that's when I started to feel weird, like not really fitting in. Lots of kids in the middle school had families with lots of money, and we didn't have that much. You could tell from the clothes they wore. I just didn't fit in with that crowd.

PSYCHOLOGIST: It sounds like middle school was a tough time for you.

DAVID: Well, it sure wasn't fun—all those smart kids and rich kids looking so cool and all. I was a pretty good student in sixth grade, though, getting mostly A's and Bs. But when seventh grade started, I figured that I just didn't want to get into a competition for grades with all those other kids. They were all growing, and I was staying short, so I figured that there was no point in trying to be like them. I didn't want to cause any trouble or anything, I just wanted to do my own thing.

PSYCHOLOGIST: Is that when you came up with the idea for the trench coat?

DAVID: Yeah, but really I saw it once in a store, and it reminded me of one of those Clint Eastwood movies, I don't know which one, but where he wore a coat like that. So I thought it would be a cool thing to wear, and nobody else was wearing one. But then those two Columbine jerks had to wear one and ruin it for me.

PSYCHOLOGIST: So the coat has become your unique trademark, is that right?

DAVID: Yeah, I guess you could say that. But I never caused any trouble at all in school. Ask my teachers, they're all cool. I know that I don't do a lot of work or anything, but I never cause trouble.

PSYCHOLOGIST: It sounds like not doing work, even though you know you can, is as much a trademark for you as your coat. Is that right?

DAVID: (Smiling) I never thought of it like that.

PSYCHOLOGIST: O.K., so let's see. Why don't we figure out how you can present your case to the principal to get permission to wear your coat again. We can practice here how to talk to him about it in a nonconfrontational way. You also may need sort of a back-up plan in the event that he refuses to grant you permission.

DAVID: Like what? Like wearing something else instead?

PSYCHOLOGIST: Sounds reasonable to me.

DAVID: I'll think about that when the time comes, but I don't want to deal with the whole thing until next week.

Case Discussion/Crisis Resolution

Unlike the other crisis case vignettes in this chapter, David's case does not suggest a danger to life or limb. Many adolescents struggle with issues of identity, and its importance as a normal developmental struggle for many individuals made it a fitting topic to address here.

David was quite agitated being without his cherished trench coat. He vacillated between anger and tears; it wasn't necessarily the loss of his trench coat that bothered him, but rather all that it represented. To him, it was as if he were asked to stroll naked throughout the school building. His coat was his protection as well as his signature attire, which set him apart from others and contributed to his identity and to his sense of self-esteem. Without it, he was bereft of any comfortable sense of who he was.

David didn't attend school for the next couple of days, despite his professed willingness to talk to the school principal. When he returned, however, he sported another long, baggy jacket of some type which served the same purpose as his original trench coat. After some time had gone by after the Columbine news and after the psychologist had intervened for David with the school principal, the trench coat ban was lifted, and David was permitted to wear it again in school. Despite his struggle with his grades, he did manage to earn his diploma. However, most people lost track of David after he graduated. Did he continue to flounder in his search for an identity that fit? Or did his experiences to date provide him more information about who he was and where he was going?

Like other adolescents who struggle with a version of Erikson's *identity crisis*, David found solace, however temporary, in the identity he had assumed and in the social group he found that accepted him. However, David still had a long way to go before he accomplished so many of the other developmental tasks enumerated by Havighurst. What can often be expected in this age group is a sense of exploration as adolescents try on one identity at a time before settling on one that feels right for them. Significant adults in their lives have to accept those identities, provided that they are not self-destructive, and allow them to "test the waters" and to experiment with different possibilities.

The psychologist followed the LAPC approach with David. He **Listened** to the verbal and non-verbal material he offered in his reaction to the trench coat ban, **Assessed** his emotional state and David's need for support and assistance in coping with this issue, came up with a **Plan** to help him address it with the principal, and asked David to **Commit** to the plan.

own identity, adolescents would be hard pressed to come up with one of their own. Difficulties arise, of course, in the reactions of teachers and caregivers to these individual "experiments." Do they try to thwart the adolescent's attempts at trying on new roles and identities and make them "toe the mark," or do they allow them some "space" in their search for that identity that seems just right for them? A social context that allows and encourages this experimentation is necessary for the adolescent.

Having the time and opportunity to experiment with these different roles is actually a prelude to the development of an identity. Erikson's version of the *identity crisis* comes during the period that he referred to as the *psychosocial moratorium*, a time when the adolescent actually delays or takes a "time out" from other excessive responsibilities before making a commitment to a particular social or occupational role (such as identity). It is during this time that the aforementioned experimentation takes place. Those who are unable to take this "time out" however, usually miss the opportunity to undertake the requisite steps to the formation of their own identity. The 16-year-old who drops out of school in order to go to work at the local factory after his father, the sole wage earner in the family, dies is not afforded the luxury of a moratorium period, nor is the young adolescent girl who finds herself pregnant and the primary caregiver of a young baby.

In addition to the moratorium stage, Erikson and others (Marcia, 1994, 1999) discussed several other *identity statuses*, or outcomes, of the search for an identity:

- **Identity foreclosure**—a very undesirable outcome, foreclosure is commitment to an identity without any exploration. Instead of considering a range of possibilities, this adolescent commits prematurely to a role usually determined by parents or other authority figures. For example, the adolescent who was predestined from childhood to follow in the family tradition and become a dentist just like his father and grandfather before him.

- **Identity diffusion**—an incoherent sense of self without any firm direction, diffusion varies in intensity from adolescent to adolescent. A sense of self-consciousness and low self-esteem makes some adolescents unable to make a decision about their lives, whereas others may become openly rebellious and simply follow whatever crowd accepts them (Kroger, 2000). Is David in this stage?

- **Identity achievement**—a healthy identity status, achievement means that a commitment is made after many options had been explored. However, since the moratorium stage has been lengthened for many adolescents by virtue of their remaining in school for undergraduate and graduate degrees, identity achievement may not be attained until several years after adolescence is assumed (or usually) over.

- **Negative identity**—an indication that there are problems in identity development. After failing to receive positive recognition and support from significant adults in their lives, adolescents assume an identity that is completely contrary to their family values and unwritten codes of conduct. In other words, being known as a "rebel" is more desirable than being known as a "nobody." The son of the local police chief breaks the law repeatedly and is known to all local law enforcement officers, or the daughter of accomplished concert pianists drops out of school to pursue a career as a rock singer against the mandates of her parents. Is David in this stage?

Identity formation is a process that takes time to unfold. The number of times that college students change their major courses of study speaks to the changing nature of the process, and it suggests that identity formation may indeed begin in adolescence but not end until after the college years are over.

ADOLESCENT SUICIDE

Even though deaths by suicide are relatively rare, suicidal thoughts and other related behaviors are much more common (Lieberman, Poland, & Cassel, 2008). Despite the best guess at the prevalence of suicide, it is important to note that the number of reported suicides may be an underestimate of the actual number (Berman, Jobes, & Silverman, 2006). Clouding the issue are those single-victim deaths in automobile accidents and in other tragic events in which the cause of death could indeed be either accidental or purposeful, yet lack enough compelling evidence to classify them as suicides.

The Center for Disease Control and Prevention (CDC) reported that there are 100–200 suicide attempts for every completed suicide among young adults ages 15 to 24. According to the CDC, 32,000 people kill themselves each year—the equivalent of 89 per day or one every 16 minutes—and another 425,000 people are treated in hospital emergency rooms for self-inflicted injuries each year. Although suicide was the eleventh leading cause of death for all ages (CDC, 2005), its mortality ranking rose markedly among 15–24 year-olds where it was considered the third leading cause of death (CDC, 2005). Males between the ages of 15–19 take their own lives at more than four times the rate of females, yet the latter group attempt suicide more frequently than males (Berman et al., 2006).

In its survey of American high school youth, the YRBSS (see above) reported some staggering statistics regarding the prevalence of those feelings and suicidal behaviors that often are precursors to a completed suicide. In the 12 months preceding the survey, adolescents reported the following:

- 28.5% felt so sad or hopeless almost every day for two weeks or more that they were unable to do some usual activities (36.7% of females made this report versus 20.4% of males)

- 16.9% had seriously considered attempting suicide (21.8% of females, 12% of males)

- 13% made a plan about how they would attempt suicide (16.2% of females, 9.9% of males)

- 8.4% actually attempted suicide one or more times (10.8% of females, 6% of males)

- 2.3% made a suicide attempt resulting in an injury, poisoning, or overdose that had to be treated by a doctor or nurse (2.9% of females, 1.8% of males)

CASE PRESENTATION: Georgia, a Threatened Suicide

Georgia was a 17-year-old high school junior. Although not an outgoing, gregarious individual, she maintained a small group of friends who tended to look out for each other. She was an average student who spoke of attending college, even though she hadn't made any overtures regarding readying applications or visiting campuses of preferred colleges. Her friends talked of going away to school and spoke in generalities about what they could see themselves doing as a career, but Georgia was always noncommittal. Her group tended to spend weekends together, seeing movies or attending parties hosted by other high school friends. No one knew much about Georgia's family, just that her mother had passed away a year earlier after a bout with stomach cancer. She and her mother had been very close.

One day two of her friends dropped in to see the school counselor at the high school, asking to see her right away because of an "emergency." The counselor sat down with the two who both expressed concern over Georgia. They told her that Georgia had been acting "standoffish" lately, preferring not to accompany the rest of the group on their weekend activities. According to them, she also started to look more sloppy than usual in her attire, something out of character for someone who always tended to her appearance with great care. Her friends went on to describe a phone call they each had received the night before from Georgia in which she told them that she wanted them to have several of her CDs of her favorite rock group. She also told them that she might not be around much longer, thus her wish for them to have the CDs. Putting all these signs together and having recently had a suicide awareness program in their Health class, they rushed to see the counselor for assistance.

Intervention

FRIENDS: Before you do anything with what we told you, please don't tell anybody else. Georgia would get real mad at us. We just wanted to find out from you what we should do.

COUNSELOR: First of all, I am ethically bound to maintain confidentiality in my interactions with my clients. However, I also am ethically bound to break that confidence in the event that I am told that someone intends to hurt themselves or somebody else or if someone is hurting them. Then I am obligated to tell those who are in a position to provide help and protection in order to ensure the safety of the individual. That is the case here with your friend, Georgia. You have done the right thing to come to me with your concerns. I agree with you that these concerns are real ones.

FRIENDS: But you're not going to tell her that we were the ones who told you, are you? She really will be mad at us!

COUNSELOR: No, I won't tell her who alerted me to this situation, but my experience tells me that when I speak with her, she will know who gave me her name. But wouldn't you rather have a friend who is alive to be mad at you rather than one whose obituary you read about in tomorrow's newspaper?

FRIENDS: O.K. You're right.

As soon as the students left her office, the counselor went to Georgia's classroom and asked her to accompany her to her office.

COUNSELOR: Hello, Georgia. I haven't seen you since the semester began. I saw that you were working in groups in class just now. What was it you were working on?

GEORGIA: (Looking down at the floor as she spoke in a low monotone) It was social studies class; and we were working on analyzing the major causes of the civil war.

COUNSELOR: It sounds like you weren't really into it.

GEORGIA: It was boring and stupid. The other three people in the group talked too much. I just didn't want to be there. It's just stupid; the civil war is over, anyway, so why go over it again?

COUNSELOR: I'm concerned that you seem pretty down right now. In fact, that's the reason I wanted to see you today. Some of your friends came to see me earlier today to tell me that they were very worried about you.

GEORGIA: (Interrupting angrily) I know, it was (names both students)! I told them not to tell anybody! I knew that I shouldn't have come to school today!

COUNSELOR: I know that you are angry with them; they were afraid that you might be angry with them for coming to me, but what they did was out of a great concern for you. They like you and value your friendship. They did the right thing by coming to me. That's why I wanted to see you, because what they told me concerned me a great deal. You are certainly not in any trouble, but you do seem down.

GEORGIA: (No acknowledgment, only silence and staring at the floor)

COUNSELOR: Tell me Georgia, have you thought about killing yourself?

GEORGIA: (Mumbling) Yeah.

COUNSELOR: About how many times have you thought about it?

GEORGIA: I don't know, a bunch, maybe 10 to 12 times.

COUNSELOR: O.K., so you really have been feeling pretty down for a while now. Am I right? Tell me the last time you thought about it.

GEORGIA: I guess I've thinking about it this week.

COUNSELOR: Has anything been going on in your life recently that might have something to do with your thoughts of suicide?

GEORGIA: I don't know, since my mother died, I've been kinda lonely. And all this talk of going away to college (her voice trails off).

COUNSELOR: And going away to college is not something that appeals to you at this time?

GEORGIA: Not now. I just wish that everybody else would just let everyone do what they want to do.

COUNSELOR: Let's go back again to what you told me before, that you were thinking about killing yourself. You said that you have been thinking about it as recently as this past week. How did you plan to do it?

GEORGIA: Well, there are lots of pills and things in my bathroom medicine cabinet. My dad is on antidepressants, and there are different kinds of pills left over from when my mother had cancer. My father doesn't do much to throw the old pills away, so I figured that I could take a whole bunch of them and do the job.

(continued)

CASE PRESENTATION: Georgia, a Threatened Suicide (*continued*)

COUNSELOR: Why have you decided not to take these pills up until now? I mean, you knew where to get them, right?

GEORGIA: Of course I know where to get them.

COUNSELOR: I am glad that you did nothing about those pills and that you told your friends instead. What stopped you from taking them?

GEORGIA: Well, I did try taking a bunch of the pills a few weeks ago, but all it did was put me to sleep; I woke up real groggy and dizzy, but everyone thought that it was because I was hungover from the night before. No one knew that I took them to try to kill myself. I thought about it again, but then I thought that my dad would be so upset, first with my mom dying, and then me! I couldn't bear to have him that upset again.

COUNSELOR: So it sounds as if you have some mixed feelings here, wanting to die, yet not wanting to because of what it would do to your father, right?

GEORGIA: I guess so.

COUNSELOR: Have you thought about taking these pills again? Or doing something else to kill yourself?

GEORGIA: I don't know anymore, but maybe.

COUNSELOR: Georgia, I am still concerned about you. Since I want to make sure that you are safe, even after you leave here, I have to call your father. I am concerned that, once you are home, you may have those thoughts again. I want your father to take you to see some other counselors who will decide if you need to talk to someone else about these feelings of yours.

GEORGIA: Whatever.

Case Discussion/Crisis Resolution

The counselor considered Georgia to be at a high risk for another suicide attempt. She had already made a previous attempt, she had access to the methods she needed to kill herself, and she sent out clear indicators that she intended to complete the act. That is, she essentially said "good-bye" to her friends and had sent out other signals (giving away her favorite CDs) that she would not see them much longer. Her friends also were able to describe changes in her behavior, and her admitted sense of loneliness upon the death of her mother also was alarming to the counselor. Another major life

---

Common risk factors for suicide include symptoms of depression, such as feelings of sadness, helplessness, and hopelessness (Brock, Sandoval, & Hart, 2006). The CDC also included among its list of risk factors:

- previous suicide attempts
- history of mental illness
- alcohol or drug abuse
- family history of suicide or violence

transition, the possibility of going away to college or of her friends all leaving her for college, was a frightening prospect for her. Georgia also did not convince the counselor that she would not make another attempt on her life, making it clear that she could do so at any time.

Whether a high risk or not, the counselor explained to Georgia that she was obligated to call her father to notify him of the danger and to have him take her to the local emergency psychiatric screening unit. Although Georgia was not pleased when the counselor told her that she was going to call her father, she did not resist the notion, as if secretly relieved. She requested to be allowed to go back to her next class while awaiting the arrival of her father at school, but the need for close supervision made the counselor deny this request. Instead, Georgia remained in the counselor's office, and the counselor also accompanied her on a visit to the women's room an hour later.

Although her father seemed somewhat resistant to leaving work early to come to school and pick up his daughter for a trip to the local crisis unit, he eventually agreed to do so when the counselor told him that, in his absence, she would be obligated to contact the local Child Protective Services unit to take her instead. When her father appeared in the high school, the counselor explained in detail her concerns and made sure that he understood the importance of making his home "suicide proof" by removing all medications in the medicine chest or in other places that Georgia might access. He agreed to do so, and he signed an agreement with the counselor that he would bring Georgia to the unit and would follow up on its recommendations for additional help or treatment. The counselor promised to keep track of Georgia's progress and to develop a plan for her to return to school with the appropriate services.

It was important for the counselor to make a carefully considered intervention once Georgia's friends brought their concerns to her attention. She was able to follow the **LAPC** model and to **Listen,** both to what her friends said and to what Georgia answered, both verbally and nonverbally, to her questions. She remained nonjudgmental, used active listening, and was able to **Assess** the fact that she was at a high risk for another suicide attempt. The **Plan** was to contact the father, have her screened by the local crisis unit, and create a follow-up system when Georgia returned to school. Although Georgia appeared quite depressed and lethargic and was not willing to **Commit** to the plan, her father did so. Georgia's sense of relief that her suicidal thoughts were finally addressed was palpable.

- physical illness
- feeling alone, depressed
- feelings of helplessness and hopelessness

Although situational factors such as physical abuse, legal troubles, the breakup with a boyfriend or girlfriend, academic failure, bullying or victimization, the death of someone significant, and knowing someone who died by suicide may serve as precipitants to suicidal behavior, they only lead to suicide among those individuals who also satisfy a host of other risk factors as well.

Guidelines for Dealing with a Suicidal Adolescent

Whenever in doubt about whether or not a seemingly depressed adolescent poses a suicide risk, the best thing to do is to ask them directly if they have thoughts of hurting or killing themselves. Of course, if they answer in the affirmative, the adult who posed the question must be able to make the appropriate intervention or provide the right referral for help. Once identified, they must also be monitored closely until the proper help is provided. Not all depressed adolescents are suicidal, but if they satisfy many of the risk factors described above, the potential for suicidal behavior increases considerably.

Perhaps the best way to make sure that suicidal adolescents are identified and treated is to be proactive and preventive in nature. Providing education for those who regularly come into contact with adolescents regarding the warning signs of suicidal thoughts or behaviors is an important step. Teachers, parents, coaches, mentors, community groups, and even other adolescents would all benefit from some form of training in recognizing the warning signs of a depressed and potentially suicidal adolescent. Educating these individuals and groups about what to do and whom to tell about their concerns is of equal importance in this training.

Many of these warning signs were present in Georgia's case: a previous attempt, making final arrangements, having access to the means of suicide, the loss of a parent, the beginning of a major life transition (college), and depression. Those who were in a position to observe these signs, including her loss of interest in all the social things that she once participated in, were able to report their concerns to the appropriate person, Georgia's school counselor. One such school-based program is Signs of Suicide, designed for middle and high schools students. It involves training in the warning signs of suicide in addition to a depression screening for the individuals involved. Parents, school staff, and students themselves go through this training program and are able to contribute to the prevention of adolescent suicide by learning the warning signs and the appropriate means of intervention (Lieberman, Poland, & Cassel, 2008).

ADOLESCENTS WHO SELF-MUTILATE:

AN OVERVIEW

It is difficult to address the issue of adolescent suicidal behavior without also addressing one of the least understood behaviors of adolescence, which appears to be increasing at an alarming rate: self-mutilation. Those who engage in this behavior, also known as "cutters," engage in direct, intentional, repetitive behavior that results in mild to moderate physical injury (McVey-Noble, Khemlani-Patel, & Neziroglu, 2006). Officially known as Repetitive Self-Mutilation Syndrome (RSM), it also is referred to as Self-Injurious Behavior (SIB), parasuicidal behavior, and deliberate self-harm (Lieberman, 2004).

They use knives, razors, the metal scraper from the plastic pencil sharpener, thumb tacks, or any other sharp instruments to make slices in their skin, usually in some little-noticed body part, like the inner thighs, the abdomen, or the inside of their upper arms (Zila & Kiselica, 2001), all the areas that can be concealed easily from others. However, their attempts at keeping these marks secret don't always escape the watchful eye of gym teachers, parents, or sports coaches. They tend to engage in these cutting behaviors secretively; they may also do so in the school bathrooms, locker rooms, or other isolated and secluded areas. Although cutting is the most common form of self-injury, other self injurious behaviors are scratching, burning oneself, hitting oneself (head against the wall), picking at old wounds, and hair pulling (trichotillomania) (Winkler, 2003).

For every 100,000 adolescents, the estimates are that approximately 750–1,800 of them will engage in self-injurious behaviors (Suyemoto & Kountz, 2002), approximately 150,000–360,000 adolescents around the country; more than 70% are female. Almost all of those who engage in self-injurious behaviors (90%) begin in adolescence (Bowman & Randall, 2004). Some also think that 13% of adolescents engage in these behaviors (Ross & Heath, 2002), although it is difficult to determine the actual number due to the secrecy attached to these behaviors.

There is a common misconception that adolescents who engage in self-injurious behavior such as cutting are doing so in a conscious attempt to commit suicide. The difference, however, is that adolescents who cut themselves seek to feel better as if to ward off suicidal feelings, whereas the truly suicidal adolescent seeks to end all feelings of pain (Favazza, 1998). In fact, there appears to be no conscious suicidal intent on the part of the cutter; it is as if they are cutting themselves so that they do not kill themselves. Even the wounds they inflict on themselves are relatively superficial and not life-threatening like slitting the wrists in a true suicide attempt. It is primarily the skin that is damaged, and not the veins, arteries, or ligaments, so the long-term harm is limited to scarring (Levenkron, 1998).

They may be engaging in self-injurious behavior like cutting because self-mutilation may actually create a sense of relief, calm, and satisfaction due to the release of the brain's natural antidepressants, endorphins. For this reason it is considered an impulse disorder not unlike eating disorders, shoplifting, and substance abuse. The behavior is controlling them; they are not controlling the behavior.

Although not a sign of a suicidal attempt, adolescents who self-injure are troubled and are crying out for help, and are not to be taken lightly. It is as if they are putting into practice what they cannot put into words; they convert the emotional pain that they cannot express into physical pain, a form of self-punishment to help them gain greater control over their own emotions (Lieberman, 2004). Other functions of self-injury (Kress, Gibson, & Reynolds, 2004) include:

- feeling concrete pain when psychic pain is too overwhelming
- reducing numbness and promoting a sense of being real
- keeping traumatic memories from intruding
- modulating affect

C A S E   P R E S E N T A T I O N : A Case of Self-Injury: Cutting

---

Jessica was a cheerleader for her local high school basketball team. She was active in the squad as well as in other school activities. Several of her teachers thought that she ran with the wrong crowd, but she was well liked by the staff, nevertheless. She was not a very talkative individual, although her grades were acceptable. She tended to keep to herself except for the cheerleading activity that she appeared to enjoy as much as she enjoyed her friends who were on the squad with her. They were a cohesive group of adolescents, both on and off the court.

One day the cheerleader coach called Jessica aside to share her concerns. During several of the practices, she had noticed numerous cuts along Jessica's stomach as she jumped high in a routine with a short, waist-length jersey that easily leaped up, exposing her abdomen. Since the faculty had recently had an in-service workshop on the issue of cutting, the coach was immediately suspicious, thus her explanation to Jessica for pulling her aside. Even though Jessica told her that it was "nothing," that all the girls were doing it, the coach nevertheless brought her concerns to the school psychologist and to Jessica's parents. Her parents were vaguely familiar with the phenomenon of cutting and decided to seek out a therapist in the community.

Intervention

COUNSELOR: Jessica, how are you feeling? You know that you are here because your parents had concerns about you.

JESSICA: I know, I know, but this is stupid! My coach told them that I had cut myself, but it's not a big deal. She should mind her own business, anyway; it's none of her business what I do with my body.

COUNSELOR: Jessica, you are not in trouble here. I know other young women like you who started cutting themselves. I know that many of them were hurting and came here for help.

JESSICA: What do you mean, help?

COUNSELOR: Well, they were hurting for different kinds of reasons. They came for help. I am wondering if you are hurting or upset about something also. If I can't help, I can find someone else for you to talk to.

JESSICA: I just feel so weird being here for this, talking to you about some cuts on my stomach. I mean, it's embarrassing!

- receiving support and caring from others
- discharging anger, anxiety, despair, or disappointment
- self-punishing
- gaining a sense of control

Another phenomenon with regard to self-injury is the issue of contagion, the imitation of the behavior of others in the environment. That is, having a friend or relative who self-injures raises the likelihood of the same imitative behavior in another adolescent. Such behaviors often spread through peer groups, grade levels, and campus clubs, serving as a "rite of togetherness" to consolidate certain friendships and romances (Froeschle & Moyer, 2004). Nevertheless, many

COUNSELOR: There is nothing to be ashamed of here. Sometimes hurting yourself is the best way to deal with your feelings. And sometimes hurting yourself is a sign of other things. Tell me, have you ever had thoughts of suicide?

JESSICA: (Immediately) No! That's got nothing to do with my cutting.

COUNSELOR: So you haven't had those thoughts?

JESSICA: No! I definitely don't want to die. I just get so stressed out sometimes, with all the practices and the school work, and all the stuff going on at home, that I just need a relief, so I started slicing my stomach one night when I was shaving my legs. In a weird way, it actually felt good. I don't know what it is, but it took a lot of my stress away.

COUNSELOR: Others have also said that cutting helps them deal with their stress, but there are other ways of dealing with those things without having to hurt yourself.

JESSICA: What kinds of ways?

Crisis Discussion/Crisis Resolution

Like many individuals who self-injure, Jessica did not appear to be at risk for any suicidal intent. What she did highlight, however, was her shame and embarrassment over being "caught" for what she had done. What also was important, though, was that the counselor did not react in a directive, judgmental way but rather reassured her that there was nothing to be ashamed of and that she knew of many other adolescents who engaged in the same behavior.

In this very early stage of the counseling relationship, the counselor used active listening in an attempt to engage Jessica in a therapeutic relationship. She used these techniques to **Listen** to her thoughts and feelings about the cutting, she used these observations to **Assess** her feeling-state and her level of potential suicidality, and her **Plan** was to either refer Jessica to another helping professional or to present to her other ways of coping with her life stresses. Finally, the counselor's last step would be to get Jessica to **Commit** to working on this very plan.

students who self-injure will invariably be assessed at low risk for suicide and will not demonstrate any overt emotional disturbance.

Guidelines for Treating an Adolescent for Self-Injury

Despite what, to most people, is the unsettling practice of purposefully cutting oneself, it is important to avoid alienating the adolescent by reacting with shock, disgust, or disbelief. Rather, building trust is critical, since the cutter is someone in pain and in need of a nonjudgmental professional.

As can be seen in the case above, once a cutter has been identified and referred to the appropriate professional, an assessment should be made regarding whether or not they are safe. Many of those who self-injure are not suicidal, but it should be ruled out by a trained professional. This assessment would determine whether or not the individual was safe or in need of additional emergency services. Whether suicidal or not, those who self-injure are looking for a way to cope with their psychic pain. For Jessica, this pain was related to the many stressors in her life for which cutting provided considerable relief. Acknowledging not only these feelings but also their use of cutting as a means of coping with them is reassuring and soothing for cutters. Providing Jessica with more appropriate means of stress reduction and with better problem-solving and coping skills would be the direction therapeutic intervention would take.

RECOMMENDATIONS FOR CHAPTER ENRICHMENT

SUGGESTED FILMS

Thirteen (2003) Tracy is at the precipice of adolescence. A straight-A student, she eventually befriends Evie, the most popular and beautiful girl in school, who leads her down the path of sex, drugs, and small-time crime. Tracy transforms herself and adopts a new identity, putting her at odds with all who knew her, especially her mother, her teachers, and her old friends.

The Breakfast Club (1985) Trapped in a day-long Saturday detention in their high school library, a group of five adolescents, strangers to each other at the start of the day, bond together in response to the villainous school principal. Each of the five students represents a social group within the school's "caste" system: the princess, the jock, the criminal, the brain, and the basket case. Commonalities among them emerge throughout the course of the day, however, as they discuss issues about their lives, their relationships, and their views of the adults in their lives.

The Virgin Suicides (1999) The Lisbon family seemed ordinary enough. The father was a math teacher at the local high school, and the mother was a woman of great religious faith. Their five daughters ranged in age from 13 to 17. Their lives all changed, however, when the youngest daughter, Cecelia, falls into a deep depression and makes a suicide attempt. Family adjustments to the event and the advice of a psychiatrist are to no avail, as Cecilia eventually makes good on her decision to kill herself. The film depicts how the family is changed in dramatic ways.

Dead Poet's Society (1989) Depicts the suicide death of a young teenager who feels trapped by his father's expectations of him.

SUGGESTED ACTIVITIES

1. Seek out a mental health counselor in your local middle or high school; perhaps a school psychologist, social worker, school counselor, or substance abuse counselor. Ask about the prevalence of suicide attempts or

completions experienced in his or her career. Discuss what is involved in a suicide assessment. Inquire also about the themes involved in these cases (precipitating events, risk factors present, and so on).

2. Contact a school administrator with many years of experience in either a middle school or high school. Discuss his or her perceptions of how the typical adolescent has changed since beginning to work in education. That is, in what ways have adolescents changed over the years? Are contemporary issues for them different from their issues 10 years ago? 20 years ago?

3. Look up the 10 most popular movies among adolescents from each of the last few decades (1970s, 1980s, 1990s, 2000s). Compare and contrast them according to themes and main characters. Are there discernable differences among these different eras in the way adolescents, families, or school personnel are portrayed?

4

Crisis at Midlife

DISCUSSION QUESTIONS

Conduct an informal survey of your parents' friends, assuming that they fall somewhere in the "Baby Boomer" age range (44–62). Have they changed jobs or have they stayed with the same position for an extended period? Have they been married for a long time?

What kinds of crises would you anticipate during the middle years of life? Why?

Are there any differences in the values or beliefs between you and your parents? In what areas are these differences most pronounced? Which values or beliefs are most similar?

INTRODUCTION

Does a midlife crisis just happen at midlife? Are midlifers any more prone to stage-specific crises than those in other life stages? Is midlife real, a popular myth, or truly a stage to enter with trepidation? The word *midlife* first appeared in Funk and Wagnall's Standard Dictionary in 1895 as "the part of life between youth and old age" (Lachman, 2004). The term *midlife crisis* itself has been attributed to Jacques (1965), who concluded that the crisis occurs during this life stage due to people's growing awareness of their own mortality and to a change in their reference point from the "time since birth" to the "time left to live." Famed psychiatrist Carl Jung (1933) described midlife as "the afternoon of life."

Research into midlife is also relatively new. Just a little over 20 years ago, Levinson (1986) claimed that the study of adult development was in its infancy, and he attributed an increase in interest in the topic to the writings of the developmental theorist Erik Erikson (see page 68). Brim (1992) also described the middle years as the "last uncharted territory in human development." Even though there has been a recent increase in research activity on the middle years, Lachman (2004) claimed that "still less is known about this period than about other age periods such as infancy, childhood, adolescence, or old age." The study of the middle years, she continued, is critical, considering the large numbers of adults currently in this stage and the large portion of the lifespan covered by this period.

Despite the dearth of research into the reality of *midlife crisis*, "If you ask people of all ages to free associate to the word 'midlife,' usually a large percentage will quickly offer the word 'crisis'" (Lachman, 2004). This tendency undoubtedly represents little more than a cultural stereotype about this period rather than an accurate portrayal, since only a small percentage of individuals seem to experience a crisis (Wethington, Kessler, & Pixley, 2004). Nevertheless, the popular notions of *midlife* and of *midlife crisis* underscore the importance of the need for accurate definitions of these terms. In general, midlife itself is not a crisis; the cases represented later in this chapter happened during midlife but are not the result of entering midlife.

DEFINITIONAL CONSIDERATIONS

The use of chronological age as the only determinant of midlife may not be sufficient, considering that the upper end of midlife is stretched further and further as people live longer and remain healthier for a greater proportion of the lifespan (Lachman, 2004). Gail Sheehy, the author of the best-selling books *Passages* and *New Passages*, which explored the topic of adult life stages, referred to midlife as "the mid-forties to mid-sixties, the most unrevealed portion of adult life" (1995, p. ix). Oliver Brim, the director of arguably the longest study of aging in the world, Harvard University's *Study of Adult Development*, considered midlife as "the years between 30 and 70, with 40 to 60 at its core, perhaps the least studied and most ill-defined of any period in life."

The National Council on Aging (2000) reported that nearly half of those aged 65 to 69 who responded to its survey on aging considered themselves to be middle-aged, as did one-third of respondents in their seventies. Despite the fact that most people consider the modal entry and exit ages of midlife to be 40 and 60, respectively, it is not uncommon for some to consider midlife to span the years 30 to 75 (Lachman, 2001).

The group commonly known as the "Baby Boomers"—those babies born between 1946 and 1964 in a never-before-seen population explosion after World War II, is a group that Lachman (2004) reported "is moving through midlife in record numbers." The period began in 1946 with the American soldiers' return home after World War II and ended after 1964 when the number of births fell below four million for the first time in the last 11 of the Boomer years. In all, 75.8 million Americans were born during this period, and Boomers today represent approximately 30% of the U.S. population (U.S. Census Bureau, 2000). Today, the Baby Boomers range from age 45 to 63.

The notion of *midlife crisis* is also hard to define because different definitions of the term abound and the issue itself is "beset with conceptual difficulties" (Shek, 1996). Problems with defining the term have resulted in conflicting findings over the years. Even the very nature of midlife varies according to multiple factors such as gender, socioeconomic status (SES), race, ethnicity, culture, region of the country, personality, marital status, parental status, employment status, and health status (Lachman, 2004).

Despite the common expectations of a crisis at midlife, the research does not support this belief. The inconsistent data collected regarding the existence of a crisis specific to midlife raises questions as to whether a crisis is indeed unique to midlife or to any one of several precipitating events such as job loss, financial problems, or illness, which can occur at any time in adulthood (Wethington et al., 2004). Still others (Lachman, 2004) suggest that the predicaments of being in the middle of life may be an impetus for change but not necessarily a crisis (i.e., the cultural emphasis on youthful appearance and the anticipated decline in cognitive and physical functioning). The research in this area will be discussed later in this chapter.

MIDDLE LIFE THEORY

Erik Erikson (see Chapter 3), one of the premier developmental theorists, addressed the midlife years in his seventh stage—the middle adult years from the late 20s though retirement, in which the crisis centers around *generativity versus stagnation.*

Individuals in this stage, he proposed, ask whether or not they have been productive and creative, leaving something important and meaningful behind (children, work, and so on). If they feel that they have not done so, they encounter the *midlife crisis.*

Psychiatrist Carl Jung (1875–1961) maintained that people's experiences with the stages of midlife transition vary from individual to individual; for some it may be a painful process, whereas for others it may be as smooth as earlier life transitions. Some people welcome such changes, and still others prefer not to remove their *personae* and take a good look at themselves.

Levinson (1986) conceived of the life cycle as a sequence of *eras*, each with its own special character and with its distinctive contribution to the whole. He referred to a *midlife transition* period, roughly ages 40 to 45, in which individuals leave the era of early adulthood and enter middle adulthood. It is during this transition period that individuals begin a new step in individuation and begin to prepare for the rest of their lives while setting new goals for themselves.

His third era, middle adulthood, spans the ages of 40 to 65. Although physical health and strength may be on the wane, individuals in this stage nevertheless can become more accepting of themselves and continue to maintain an active personal and professional life. This transition, however, can indeed be a crisis for some people, a time of great struggle and of feeling limited by uncontrollable life events. The anxiety that they experience while approaching this stage is more of a crisis than a transition for them.

WHAT THE RESEARCH SAYS

Research involving the reality of crisis at midlife is equivocal. Recent research has cast significant doubts on the belief that crisis is inevitable during this time more often than at other times in life. Older research, however, suggested that midlife was indeed a time of great turmoil and stress. For example, some (Levinson, Darrow, Klein, Levinson, & McKee, 1978) have found that 80% of the participants in their study had experienced midlife crisis and Ciernia (1985) found crises present in 70% of the men studied.

On the other hand, there is the view that midlife is a period of peak functioning for the individual (Neugarten, 1968) and an age period with desirable characteristics. Others (Wethington et al., 2004) support this notion, reporting that only a small minority (26%) of their study participants experienced a midlife crisis.

There are several problems which confound the study of this topic (Shek, 1996; Lachman, 2004). Included among the problems associated with this research are the following:

- reliance on questionnaires and psychological scales for data collection are unreliable and unproven as accurate measures
- regarding the midlife crisis as a one-dimensional concept and not one with multiple facets
- reliance on information regarding midlife crisis from the accounts of clinician's work with middle-aged clients who already had problems and sought therapy

Researchers are concerned with the inaccurate picture of individuals at midlife that the use of flawed measurement techniques may create. The more unreliable the techniques used, the most disparate the results, with midlife portrayed as either a bane or a boon to the individual.

A more balanced view has been proposed, one designed to reconcile the disparate views of midlife (Lachman, 2004). Lachman proposed four perspectives as alternatives for exploring the paradox of midlife, offering reasons why there have been so many differences in research findings into this age group. She suggested the following:

1. The differing findings about life at midlife represent two extremes along the same continuum, with most people falling somewhere in the middle and doing fine without a crisis, and a few others falling at either extreme end of this continuum.

2. The portrayals of midlife may describe individual differences only, with some people doing well and others who are not.

3. There is a sequential relationship between crisis and peak, with crisis having an adaptive quality that promotes a positive response and leads to a period of growth—a peak in performance or status.

4. People show different outcomes in various domains of life, with crises appearing in one area (work) but not in others (family, social).

The following table summarizes those research findings which illustrate the different patterns of midlife functioning (Lachman, 2004):

Function	What We Know
Cognitive Functioning	Research does not support the popular belief that cognitive functions (such as memory and reasoning) deteriorate in this life stage. If anything, verbal memory seems to peak at midlife, as does vocabulary and inductive reasoning.
Personality and the Self	Although personality seems to be set in young adulthood and to remain stable throughout life, there also is evidence that personality does change during adulthood. Different traits also follow different patterns of change, with some showing an increase (agreeableness) and some a decline (neuroticism).
	Most midlifers with a well-established sense of identity function well psychologically and easily cope with change and with the stressors of everyday life. Evidence suggests that midlife is generally a time of increased well-being, although this may vary by social class.
Emotional Development	The affect of midlifers is more like that of younger, rather than older adults. Major depression decreases with age, although marital separation or divorce elevates the risk for depression, with men suffering from these events more than women. People during this stage also regulate emotions more effectively than younger or older adults.
Social Relationships	Midlifers reported that family was the most important and satisfying area of their lives. Even those in the "sandwich generation," the state of existing in the dual role of raising adolescent children and caring for their own aging parents, considered this role to be a "squeeze" but not a stress. Those with children reported more distress than those without, but also greater psychological wellness and generativity.
Work	The role of work is central during this period. The impact of job instability depends on the person's age and the state of the economy. As a transition period before retirement, this phase can be either a welcome precursor to retirement or something to be avoided.
Health & Physical Changes	For most midlifers, health is generally good and most physical changes are not disabling, even if they do raise concerns about the aging process. Individual differences in aging are broad and are influenced by such things as heredity and lifestyle. Health-related behaviors such as exercise and vitamin-use decline with age. There also is no evidence for a universal experience of distress for women due to menopause.

A MacArthur Foundation–sponsored study *Midlife in the U.S.* (MIDUS) surveyed approximately 15,000 people over almost a decade and concluded that the idea of an inevitable midlife crisis was largely a myth and no more likely at midlife than it was at any other life stage. The commonly held belief that the "empty nest" syndrome created when the last child leaves home permanently creates its own distressing aftermath is also misleading because this event actually creates the advantages of more freedom, breathing space, and opportunity.

The American Association of Retired Persons (AARP) commissioned a study, *Boomers at Midlife 2004*, designed to investigate what people born between 1946 and 1964 had to say about their lives. Approximately 2,500 individuals at middle age participated in a telephone survey examining seven broad life areas: family and friend relationships, personal finances, religious or spiritual life, work or career, physical health, mental health, and leisure activities. Below are some of the survey findings that Boomers are:

- more similar to younger than older individuals; differences tend to be related to social or political issues rather than to personal life assessments
- satisfied with their lives overall
- most satisfied with relationships with family and friends
- very satisfied with their mental health
- least satisfied with their personal finances and their work lives (23% reported that their financial life was the worst thing in their lives; only 40% were very satisfied with their work or career)
- not very satisfied with their leisure activities (only 30% reported being very satisfied)
- satisfied with their religious or spiritual lives (48%)

These findings were similar to those from two earlier surveys conducted by the AARP. Some differences were noted, however, in gender, race and ethnicity, income, and education level. Some of these differences are listed below:

Gender Differences Among Boomers

- Men (43%) were more satisfied with where the country was going than women (29%)
- Women placed greater importance on (58% vs 36%) and gained satisfaction with (53% vs 42%) their spiritual/religious lives than men do
- Women were more likely than men (41% vs 35%) to name family and friends as the best thing in their lives

Race/Ethnicity Differences Among Boomers

- African Americans were most likely to pick their religious/spiritual life as most important to them (38%), whereas white boomers chose family and friends as most important (43%)
- African Americans (44%) were more likely than white (29%) or Hispanic boomers (26%) to claim that they were worse off than expected

Income Differences

- Higher-earning boomers (income of $75,000 or more) were more satisfied with their lives in general than low-income boomers (less than $25,000) (91% vs 68%)
- Low-income boomers rated their health status lower than higher-income boomers
- High-income boomers (37%) were more likely to plan their future in detail than low-income boomers who tended to be spontaneous and have no detailed plans for the future (63%)

Education Differences

- College-educated boomers were more likely to be more satisfied than those without a college degree with their lives in general (86% vs 80%), their mental health (65% vs 57%), personal finances (27% vs 20%), and their work/career lives (48% vs 36%)

CASE PRESENTATION: Brad and Season's End

Brad had been married to his wife, Sarah, for almost 23 years. College sweethearts who dated for several years before marrying a year after graduation, Brad, a marketing major, and Sarah, an education major, accepted jobs soon after graduation. Each eventually went on to obtain master's degrees in their respective fields. Always a very competitive, driven individual, Brad prided himself on his physical fitness and on his ability to continue to compete in a variety of athletic events. In addition to playing in numerous adult basketball leagues, he also participated on baseball and softball teams whenever he had the time. Brad was always interested in winning, arguing every referee's or umpire's decision that he thought was unfair. While others played the games just for the camaraderie and the physical fitness benefits the competition afforded them, Brad was in the game to win.

Sarah, on the other hand, humored what she referred to as Brad's obsession with sports. She maintained an active professional life, moving into an administrative position as Human Resources Director of a large public school district after spending several years as an elementary teacher. Brad changed jobs several times when the marketing divisions of his companies either downsized or closed entirely. Nevertheless, financial considerations were never a serious concern for the couple.

Brad and Sarah eventually had two sons, three years apart. The proud father didn't wait too long until he introduced them to all sports. Before they were age-eligible to enroll in the town's organized sports programs, he had them on the front lawn and at the local fields and courts throwing, catching, hitting, and shooting balls

(continued)

C A S E   P R E S E N T A T I O N : Brad and Season's End (*continued*)

---

of all kinds. Sarah attended as many games as she could while balancing her busy professional life. "As I look back at it now," she said, "what Brad and I had in common were the kids and sports."

Both sons went on to play organized sports through their middle and high school years, gaining some acclaim along the way for their talents. Brad and Sarah gained some vicarious fame of their own as their sons' parents. One of their friends commented, "I always thought that it was odd that in most of the games they (Brad and Sarah) attended as fans, they hardly ever sat together. Brad sat with his friends and Sarah with hers."

Then the second of their two sons graduated from high school and moved away to college. For him, sports were a thing of the past; for Brad and Sarah, so was their marriage. The break-up was a slow, insidious process. "It probably started long before Brad left," Sarah mused one day. "We had spent so much time involved with the boys' sports activities that we never learned how to deal with just each other." After both boys had departed for college, Brad and Sarah continued with their individual pursuits, both personal and professional. Brad remained in the house but moved to a bedroom away from Sarah; they agreed upon the sharing of the household responsibilities and finances but little else.

Sarah asked Brad repeatedly for the two of them to see a marriage counselor, but he refused, claiming that the current arrangements fit him. After approximately two years of this solitary existence under the same roof, however, Brad decided to leave. Rumors abounded that he had been seen in the company of a much younger woman several times in neighboring communities. Sarah also reported that he had increased his visits to the local gym and had lost close to 20 pounds. "If ever there was such a thing as a midlife crisis, Brad is the poster boy. I don't know if he ever grew up; he always played games, and those games are what made him smile. I just wish I knew then what I know now."

Case Discussion/Crisis Resolution

Although cases such as this one often reinforce the popular notion of the midlife crisis, the prevailing belief is that midlife alone does not bring with it the inevitability of problems. Major life transitions create crisis, and these transitions create an impact on any of the stages of life. The transition for Brad and Sarah came when their second son left home for college, forcing them to address long-standing communication deficits in their marriage. The fact that this occurred as they both entered the midlife years was more a function of their son's departure than of midlife itself. His departure at any other life stage would undoubtedly have triggered a similar marital split.

Brad's decision to leave Sarah also goes against the trend found by the AARP in its groundbreaking survey *The Divorce Experience: A Study of Divorce at Midlife and Beyond*. In its survey of 1,147 men and women who experienced a divorce in their 40s, 50s, or 60s, it found that the majority of midlife divorces were initiated by women; 66% of the women surveyed said that they had been the initiator, compared to only 41% of the men. The study also revealed that, regardless of who began the divorce process, three in four respondents (76%) said that they made the right decision, citing freedom, self-identity, and fulfillment as their greatest gains from the divorce.

CASE PRESENTATION: Mary and Her New Life

Mary was 38 years old when she entered the work force. Born into a traditional family structure for its day, she was the youngest of three children, all girls, who were raised by a stay-at-home mother and a father who was a police officer by day and a handyman during his off-hours to bring in some extra income. College for the girls was neither discouraged nor encouraged, since there was an unspoken expectation that marriage and motherhood were in their future. Mary's oldest sister was married at the age of 19 to a police officer, the son of her father's friend. The sister next in line became a dental hygienist, worked for a few years before marrying a dentist, and stayed at home to raise her growing family.

Mary always had other plans for herself, despite following the path that she thought was her legacy: finish high school, consider college as a second option only, get married, and stay at home to raise a family. "Being a dutiful daughter," she explained, "I met my Al, my future husband, while taking courses at the local community college and put my own plans on hold in order to follow what I thought had been preordained for me." Both her parents encouraged her to pursue a relationship with her boyfriend, a criminal justice major with plans for a career in law enforcement, claiming that the stability of a job as a police officer and the pension it would offer her were of primary importance. Any talk of attending a four-year college to complete a degree in business, Mary's personal goal, her parents ignored completely.

Mary eventually finished her two-year degree. Her part-time work in the business field during her community college years introduced her to a world that she knew was for her. However, she found herself pregnant before she had the opportunity to explore this career path more fully. A quick marriage followed, as did three children over the next six years. Now 26 years old, Mary began taking courses on a very part-time basis at a local college; business administration remained her passion. It took her five more years, but she eventually earned her bachelor's degree.

Her entry into the workforce, however, had to wait. "I can't say that Al discouraged me from working, but, as I look back on it, he more or less just humored me in my talk of working full-time," she claimed. Al was happy to have her home except for the few part-time hours she worked at the personnel department of a nearby department store, a favor granted her by the contacts she had made years earlier in

---

CASE PRESENTATION: Bill's Crisis or Opportunity?

Bill was 52 years old when he knew that it was time for a change. A former high school teacher and school counselor in public education for almost 30 years, he began to think, as he entered his 50s, that there was life beyond his comfortable professional existence. His friends and family members referred to his talk of a career change as a midlife crisis. His wife, Debbie, worried about the stability of other employment positions as well as of the impact on his pension that retirement before the age of 55 would create, needed significant reassurances before she reluctantly supported the plan.

Bill knew that there would be opportunities out there, since he held a doctorate degree in psychology, making him eligible for different kinds of positions in the private and public sector. His primary concern, however, was related to his age: Would prospective employers shy away from someone in his 50s beginning a new career? Despite suggestions from friends that he exclude from his resume the actual years marking the granting of his different degrees to avoid indication of his age, Bill decided to keep the years in the document. His first interest was in college teaching, so out went the resumes. His fear of his age getting in the way of employment was realized when, a year after losing an assistant professor position to another finalist, the search committee chairperson told him it was "because the other person was

her previous work experience. "When a full-time position opened up, my boss told me that the job was mine if I wanted it. That's all I needed to know," Mary said.

Al argued against Mary entering the work force on a full-time basis, citing childcare needs and their stable financial status with only her part-time position. Nevertheless, Mary asserted herself, made arrangements for childcare and other household needs, and took the position. "The first few years weren't easy, especially with Al's passive resistance to my working. He never said anything outright, but it was clear to me that he resented my working full time."

Four years into her job Mary told Al that she wanted to separate. The increasing stress of managing both job and family and of coping with growing strains in the marriage due, in large part, to Al's lack of support for his wife made the split inevitable. She thought about it for several years before she did it, wanting to work things out for the benefit of her children who now ranged in age from 16 to 21 years. Although they have not yet filed for divorce, Mary remains steadfast in her belief that the split was for the better.

Case Discussion/Crisis Resolution

Mary's case was a composite of several individuals who appear to match some of the AARP findings. Marital discontent often festers for years, and a third of the women in the AARP survey reported that they started contemplating separation and divorce about two years before they initiated it. Women in the Baby Boomer generation, those in the workplace in their 40s, 50s, and 60s, tend to find a whole network of people who are sympathetic to their plight regarding a failing marriage.

Even though many bad marriages stay intact for the sake of the emotional lives of the children involved, according to the AARP, many more men than women worry about their post-divorce relationship with their children. Forty-two percent of the men surveyed said that they feared losing contact with them, whereas only 15% of women had these same fears. Finally, despite claims against remarriage, 75% of women surveyed enjoyed a serious relationship after divorce, usually within two years, as did 81% of men.

younger, and we thought that he would be with us longer." The chairperson then greeted Bill's mention of age discrimination with stunned silence. Bill eventually secured a teaching position at the university level, however, where he remains a tenured associate professor to this day.

Case Discussion/Crisis Resolution

Bill never viewed this career change, albeit a change that kept him in the same general field, as the result of a midlife crisis. A transition for sure, but it only came at midlife because the 30 years he spent in public education placed him at that life stage with the awareness of wanting to do something different. Were it not for these years of experience, he undoubtedly would not have chosen this change. Driven by the opportunity to give something back to the profession and by the wish to exercise an entirely different set of skills, Bill looks back at his transition with a sense of satisfaction that it was indeed the right thing for him to do at the time. So was this a crisis or a transition? For Bill, this transition never reached crisis proportions; rather, he is reminded of Erikson's (see page 68) challenge of the middle years, *generativity versus stagnation*, as he opted for the former.

RECOMMENDATIONS FOR CHAPTER ENRICHMENT

SUGGESTED FILMS

American Beauty **(1999)** Earning the Oscar for best picture, the movie tells the story of a man who, at midlife, finds himself unemployed and spiraling into a serious midlife crisis. He discovers that his wife is having an affair with a coworker and that his daughter has sought companionship with a neighbor, while he finds himself lusting after his daughter's teenage friend.

Wonder Boys **(2000)** Lost in a sea of indecision, an award-winning writer and professor at a small Pennsylvania college is unable to complete his newest novel, despite the insistence of his earnest editor. His 2,611 pages already written provide no hint of bringing the project to closure. His wife leaves him, and he begins an affair with the wife of the department chair.

10 **(1979)** A popular comedy when it was released, *10* provides a somewhat stereotypical view of a midlife crisis as a male-only experience. A songwriter who is very restless in his less-than-fulfilling marriage has a chance encounter on the beach with a young and very beautiful woman. Longing to reaffirm his sexual vitality, he pursues her.

SUGGESTED ACTIVITIES

1. Visit a local bookstore. Browse through those sections usually labeled as "Self Help" or some such equivalent. Calculate the approximate percentage of those books designed for people at midlife.

2. Pick five people at midlife and interview them about the areas in their lives similar to those surveyed in the AARP study, *Boomers at Midlife 2004*. Have they experienced anything that might constitute a crisis? Was the crisis due to midlife or to some other event that happened to coincide with midlife?

3. Contact a local plastic surgeon. Ask them about the ages of the patients for whom they perform cosmetic surgery. How many are in middle age? men? women? Inquire also about any changes or trends over the last 10 years or so in the ages of those seeking elective plastic surgery.

5

Intimate Partner Violence and Domestic Violence

DISCUSSION QUESTIONS

Usually when people hear the term *domestic violence* they think of physical abuse that occurs when a husband beats his wife, but this is just one variation of intimate partner violence. What are some other types of abusive relationships?

It is common when you hear of someone who is involved in an abusive relationship to think, "Why don't they just leave?" Why is this often "easier said than done"?

What causes people to become batterers? What do you think motivates this type of behavior?

There's been controversy regarding mandatory reporting of intimate partner violence. Some states have laws that mandate that police make an arrest whenever they are called to intervene in a domestic violence incident. Some states have laws similar to child abuse reporting laws that mandate that medical and human service staff report any instance where they suspect intimate partner abuse. What do you think are some of the advantages and disadvantages of these laws?

INTRODUCTION

This chapter explores a variety of cases designed to demonstrate some aspect of intimate partner violence and/or domestic violence. These terms are used somewhat interchangeably although domestic violence has traditionally been used to denote physical abuse within a marital relationship. Today, it is widely known that violence can occur in any relationship whether it be between nonmarried heterosexual couples (either dating or living together), gay or lesbian couples (either dating or living together), and adult child-parent relationships. The term *intimate partner violence* is preferable because it encompasses both emotional and verbal abuse, as well as physical and sexual abuse. Emotional and verbal abuse can be as devastating as physical abuse.

It is important that intimate partner violence be included in the training of crisis intervention counselors, human service workers, law enforcement and medical personnel. An abuse incident, whether it be physical, verbal, or emotional, is often the culmination of several incidents of abuse that occur over the course of time. It is often when violence escalates that it throw's the abuse victim into a state of crisis, such as when the abuse results in physical injury requiring medical intervention.

Recent trends in intimate partner violence indicate that there has been a decline in the number of reported incidents between 2001 and 2005, however, it is widely accepted that intimate partner violence is underreported. On average, non-fatal intimate partner violence accounts for 22% of violent victimization of girls and women 12 years and older. For homicide, intimate partner violence accounts for 30% of women and 5% of men. With regards to marital status, women who are separated from their husbands report the highest incidence of intimate partner violence. Racial and ethnic factors must also be taken into account when looking at the statistics pertaining to intimate partner violence. Between 2004 and 2005, it appears that rates of intimate partner violence remained stable for European American women and African–American women but rates were generally higher for Native American and Alaskan Native women. From 1993 to 2005 the rates of intimate partner violence fell by two thirds for women of Hispanic origin (Bureau of Justice, 2009).

Much of the literature pertaining to partner violence points to a pattern of abuse that tends to be cyclical, rather than random acts of malevolence. Lenore Walker's Cycle Theory of Violence (1980) indicates that there are usually three phases in the partner violence sequence: 1) The Tension Building phase, 2) The Acute Battering phase, and 3) The Loving Contrition phase. The Tension Building Phase is often characterized by a gradual escalation of tense emotions between the partners. Potential victims may try to placate their partners, agreeing with them or doing things to try to please them in an attempt to diffuse their anger. Some of these attempts may work momentarily. This begins the Acute Battering phase in which batterers "typically unleash a barrage of verbal and physical aggression that often leaves the woman severely shaken and injured" (Walker, 2000, pp. 126–127). This is the phase where physical injuries occur and police intervention may take place: the pinnacle of the crisis. This phase ends when the battering incident has stopped. Batterers often experience a reduction in tension and anger, a feeling of calm or relief that unfortunately only serves to reinforce the violent behavior. Victims are left feeling physically and emotionally bruised and battered, as well as helpless. In the Loving-Contrition phase, the batterers often apologize for their behavior, promise they will never do this type of thing again, and express regret or guilt for their behavior. In many instances, according to Walker, this phase is accompanied by a reduction in tension, however, this can also be the time at which lethality is at its greatest, especially in the absence of any contrition or remorse.

For crisis counselors working with battering victims, it is not unusual to observe signs of depression that often result from feelings of learned helplessness (such as, "no matter what I do or say, it will not stop the beatings") and feelings of hopelessness. With ongoing counseling however, the research literature indicates that the majority of battered partners will leave their abusers. The point of initial contact that brings battered partners into crisis counseling is therefore a crucial time to engage them into the treatment process. It is therefore important that crisis counselors be empathetic, understanding, and above all, nonjudgmental. The following cases will describe various types of intimacy partner violence.

CASE PRESENTATION: Physical and Verbal Abuse in a College Couple

Verbally and physically abusive relationships are common among teenage and college-age populations as shown in the following case.

Jamie and Nick are college sophomores who have been dating for the past year. They met in their freshman year at a fraternity party and have been seeing each other exclusively ever since. After coming back to school from winter break, Jamie decided that she wanted to take a break from the relationship so she could see other guys. She felt that Nick was monopolizing too much of her time and was becoming too possessive. Nick did not take the news very well. He planned on spending spring break with Jamie and had already made arrangements for them to go to Florida. Jamie felt bad about backing out of their spring break plans but she felt it would not be fair to Nick to go with him, given her change of heart. Nick tried to convince Jamie to reconsider, resume the relationship and go to Florida with him but she was firm in her decision. Nick began to stalk Jamie and was constantly calling her and leaving angry and threatening messages on her cell phone. One Thursday evening Jamie went to a party with some of her friends. Nick found her there and began to yell and scream at her, then hit her, giving her a black eye. Jamie left the party crying and returned to her dorm feeling depressed and blaming herself for going to a party where Nick could be. Her Resident Advisor (RA) convinced her to see the counselor in the college's counseling center.

In exploring the safety aspects of this case, it is important that the counselor have a clear understanding of what took place and the history of Jamie's relationship with Nick. It is also important that the counselor take every possible step to ensure Jamie's safety given the recent incident. In order to accomplish this task, the counselor explores whether or not Jamie is willing to file a restraining order against Nick.

Intervention

The following is an excerpt from the initial session with Jamie at the college counseling center:

COUNSELOR: When your RA convinced you to call the hotline earlier you sounded very upset. I'm glad you chose to come in right away. Did you find the office O.K.?

JAMIE: Yes, the directions were fine. Thank you.

(continued)

CASE PRESENTATION: Physical and Verbal Abuse in a College Couple *(continued)*

COUNSELOR: Have you had your eye looked at?

JAMIE: Yeah, the RA brought me to the student health center before bringing me here. They said I would be O.K.

COUNSELOR: That's good. Could you tell me what happened? Start from the beginning.

JAMIE: Last year was my freshman year and I met this guy Nick at a frat party. We hit it off and began dating and I guess as the spring semester came around, we got more serious. We saw each other a few times over the summer but we were both working a lot. When we got back to school things were okay, at first, but I felt like Nick was getting too needy and possessive. I suggested we take a break and he went ballistic on me. So, I just stuck it out until winter break. But all semester he got more and more pissed at me and kept accusing me of hooking up with other guys.

COUNSELOR: Did you get into arguments often?

JAMIE: Yeah. It seemed like all we did was fight. So, I told him again that I needed a break and that this time I meant it. He went ballistic again but I stood my ground. Then Nick started leaving really nasty messages on my cell phone. I also found him following me one time, but I didn't confront him. I figured the less attention I paid him the better. Earlier tonight though I went to a party with some of my friends and Nick showed up and started a scene. He was yelling and screaming at me in front of everyone and then he hit me. A bunch of guys dragged him outside. That was the last I saw of him. Someone said they were going to call the campus police but because of the keg there, they decided not to. So I went back to the dorm with one of my suitemates. She was the one who brought me to the RA.

COUNSELOR: This has really been an ordeal for you. How are you feeling right now?

JAMIE: I'm still shaken up I guess. I'm glad to be back at the dorm though. I'm just not sure what to do next? I don't feel safe after what happened tonight.

COUNSELOR: Do you mean staying in the dorm?

JAMIE: No, I'm okay going back to the dorm. I feel safe enough there. I mean in general. Now I don't know what Nick will do next. If he'll do something like this again?

COUNSELOR: Had there been other instances of violence in your relationship?

JAMIE: No, not really. It was more Nick yelling at me or threatening that if I he caught me with another guy, he would beat him up, stuff like that.

COUNSELOR: Did Nick ever threaten to hurt you?

JAMIE: No, not directly. It was more implied. It was actually the angry look on his face.

COUNSELOR: Jamie, one of the options you have is to file a restraining order against Nick. This will help to keep him away from you and from hurting you again.

JAMIE: A friend of mine filed a restraining order against her ex-boyfriend. How would it work given that we both go to school here?

COUNSELOR: Is Nick in any of your classes?

JAMIE: No, not this semester.

COUNSELOR: It would mean that he could not come within 500 feet of your dorm and he could not call, write, or send you e-mails.

JAMIE: What if he does? I know he wouldn't follow those rules.

COUNSELOR: If he contacts you, it would be considered a violation of the court order and he would have to appear before the county judge. The judge could put him jail.

JAMIE: I don't want to get Nick in trouble. I just want him to leave me alone.

COUNSELOR: That's understandable; this is a tough step to take. (It's important that the counselor not pressure Jamie into making a decision so that Jamie feels that she has control over the situation. The counselor decides to revisit this issue later in the meeting.)

COUNSELOR: The other thing that will happen, given that the incident took place at one of the fraternities, is that Nick will have to appear before the college's Disciplinary Committee. Usually the Committee makes some recommendations in order to try to prevent future incidents.

JAMIE: What type of recommendations would they make?

COUNSELOR: Well for starters they would probably have Nick go for a psychological evaluation. They might also have him go to anger management training and counseling.

Case Conceptualization/Crisis Resolution

After this initial session, Jamie and Nick would move into individual crisis counseling. It is common that crisis counseling may take place over the course of several sessions, depending on the nature of the crisis and person's response. Jamie would be encouraged to express and process her feelings about the abusive incidents in the relationship. As alluded to earlier, it is common for many abused partners to diminish these incidents or to downplay their significance, thereby creating a more favorable image of the relationship. It is important for the counselor to question how Jamie felt about these incidents. Here, the "Four-Incident Technique" described by Lenore Walker may be particularly useful. The counselor would also focus on *behavioral adjustments* that Jamie could make. For example, Jamie might be encouraged to spend time with her friends or to refrain from responding to Nick's attempts to contact her. She may also be encouraged to develop a safety plan whereby she would be able to stay with a friend if she felt threatened. This phase of counseling would also focus on *cognitive mastery*. As was mentioned in the vignette, Jamie initially blamed herself for Nick's violent reaction. Jamie would be encouraged to stop taking responsibility for Nick's behavior and to realize that she did not make him abusive—only he can make that decision and only he can be responsible for whether or not he becomes abusive. In order to provide Jamie with some immediate skills, she may be encouraged to do some reading on abusive relationships.

CASE PRESENTATION: A Verbal and Emotionally
Abusive Relationship

In the case of Tyrone and Cherie, a classic picture of a verbally abusive relationship is presented. Tyrone displays many of the characteristics of verbally abusive men.

Tyrone and Cherie have been married for thirteen years. Tyrone had always been very critical of Cherie, almost from the beginning of their relationship. If she made an error in the checkbook, he called "stupid" or "retarded." He constantly criticized her appearance. If she tried to look nice for Tyrone, he called her a "slut." When she put on weight after having their first child, Tyrone referred to her as "the mother cow" or said she looked like, "a Mack Truck." At first, the name-calling was confined to the home, but Tyrone soon began to call Cherie names in public or around friends and family members. He would get very jealous if she spent time on the phone with her mother or sister and would go into a rage if she spent any time talking with her girl-friends. Tyrone also had threatened to cut the phone line and to take their checkbook and credit cards away from her. Cherie felt like a prisoner within her home and felt that Tyrone was constantly beating her down with his temper tantrums and criticisms.

Intervention

Tyrone is threatening, controlling, critical, and intimidating toward Cherie. Although abusive patterns like this often go on for years, it is also likely that they can erupt into physical violence. Assuming that there have been no instances of physical violence and also assuming that Tyrone would not come in for counseling either with Cherie or individually, it is most likely that Cherie would seek counseling alone. It is also common, however, that Cherie would be too fearful to initiate counseling herself, so let's assume that Cherie was referred for counseling by her physician who noted symptoms of depression. In such a case, the session might go as follows:

COUNSELOR: Hello, Cherie, I understand you have been referred here by your internist, Dr. Rodriquez. Is that correct?

CHERIE: Yes, I went to see her because I was having trouble sleeping. I thought she would give me a sleeping pill, I didn't think she would refer me to a psychologist.

COUNSELOR: Why did she?

CHERIE: Well, I guess as I was explaining why I couldn't sleep, she said it sounded like depression, so she referred me here.

COUNSELOR: Would it be all right for me to talk with Dr. Rodriquez? If that's OK, I will have you sign a release form, allowing us to talk.

CHERIE: Sure, I'm fine with that. I guess.

COUNSELOR: So, Cherie, it has been my experience that when people are having trouble sleeping because of depression, that the depression can be caused by a number of things. It can be biologically related, as in the case of heredity where certain kinds of depression will run in families. Or it can be hormonally related, as would be the case with certain kinds of thyroid problems. Depression can also be linked to situations going on in one's life, as would be the case when someone experiences a traumatic loss, or is going through a situation over which they feel they have little or no control. Do any of these things seem to apply to you, Cherie?

CHERIE: Well, no one in my family has ever suffered from depression that I know of. Dr. Rodriquez mentioned that all of my tests came back negative, so there doesn't seem to be anything medical going on. She asked me if anything was going on in my personal life. I did mention that I was having some stress at home.

COUNSELOR: What kind of stress?

CHERIE: Well, Tyrone and I have been married for thirteen years and we have two children. Things between us haven't been too good lately. Tyrone thinks I spend too much money and even though I work full-time, we just can't seem to make ends meet.

COUNSELOR: What has been happening between you and Tyrone because of these financial worries?

CHERIE: Tyrone gets very angry. He doesn't hit me or anything, I don't want you to get the idea that he is abusive, but he can really get going when he's mad. He'll yell at me and the kids and I guess I get really stressed out over it.

(Here it is important for the counselor to cautiously explore some of the types of verbal abuse such as those put forth by Evans in her book, *The Verbally Abusive Relationship* (Evans, 1992), or to explore some of the items listed by Tolman (1989) in his assessment scale called *The Psychological Maltreatment of Women Scale*. It is also important that the Counselor not launch into an attack of Tyrone, as this would only alienate Cherie or add to her feelings of guilt or responsibility.)

COUNSELOR: So, it sounds like things can get pretty stressful at home. How do you cope with the stress?

CHERIE: I try to talk with my girlfriends on the phone or with my sister, but... (hesitates).

COUNSELOR: What were you going to say?

CHERIE: Well, Tyrone gets angry if I talk on the phone. One time, he threatened to pull the phone out of the wall. He gets really mad when I'm on the phone with anyone.

COUNSELOR: Is there anything else that Tyrone gets angry with you about?

CHERIE: No, mostly the credit cards and the phone. He gets really mad.

COUNSELOR: What do you do when he gets angry?

CHERIE: I just try to calm him down. I don't like him yelling in front of the children. Or I'll try to find ways to keep him from getting angry like cooking his favorite meals or making sure his newspaper is ready for him when he gets home, stuff like that.

COUNSELOR: It sounds like you have been coping with the stress for a long time.

CHERIE: Tyrone wasn't too bad in the beginning of our marriage, but then he got worse after our baby was born. Things went really downhill from there.

COUNSELOR: Is there anything you can do to change your situation? Are there any options you can use to cope with the stress?

CHERIE: No, not really. Divorce is against our religious beliefs and my mother has already told me not to expect any support from her. She was against my marrying Tyrone because she said he was too possessive. Tyrone would never come in for counseling either.

(*continued*)

CASE PRESENTATION: A Verbal and Emotionally Abusive Relationship *(continued)*

COUNSELOR: Does Tyrone know you were referred here?

CHERIE: Yes, but he thinks it is part of my medical problems. Plus Tyrone says I need a "shrink" anyway because he says that I'm crazy. He's threatened to have me committed and says he'll take the children away from me.

COUNSELOR: What makes him say these things?

CHERIE: Oh, it's usually something I've done. Like I spent too much money on food or I bought the kids new sneakers.

COUNSELOR: Cherie, it doesn't sound like these purchases are irresponsible. Is it possible that Tyrone is the one with the problem? It sounds like he can be really tough to deal with?

CHERIE: Yeah, I guess you could say that. I guess it's just his nature.

COUNSELOR: Cherie, tell me something nice about Tyrone?

CHERIE: Well, he is really good with our son. He takes him fishing with him all the time. Last year they caught ten fluke down at the river. They came home laughing and we had a great time, eating the fish they caught.

CASE PRESENTATION: A Case of Physical and Verbal Abuse

The case example of Stacy and Mike represents a classic illustration of physical and verbal battering. Mike represents an insecure batterer, or a "Pitbull" (Jacobson & Gottman, 1998), who constantly uses verbal and physical intimidation to "keep Stacy in her place." It is unlikely that individuals like Mike will present to treatment on their own and usually will only do so when mandated into treatment by the courts. It is also common for batterers to project blame for their explosive anger on their spouses or partners. Stacy finds herself constantly "walking on eggshells" in fear that something she will say or do will incite Mike's rage.

Stacy and Mike have been living together for three years. They had dated for six months before moving in together, which Stacy's mother had very much objected to. She felt that Mike was "no good" and that there was something about him that she just didn't like. Stacy felt that no matter who she went out with, in her mother's eyes he wouldn't be good enough for her. Stacy and Mike often got into heated arguments, usually about his spending time with friends at the local sports bar. She felt he was drinking too much and spending too much money on sports gambling. Whenever she confronted Mike, he would go into a tirade and would storm around the house, sometimes breaking things. In one of these arguments, Mike hit Stacy and then stormed out of the house to "cool off." He came a few hours later with flowers for Stacy and told her he was sorry and that it "would never happen again." Unfortunately, four weeks later, one of Mike's favorite teams lost a playoff game and he lost a lot of money. When he came home Stacy was angry with him, as they had

Case Conceptualization/Crisis Resolution

This case provides many examples of a verbally abusive relationship. From Cherie's description, Tyrone tries to control just about every aspect of her life. Cherie plays the dutiful codependent as she tries to placate Tyrone out of fear that his anger will explode. However, no matter what Cherie does, Tyrone continues to use his temper as a means to control and manipulate Cherie. This is a common characteristic of verbally abusive relationships. Victims of verbal abuse often become brainwashed into believing that nothing they do is right, and develop a sense of learned helplessness (no matter what I do, it won't make a difference). This is one of the reasons that victims so often present with depressive symptoms, as Cherie did when she sought help from her physician.

Evans (1992) makes several recommendations for individuals who find themselves in verbally abusive relationships. She suggests that it is first important for partners to know when they are being put down, ordered around, or yelled at. They also need to develop awareness that they are dealing with an abusive partner who is trying to dominate or control them, but that there is nothing that they have done to cause the abuse. Finally, she suggests that partners take a firm, authoritative tone in dealing with verbal abuse, so as to convey that this type of verbal behavior will not be tolerated. Hopefully, Cherie will continue in counseling beyond this crisis phase and will be open to exploring the issues that Evans recommends.

planned to go over to her mother's house for dinner. She told Mike to pack his things. Instead, he started turning over furniture and then hitting her, telling her "No one is going to tell me what to do."

Most beginning counselors make the mistake of assuming that reasoning and rational explanation is all that is needed to get Stacy to leave. Usually, women in Stacy's situation will keep the abuse a secret from their friends and family because they don't want to hear those dreaded words, "Why don't you just leave him?" This would especially be true if Stacy were to tell her mother about the abuse. Stacy may feel invested in making the relationship work or want to prove to her mother that Mike is "not such a bad guy." As indicated earlier, however, there are many reasons why battered women stay in the relationship, so it is best that counselors listen for these various reasons in a nonjudgmental manner. Again, it is best to ask open-ended questions and to stifle the impulse to criticize Mike and his abusive behavior. In conceptualizing abuse cases like this from the viewpoint of modern crisis intervention models such as those developed by Roberts (1998), the most important step is that of Assessing Lethality or Ensuring Safety. As the Nicole Brown Simpson case suggests, verbal and physical battering, and sexual jealousy, often go hand-in-hand.

In the following case transcription, excerpts from an initial session with Stacy will be presented. As the case is presented, see if you can pick out how some of this ties in with suggested format questions used in Survivor Therapy (Walker, 2000).

(continued)

C A S E P R E S E N T A T I O N : A Case of Physical and Verbal Abuse *(continued)*

Intervention

COUNSELOR: Stacy, I understand that your sister referred you here. Why did she suggest that you come to Women's Center?

STACY: Oh, she has it in her head that my boyfriend, Mike is abusive or something. I agreed to come, mostly to get her off my back. No offense to you, I just don't see why my sister gets so upset.

COUNSELOR: Had something happened that caused her to be concerned? (Although the counselor notices some bruising, she refrains from asking about this too early in the session. Her goal at this point is to help Stacy feel comfortable with having come to the Center. This is usually a big step, although it is not uncommon for the battered spouse to deny the importance of having taken this step. Often they may feel that others are beaten or abused more severely than they are, therefore, they do not deserve to access counseling services. Stacy goes on to explain the incident described in the vignette at the beginning of the chapter.)

COUNSELOR: The incident you described sounds really frightening. How did you feel?

STACY: Yeah, I guess I was afraid, but I can usually get Mike to calm down or if he does go for a walk or goes down to the bar, he usually will calm himself down.

COUNSELOR: What was Mike like when he came home?

STACY: Well, he was checking for phone messages and was snooping around to see if I had been talking to anyone or if I had anyone over. He does get kind of crazy, thinking that I'm fooling around. (Remember, it is not unusual for male batterers to display a great deal of sexual jealousy, some of which may border on paranoid-like suspiciousness.)

COUNSELOR: How did you feel at that point?

STACY: I was really, really afraid. Usually, when he gets crazy like that, it means he is going to blow up. I just try to lay low and not argue with him, but that only lasts for so long. (Stacy is describing the "tension building" phase, which often precedes explosive physical violence. It is not unusual for many abused women to try to placate their abuser in order to try to reduce the tension. The counselor's goal at this point in the session is to get Stacy to explain as much of what she can remember and to elicit her feelings and reactions.)

COUNSELOR: What happened then?

STACY: Well, I told Mike I wanted him to leave and that's when he really blew up. He started throwing furniture and then he started hitting me. He finally left and I called my girlfriend, Jennifer. I think she was the one that told my sister what happened.

COUNSELOR: Why do you think Jennifer did that?

STACY: Well, I guess she thought she was helping me or something. I was really pissed at her, but then I realized she was trying to help.

COUNSELOR: And what was your sister's reaction?

STACY: She was really angry. She and Mike never got along, but I thought it was because our mother never liked Mike.

COUNSELOR: How did you feel about your sister's reaction?

STACY: Well, I guess I could see her point, I think she's overreacting though by wanting me to come to a women's crisis center. It's not like I'm an abused woman or something.

COUNSELOR: Stacy, could you tell me about the first time that Mike lost his temper with you? Everything you've told me so far, is very similar to the stories of women who seek help here at the Women's Center. Is it possible that you are an abused woman? (At this point, the counselor will begin to get some information using Walker's (1994b) Four-Incident Technique (the first abuse incident, the most recent, the worst incident, and a typical incident). Stacy relates other incidents similar to this one.)

STACY: I guess, as I was listening to myself recall all those incidents with Mike, I began thinking that maybe I am, or that you're thinking that I'm some kind of nut case for staying with him.

COUNSELOR: Not at all, I don't think you're a "nut case." It sounds like you've tried many different things to try to survive a very difficult situation. I'd like to talk about what you would like at this point. What are your goals?

At this point in the session, the counselor provides Stacy with feedback about her situation. It is not uncommon for women to vehemently deny that they are abused, or to compare themselves to other battered women they know or know of and rationalize that their situation is not nearly so bad. This minimization sometimes is used as the rationale for why they haven't sought help ("their situation is so much worse than mine"). Here it is important to reinforce that any woman who is verbally, emotionally, or physically abused should have access to counseling no matter what type of abuse or how severe the abuse may have been. It is important that the counselor gather information about Stacy and her relationship with Mike in a nonjudgmental manner. It is also important to keep the focus on the here-and-now. This is not a time for exploration of prior relationships or family history. The emphasis is purely on the abusive relationship and how to ensure that Stacy will be safe in the future.

Case Conceptualization/Crisis Resolution

Although the aforementioned case focuses on Stacy and her reactions to the abuse incidents that resulted in her sister bringing her for crisis counseling, it is important to keep in mind that batterers also need to be referred for ongoing treatment. In working with Mike (and batterers in general), there are usually four main goals that become the focus of this treatment: 1) to ensure the safety of the victimized partner, 2) to alter the batterer's attitudes toward relationship violence, 3) to increase the batterer's sense of personal responsibility rather than to project blame on the victimized partner, and 4) to learn nonviolent alternatives to dealing with conflict in order to change past behavior (Edleson & Tolman, 1992). Generally, couples counseling is contraindicated because it may place the victim at greater risk for battering. For example, if the battered partner were to bring something up in counseling that angers the batterer, this could then lead to a battering incident once they leave the office. What is considered "best practice" is to treat the couple separately and to continue to do so until the battered partner either safely leaves the relationship or until such time as all parties agree the batterer has demonstrated sufficient progress in their own treatment, that they no longer pose a risk for becoming either emotionally or physically abusive.

Some General Guidelines for Crisis Counseling with Couples Exhibiting Intimate Partner Violence

Battered women may present for crisis counseling in a variety of settings. They may be first seen in criminal justice settings by judges or court personnel involved with the legal aspect of the battering situation, such as when the police make an arrest or when the battered spouse applies for a restraining order for protection. The battered partner may seek assistance at a shelter for battered women and their children. The battered spouse may appear in an emergency room with broken bones, a broken nose, bruises, or similar physical trauma. They may also seek help in a mental health clinic for Posttraumatic Stress Disorder (PTSD) symptoms or for treatment for some other anxiety disorder, depression, or alcohol or drug abuse. It is also possible that the battered spouse may seek help from a clergy member with hopes of obtaining marital counseling to help preserve the marriage or with hopes that the priest, minister, or rabbi will admonish the batterer for their abusive behavior and in doing so, somehow get them to stop. The battered spouse may reach out to other family members or friends for help. They may seek financial help, a place to stay, or just emotional support. Whatever the point of entry into the crisis intervention delivery system, there are certain "givens" that effective crisis counselors must take into consideration in any of these cases.

1) It is common that the battered partner will not identify their crisis domestic violence or intimate partner violence. Perhaps the only two exceptions to this may be in instances where the battered partner seeks a restraining order from the courts or specifically seeks assistance at a battered women's shelter. In those instances, the woman must have been victim to an unusually violent threat or suffered intense physical harm in order to access those services. Although there may still be evidence of denial as to the nature and extent of the intimate partner abuse (for example, the woman may blame herself for her injuries), there is usually less likelihood that the abuse will be denied altogether. In the other points of entry, the battered partner may deny that their injuries are the result of their partner's abusive, violent behavior. This is not unusual, because the abused partner may be fearful of being discovered. They may fear retaliation or that they will have neither a place to go nor the financial means to support and protect their children.

2) It is important that crisis counselors take into account that they may be working with an abused partner who is in denial that they are in an abusive relationship, or they may present with other symptoms that can lead the crisis counselor down the wrong path by assessing the crisis as something other than a domestic violence situation.

3) If abuse is suspected, do not interview the partners together. This is suggested for two reasons. First, it is unlikely that abused partners will give up much information while under the watchful, threatening eye of their abusive partner. In many instances, abusers coach their abuse victims in terms of what to say and what not to say. Therefore, it is better to conduct a separate interview if the abusive partner is present. The second reason also pertains to

outpatient counseling centers; if the counselor suspects abuse, they should refrain from doing any couples or marital counseling. Even in couples counseling, once abuse is discovered in the relationship, it is a basic tenet **NOT** to treat the couple together, but rather to work with the each individual separately. The prevailing theory is that by working with the couple together, it puts the battered partner in too much danger. For example, if that partner were to say or do "the wrong thing" within the session, the likelihood of abuse once the session is over is greatly increased.

4) It is of utmost importance to ensure the safety of the battered partner (Roberts, 1998). No matter what setting this individual presents in, it is imperative that the crisis worker has explored every possible alternative to make certain that the battered partner cannot be revictimized. This usually means that legal charges are pressed against the batterer and that the abused partner has a safe place to go, preferably one that the batterer is unaware of or does not have access to. Just as locks are only effective with honest people, so too do restraining orders have their limitations if not effectively enforced. The police cannot be in all places at all times. It is common for batterers to defy restraining orders by trying to establish phone contact with their partners in order to pressure them into dropping the restraining order. Although restraining orders make provisions that there is to be no phone, written contact, or face-to-face contact, this part of the court order cannot be enforced if the abused partner falls unwittingly into the trap of the abuser ("see you broke the law by taking my call, you're as guilty as I am"). Some treatment providers and those working in shelters for battered women feel that a restraining order can sometimes represent a challenge to the masculinity of the batterer and therefore some batterers will purposely defy the court order or may escalate their level of violence. Lethality increases when a restraining order is initially filed. It is important to take collaborative steps to help ensure the battered partner's safety. Although it is difficult to predict the next act of violence, in order to assess the immediate danger that the battered partner may be in, it is important to take into account the history of the batterer, frequency and severity of violence, frequency of intoxication and drug use, threats to kill, threats to harm the children, access to weapons, current stressors in his or her life, attitudes toward violence, any reports of psychiatric impairment, forced sexual acts, and the battered partner's prior suicide threats or attempts (Sonkin & Durphy, 1993; Walker, 1994). It is important for crisis counselors to provide the battered partner with phone numbers of domestic violence shelters as well as other emergency numbers.

5) In working with intimate partner violence victims, it is important that the counselor not judge, preach or blame, nor should they force the victim into choosing a course of action that they cannot or are not willing to follow. It is important that the crisis counselor convey acceptance. Since most abused partners often understate their cases, it is also important that counselors believe what the victims have to say and that questions pertaining to the abuse not convey disbelief about the abuse incident or a lack of understanding. The battered partner must trust the counselor and also believe that this trust will not be betrayed.

A FINAL THOUGHT

A recent *New York Times* article (Sontag, 2002) raises many important controversial issues pertaining to domestic violence and how counselors handle these cases. From a rational perspective, most counselors want to make the victims safe and to end the cycle of violence by encouraging them never to return to their batterers. However, this is not always the goal of the battered, whose lives may be inextricably intertwined with their abusers. As Sontag points out, "Well-meaning professionals often find themselves in an uncomfortable and sometimes adversarial relationship with victims. Prosecutors especially, become frustrated by the many women who balk at testifying against their boyfriends or husbands.... As Ruth Schulder, a social worker in the Bronx, says: "Nobody has the right to say to a woman, 'You can't be with this guy.' So we have to deal with the reality." As indicated in the Discussion Questions, it is often easy to recommend that someone leave an abusive relationship and to provide referrals to women's shelters, however, the reality of taking this step is extremely difficult and involves many factors. Crisis counselors must be able to offer options to battered victims even with the realization that they may choose not to exercise these options at this particular point in time. Therefore, as mentioned earlier, it is of utmost importance that crisis counselors be nonjudgmental in discussing these alternatives.

RECOMMENDATIONS FOR CHAPTER ENRICHMENT

SUGGESTED FILMS

The Burning Bed (1984) This film is based on the true story of Francine Hughes who is imprisoned within a marriage with a husband who beats her viciously while in uncontrollable rages. Eventually, she sets fire to her house, killing her ex-husband. This film provides an accurate depiction of battered women's syndrome and the devastating impact of abuse on victims and families. It also portrays an accurate depiction of the "Pitbull" type of abuser, as described by Jacobson and Gottman (1998).

Sleeping with the Enemy (1991) This film portrays intimate partner violence in a married couple where the husband is compulsive, controlling, and dangerously violent. The husband accurately portrays the "Cobra" type of batterer as described by Jacobson and Gottman (1998).

This Boy's Life (1993) This film portrays a single mother who leaves a relationship with an abusive boyfriend only to end up in a marriage that starts out noncontentious, but ends up with an abusive, controlling, alcoholic husband. This film depicts the impact of abuse on the family.

What's Love Got to Do with It (1993) This film depicts the life of Tina Turner and the abuse she suffered by her husband, Ike Turner. This film provides a chilling and brutal depiction of intimate partner violence.

Domestic Violence: Faces of Fear **(1996)** This documentary, narrated by Diane Sawyer, provides excellent background information into the issues surrounding intimate partner abuse. There are several interviews with survivors of intimate partner abuse and various professionals who deal with partner abuse on a day-to-day basis including attorneys, counselors, domestic violence shelter volunteers, and counselors who work with batterers. The only problem noted is that the samples of batterers depicted are nearly all men of racial and ethnic minorities, which may give students a misperception that only men of color are batterers. With this exception, this is an excellent documentary that will provide students with a wealth of information.

SUGGESTED ACTIVITIES

1) Every county court hears cases pertaining to intimate partner violence, some on a daily basis, others establish one day of the week in which these cases are heard. These cases are heard in open court, therefore anyone can attend. Although it is inadvisable for a large group of students to attend a court session, it may be possible for a few students to attend. In many instances, judges welcome students to their court because they want future counselors, social workers, and psychologists to be aware of how devastating intimate partner violence can be. Students can report back to the class what they heard and any reactions they had to attending the court session, with strict instructions not to break the confidentiality of anyone whom they may have seen in the courtroom.

2) Students can watch one of the suggested films and then discuss how the film matches their perceptions of intimate partner violence.

3) Students can explore what resources exist for victims of intimate partner violence in their county. They can explore what kinds of hotlines, outpatient programs, and battered women's shelters are available in their area.

4) Intimate partner violence is unfortunately common among college-age students. If asked to create an awareness and prevention program on their campus, what would they include? What types of marketing might help to educate the public about intimate partner violence and to make potential victims aware of resources on or off campus?

5) Law enforcement personnel deal with intimate partner violence on a daily basis. Some statistics indicate that police officers are more at risk for injury in domestic violence disputes than in any other type of police work. Arrange to have a state, county, or local police officer come to class to talk about individual experiences with intimate partner violence. How are situations managed where a couple is accusing each other of violence? Are the police ever called to cases in which women abuse men? Is the police officer for or against mandatory arrest laws? Is it true that police are often called to intervene with the same couple or family repeatedly and if so, how are those cases approached differently?

6

The Crisis of Sexual Assault

DISCUSSION QUESTIONS

Take this simple True-False quiz testing your knowledge of sexual assault. Discuss your answers with your classmates before checking them against the correct answers, which can be found in the next section. This quiz is courtesy of *Men Against Sexual Assault* (University of Rochester):

1. She was asking for it because of the way she was dressed.

2. Use of drugs and alcohol lead to more occurrences of rape.

3. People who commit rape are usually psychopaths or stalkers who jump out of the bushes at night.

4. People can be raped even if they have had sex before.

5. If the victim has had sex with the attacker before, it is not rape.

6. When men are sexually aroused, they have to have sex.

7. If the victim does not actually fight the attacker, then it is not rape.

8. Rape is a crime of aggression and violence, motivated by anger and the desire for power and control.

9. A woman can be raped even if she willingly goes to a man's room.

10. Women rarely lie about being raped.

QUIZ ANSWERS

1.   *She was asking for it because of the way she was dressed.*
Answer: False. This belief is little more than one of those "rape myths," stereotypical beliefs about rape "that serve to deny, trivialize, or justify sexual violence exerted by men against women" (Bohner, 1998, p. 14). Acceptance of this and other rape myths

places women in a disempowered position and also is associated with greater rape proclivity in men (Malamuth & Check, 1983).

Rape myths place responsibility for sexual assault on women by attributing to them certain indecent behaviors or other instances of lapses in moral judgment that actually caused the rape to occur. Walking in a certain manner deemed seductive by the assailant, wearing provocative attire, or considering her eye contact as inviting are just some of those behaviors that assailants consider causally related to the act of sexual assault. Individuals who ascribe to rape myths truly do believe, "She asked for it by the way she was dressed and the way she looked at me." Other rape myths (Scully, 1990) are generated by beliefs that 1. women could indeed avoid rape if they really fought hard enough, 2. that victims ask for and secretly enjoy rape, and 3. that they only conjure up reports of rape to punish men for some perceived wrongdoing.

2.   *Use of drugs and alcohol lead to more occurrences of rape.*
Answer: True. Alcohol and sexual assault often occur together. More than one-third of all sexual assaults happen when the assailant is under the influence of alcohol (30%) or drugs (4%). The victim also is intoxicated in some cases. However, one must be careful not to attribute the assault to intoxication only; being inebriated does not cause the assault but rather allows the assailant to ignore sexual boundaries. A drunken victim also finds it more difficult to defend herself against an attack.

The appearance on the nightclub and dating scene in relatively recent years of what are commonly known as "date rape drugs" also has placed individuals at risk for sexual assault. The concern over the proliferation of these drugs resulted in the passage in 1996 of the Drug Induced Rape Prevention and Punishment Act making it a felony to give a controlled substance to individuals with the intent of committing sexual assault or any other crime on them.

These drugs cause the individuals to pass out, making them unable to resist an assault and unable to recall what happened the next day. Many victims of these drug-induced assaults fail to report them to the authorities, blaming themselves for being too drunk to remember any details; a state of confusion caused by the drugs, which may last for several days, also may result in the destruction of necessary evidence to charge the assailant with the crime. The most commonly used date rape drugs are rohypnol, gamma-hydroxybutyrate (GHB), and ketamine.

3.   *People who commit rape are usually psychopaths or stalkers who jump out of the bushes at night.*
Answer: False. According to the National Crime Victimization Survey (NCVS) (2005), the typical assailant is neither a psychopath nor an individual with a major psychiatric disorder. They do not hide in dark alleys or behind bushes waiting for their next victim to arrive. Rather, nonstrangers, individuals known to the victims

as family members, acquaintances, or intimate partners, accounted for almost three-fourths (73%) of all sexual assaults; 38% of the perpetrators were a friend or acquaintance of the victim; 28% were intimates of the victim; and 7% were other relatives. Only the remaining 27% of assailants were strangers unknown to the victim.

The Rape, Abuse & Incest National Network (RAINN), the nation's largest antisexual-assault organization, reported that four out of ten sexual assaults take place at the victim's own home, with another two in ten occurring in the home of a friend, neighbor, or relative.

4. *People can be raped even if they have had sex before.*
Answer: True. A victim's sexual history has nothing at all to do with a case of rape. One doesn't have to be a virgin to be a victim of a sexual assault. A victim even could have had sexual relations with the assailant at an earlier time and can still be raped by them. The major issue pertains to consent (see next section), and if the victims do not give consent, regardless of their sexual history with the assailants beforehand, a rape can still take place.

5. *If the victim has had sex with the attacker before, it is not rape.*
Answer: False. See the answer to question number four above.

6. *When men are sexually aroused, they have to have sex.*
Answer: False. A state of sexual arousal (such as an erection) is not causally connected to sexual assault. There are also no adverse physical consequences to a man if he does not have sexual relations when sexually aroused.

7. *If the victim does not actually fight the attacker, then it is not rape.*
Answer: False. There are too many reasons why a victim might not fight back during a sexual assault. Verbal threats of harm to herself or to her friends and family members, the presence of a weapon used to intimidate her, or a state of complete terror are just some of the reasons why victims sometimes remain silent during an attack.

8. *Rape is a crime of aggression and violence, motivated by anger and the desire for power and control.*
Answer: True. Although there are too many different kinds of rape for a single explanation to satisfy each of them (Cavaiola & Colford, 2006), contemporary research suggests that no more than approximately 10% of all rapes are committed for purposes of sexual pleasure (Kendall & Hammen, 1998). Other social-cultural explanations view sexual assault as an act of men's control over women in a culture that is more patriarchal in nature and that socializes males to associate power with masculinity and passivity with femininity (Odem & Clay-Warner, 1998).

9. *A woman can be raped even if she willingly goes to a man's room.*
Answer: True. If a woman does not give consent for a sexual encounter, whether she is in a public place or a private place such as a car, home, or college dormitory

room, then the sexual encounter is rape. In cases of date rape (also known as acquaintance rape), agreeing to be with a person in a dating relationship, for example,
does not imply consent for sex, and sexual contact without consent is still rape.
Another far less common rape type is spousal rape which occurs in dysfunctional
marital relationships in which there is sexual assault against a spouse. Even if committed in the couple's own home and in the context of marriage, sex without
consent is still rape.

10. *Women rarely lie about being raped.*
Answer: True. One of the reasons why so many rapes go unreported is the
victim's belief that people will not believe her. However, false reports are very
rare; only 8% of reported rapes are false.

INTRODUCTION

The exact definitions of *rape*, *sexual abuse*, *sexual assault*, and other related terms
differ by state. Some of the general guidelines from the U.S. Department of
Justice, however, describe *rape* as an act of forced sexual intercourse, including
vaginal, oral, or anal penetration by a body part or an object and *sexual assault*
as unwanted sexual contact that stops short of rape and that may include sexual
touching and fondling.

The National Women's Health Information Center (NWHIC) defines sexual assault more broadly, however, as any type of sexual activity that an individual does not consent to, including the following:

- vaginal, anal, or oral penetration
- inappropriate touching
- sexual intercourse that a person says "no" to
- rape (a common form of sexual assault)
- attempted rape
- child molestation
- anything verbal or visual that forces a person to join in unwanted sexual
  contact or attention such as voyeurism, exhibitionism, incest, and sexual
  harassment

In addition to the above forms of sexual assault, the U.S. Department of
Justice's Office on Violence Against Women also defined sexual assault as any
type of sexual contact "without the explicit consent of the recipient of the unwanted sexual activity" and added several others:

- forcing an individual to perform or receive oral sex
- forcing an individual to masturbate or to masturbate someone else
- forcing an individual to look at sexually explicit material or forcing an
  individual to pose for sexually explicit pictures

In general, state law also assumes that individuals cannot give consent to sexual activity if they are forced, threatened, unconscious, drugged, a minor, developmentally disabled, chronically mentally ill, or believe that they are undergoing a medical procedure.

STATISTICS

In the most recent Department of Justice NCVS (2005), the nation's largest crime study, there were an average of 200,780 sexual assaults in the previous two years. RAINN calculated that this number is the equivalent of approximately one sexual assault every two-and-a-half minutes. The Survey, however, does not include victims 12 years of age or younger, thus excluding this population from the total amount even though estimates are that one in six victims of sexual assault are under age 12.

Considering the fact that a staggering 59% of sexual assaults go unreported, the Survey numbers must be considered to be a minimal estimate of its prevalence. These unreported cases, however, vary depending upon the relationships of the assailant to the victim. The National Violence Against Women Survey (NVAWS) (2001) found that many more rapes and sexual assaults committed by strangers were reported to the police (41%) than those committed by intimates; for example, rapes and sexual assaults committed by a boyfriend or spouse were only reported 24% of the time. Most of these latter victims who did not report their attacks thought that the police would not or could not do anything on their behalf. Other reasons victims do not report sexual assault by an intimate (a current or former spouse, boyfriend, or girlfriend, including same-sex relationships) involved the belief that the assault was a minor, one-time incident or that silence was the best way to protect the children or the relationship with the assailant (NVAWS, 2001). Reasons for not reporting sexual assault by a stranger are more related to fear of reprisal from the perpetrator, media publicity, or fear of being blamed for the attack itself (Cavaiola & Colford, 2006).

Other findings from the NVAWS include the following:

- Three in four women who reported that they had been raped and/or physically assaulted since age 18 said that a current or former husband, cohabiting partner, or date committed the assault.

- Almost one-fifth of women (18%) reported experiencing a completed or attempted rape at some point in their lives.

- One in 33 men (3%) reported experiencing a completed or attempted rape at one time in their lives, even though the NCVS reported that 10% of sexual assaults are against males.

- Approximately 44% of rape victims are under age 18; about 15% are under age 12.

VICTIMS' REACTIONS TO SEXUAL ASSAULT

There are a multitude of factors that have a direct impact on the reactions of victims after a sexual assault. The victims' age and developmental level; the relationship to the assailant; the presence of a support system for the victim; the reactions to the assault by family, friends, the police, and medical personnel; and the severity and duration of the attack all contribute significantly to the victim's response. The National Center for Victims of Crime listed the following typical responses to a sexual assault which might apply to many, but not all, victims:

Physical Effects	Emotional/Psychological Effects
■ pain	■ shock or denial
■ injuries	■ irritability or anger
■ nausea	■ depression
■ vomiting	■ social withdrawal
■ headaches	■ numbing or apathy (detachment, loss of caring)
Physiological Effects	■ restricted affect (reduced ability to express emotions)
■ hypervigilance (always being "on your guard")	■ nightmares or flashbacks
■ insomnia	■ difficulty concentrating
■ exaggerated startle response (jumpiness)	■ diminished interest in activities or sex
■ panic attacks	■ loss of self-esteem
■ eating problems or disorders	■ loss of security or trust in others
■ self-mutilation (cutting, burning, or otherwise hurting oneself)	■ guilt or shame or embarrassment
■ sexual dysfunction (not being able to perform sexual acts)	■ impaired memory
	■ loss of appetite
■ hyperarousal (exaggerated feelings or responses to stimuli)	■ suicidal ideation
	■ substance abuse
	■ psychological disorders

A combination of any of these signs could also be part of a larger problem known as Rape Trauma Syndrome (RTS), which includes several Post-Traumatic Stress Disorder (PTSD) symptoms specific to the experience of rape or sexual assault. RAINN describes three phases to RTS:

1. **Acute phase**—occurs immediately after the assault and usually lasts a few days to several weeks. Reactions in this phase typically fall into three categories:

   - Expressed—Victims are openly emotional, appearing agitated or hysterical and suffering from crying spells or anxiety attacks.

- Controlled—Victims appear to be without emotion and act as if nothing happened; this calm may be a state of shock.

- Shocked disbelief—Victims are disoriented and suffer from difficulties in concentrating, making decisions, or doing everyday tasks; poor recall of the assault also may result.

2. **Outward adjustment phase**—Victims resume what appear to be normal lives while suffering from considerable inner turmoil. Many of the emotional and physiological symptoms listed above appear during this phase. Victims tend to use any of five coping techniques:

- Minimization—Victims pretend that "everything is fine" or that "it could have been worse."

- Dramatization—Victims are unable to stop talking about the assault; it dominates their lives.

- Suppression—Victims refuse to discuss the assault, acting as if it never happened.

- Explanation—Victims overanalyze what happened.

- Flight—Victims attempt to avoid the pain (moving, changing jobs, relationships, or appearance).

3. **Resolution phase**—The assault is no longer the central focus of the victims' lives. The rape is accepted as part of their lives, yet they move on and the pain lessens over time.

Courtney, a rape survivor herself (see page 104), summarized those similarities among the reactions of rape victims whom she currently helps to counsel:

- feeling terribly alone

- not being sure of who you are anymore

- being terrified, experiencing nightmares

- having flashbacks brought on by colors, smells, or other reminders of the assault

- feeling angry (those who can't express their anger go into deep depression)

- feeling unable to relate to other people

WHAT TO DO WHEN SEXUAL ASSAULT IS REPORTED

Although a victim is not required to report a sexual assault, the local prosecutor's office may decide to pursue prosecution with or without the victim's participation in the process. However, it also is unlikely that the prosecutor would proceed with the case without the victim's cooperation. Reasons for reporting range from the importance of prosecuting sexual offenders and "keeping them off the streets" to helping the victims regain a sense of control, an important component in their recovery.

Making a report requires a call to 911 by the victims themselves or by a friend or family member they may have called first. However, if ever there is a question of any kind regarding the process of reporting a sexual assault, victims themselves or their friends and family members can call the National Sexual Assault Hotline for free, confidential advice about anything related to the process. The 24 hour-a-day, seven-day-a-week hotline number is: **1-800-656-HOPE**. Most prosecutors' offices have an established Sexual Assault Response Team (SART) that is activated whenever a sexual assault is reported. The SART is a multidisciplinary team composed of professionals involved in the immediate response to a report. Although SART components vary by community, members typically include:

- Rape care advocates—They will be involved in initial contact with the victim via hotlines or in face-to-face meetings. Called as soon as the report is made, they may accompany the victim to the local police station, to the hospital for treatment and the collection of evidence, or simply provide any other supportive assistance requested by the victim. In most communities, the local women's shelter or rape crisis center provides these advocates.

- Forensic medical providers—A Sexual Assault Nurse Examiner (SANE) is a medical professional trained in the treatment of victims and in the collection from them of key physical evidence such as hairs, fluids, and fibers after the assault. They typically coordinate with rape care advocates to ensure that victims receive crisis intervention and support during and after the examination process. Other health care personnel may also include emergency medical technicians, gynecologists, surgeons, or other private physicians. The purpose of this forensic examination is to provide any evidence necessary to establish that a crime occurred and to help identify who the assailant was.

- Law enforcement representatives—Police officers or detectives who are assigned to investigate the report, interview the victims, and coordinate the collection of evidence to assist with the prosecution of the case. The officers assigned typically have specialized training and experience in the area of sexual assault investigations. They perform other tasks as well, like providing transportation to the local medical facility.

- Prosecutors—Their role is to decide whether or not there is sufficient evidence to prosecute the case. Some communities involve them more actively, and the Office of Violence Against Women (OVAW) in the Department of Justice suggests their full participation in SART.

The OVAW developed *A National Protocol for Sexual Assault Medical Forensic Examinations* (2004) and emphasized the importance of a timely, appropriate, sensitive, and respectful response to the disclosure of a sexual assault. The *Protocol* calls for all involved to put the needs of the victims first throughout the exam process and afterward, particularly being mindful of the victims' needs for privacy, for advocacy, and for information regarding each step of the examination and of subsequent legal steps in the possible prosecution of the case.

Eileen Allen, RN, is a certified SANE and is the coordinator of SANE/ SART services for all of Monmouth County, New Jersey's fourth most populous of its 21 counties, with a population of 655,000 people. Allen oversees a staff of 14 trained forensic nurses (SANEs) who are available 24 hours a day, seven days a week, to respond to calls from hospital emergency rooms or law enforcement personnel regarding a case of sexual assault.

The purpose of SART, Allen explained, is to help the victims "make informed choices and decisions about how to proceed." The SANE leads the

---

C A S E   P R E S E N T A T I O N : Anita, a Case of Sexual Assault

CAUTION: The following four cases provide accounts of sexual assault that are relatively graphic and descriptive. Please be advised.

Anita was an 18-year-old high school senior in a school of approximately 1,200 students in a suburb in a southern state. She was an average student who planned to attend the local community college the following year and eventually to complete a four-year bachelor's degree. Her longer-term professional plans, she told her school counselor, were unclear; all she knew, she claimed, was that she wanted to work with children in some capacity. Anita's academic record was without any significant blemish; aside from one or two Cs on her high school transcript in some of her college prep classes, she did well. Her discipline record also was unremarkable. With the exception of leaving school with a host of other students on the annual "cut day" for which she received the penalty of a detention, there were no other offenses worthy of note.

It was just after the semester break that the vice principal assigned to the senior class noticed a slight change in her performance, however. Anita started a pattern of tardiness to school in the morning, causing her to miss close to 20 minutes of English IV, her first period class. A requirement for graduation, a failure in this class would result in her inability to graduate without first making it up in the district's summer school program. The vice principal grew concerned about this possibility and spoke with Anita several times about this pattern, only to have her reassure him that she would do her best to arrival at school on time. The reasons she gave for being late were varied: oversleeping, car trouble, and having to babysit her younger stepbrother whenever her mother worked overtime in her night shift.

Always alert to the goings-on among the seniors he was responsible for, the vice principal regularly consulted with the school psychologist about those students who concerned him, particularly his seniors who hoped to graduate in June of that year. If ever he saw something in their academic or behavioral record that concerned him, he sought out the psychologist for some problem-solving feedback. And so it was with Anita; as her tardiness began to mount, he asked the psychologist if there was anything in her case that might suggest the need for psychological intervention. The psychologist, seeing nothing in her record to indicate any long-term pattern of difficulties that would threaten graduation, save for this recent collection of tardiness, simply suggested that the vice principal speak with Anita again about the risks that this pattern posed to graduation. The vice principal had a well-earned reputation as being a fair, even-tempered school administrator who gave students good advice; the psychologist knew that he would address this problem with Anita in a professional and benevolent manner. The psychologist was a virtual stranger to her, whereas the vice principal had known Anita for a year since her arrival at the school, making him the logical person to speak with her.

interview with the victims and explains the services available to them as well as the various options they have in accepting them as offered. That is, they can choose whether or not they want to proceed with the forensic medical examination, the services of a rape care advocate, and law enforcement (such as filing a report and agreeing to an interview with a police officer).

Providing victims with these choices throughout the process is intended "to empower victims to do what's in their own best interests at the moment," Allen said. Thus, they have the right to accept or reject any one or all of the services offered to them.

It was later in the week after this conversation when the vice principal left an urgent message for the psychologist to see him right away. He told the psychologist that Anita disclosed the reason for her tardiness just moments earlier; the explanation was nothing that either of these school professionals anticipated. According to Anita, her stepfather, who had moved into the home after marrying her mother about a year ago, had begun fondling her, rubbing her breasts, and placing his hands on her buttocks, usually when her mother was not around. He would laugh when she recoiled and pushed away, claiming that she was making a "big deal" over nothing. Rather than tell her mother about what was happening, she kept quiet about it, lest she upset her mother who seemed to be in love with her husband after having been a single parent for several years. Anita felt that she would be able to survive as long as she avoided being alone in the house with him; she also had planned to be out of the house and on her own after graduation just a few months later.

Anita went on to explain to the vice principal that her stepfather's job change several months ago resulted in a change in his work hours. Instead of having to leave the house to make the 6:20 a.m. train, he now was able to sleep late and catch the 7:15 train, keeping him in the home while Anita prepared herself for the start of her school day at 7:40. Part of this ritual was her morning shower. She realized at one point that her stepfather had unlocked the bathroom door and stared at her in the shower. Although she suspected that it may have been happening for several weeks, she doubted her suspicions, lacking any real evidence to confirm this awful truth. Finally, she saw him one morning looking at her through a small opening in the door; when she screamed, he claimed to be unaware that she was in the bathroom and that he only wanted to retrieve his razor from the medicine chest.

So, Anita told the vice principal, her lateness coincided with the realization of her stepfather's voyeurism. She had to wait until he left the house for work each day until she dared undress for the shower, thus her late arrival at school each day.

Intervention

The response of the psychologist and the vice principal was to call the local Child Protective Services (CPS) office to report the abuse, but Anita's age (18 years) placed her beyond the reach of CPS. The psychologist explained to her, therefore, that she had the right to contact the police, since what her stepfather had done to her constituted sexual assault.

(continued)

CASE PRESENTATION: Anita, a Case of Sexual Assault
(continued)

PSYCHOLOGIST: If you would like, Anita, you can call the police to report what your stepfather did to you.

ANITA: But why would I do that? I mean, what can they do? It's not like I have any proof or anything. What if it's just my word against his?

PSYCHOLOGIST: You're not convinced that the police will believe you?

ANITA: That's right. My stepfather has lived in this town all his life. I just moved here with my mother when they got married last year. He'll deny doing anything wrong and they'll believe him.

PSYCHOLOGIST: Have you considered talking to your mother about it?

ANITA: No way! She's really into him; she thinks he's the greatest! Besides, my mom caught me making out with my boyfriend a few weeks ago, and she went crazy, calling me all kinds of names. I wouldn't be surprised if she even blamed me for what happened.

PSYCHOLOGIST: It seems that there are so many things that you are thinking about. Would you like to talk to someone who works with young women like you who have had similar experiences? This person may have some advice for you that you might find helpful.

ANITA: Who are you talking about?

CASE PRESENTATION: Nicole, a Case of Date Rape

Nicole, a 16-year-old high school sophomore, had it all figured out. Assuming that her parents would never let her attend the end-of-season football party at the team captain's home because of the number of seniors who would be there, she concocted a plan with her friend Cherise to make it all happen. Nicole told her parents that she was going to a sleepover at Cherise's house with a few other classmates; Cherise's parents, she assured them, would be home to supervise the gathering.

Instead, both girls went to the party. Not only were the captain's parents not home at the time, but among the dozens of familiar faces were many other outsiders, older-looking young people who provided the underage partygoers with a large supply of alcohol. Nicole had a few beers, and as her inhibitions loosened, she began to take her turn atop the dining room table and dance to the loud rock music resounding through the room. After several minutes of entertaining the crowd, she stepped down from the table, woozy and unsteady on her feet, and went upstairs to use the only available bathroom.

Kevin, a 17-year-old senior who was in Nicole's biology class, followed her upstairs. As she exited the bathroom, Kevin greeted her in the hallway, pulled her into the bedroom, and fell with her onto a bed covered with the coats of the party

PSYCHOLOGIST: There is an agency nearby that provides not only shelter for victims of domestic violence and sexual assault, but also counseling and advice and other support services. There is a hotline number you can call if you wish to talk to someone there.

ANITA: But will they call the police?

PSYCHOLOGIST: The decision to call the agency is yours and yours alone. If you don't want to call, then you don't have to. The advantage in calling the hotline is for you to ask them questions about what happened and about what they might be able to do for you.

ANITA: Do they keep a record of the call?

PSYCHOLOGIST: You can call anonymously if you want; they don't need to have your name to be able to talk to you.

ANITA: O.K., then, I'll call them.

Case Discussion/Crisis Resolution

Anita spent a considerable amount of time with the advocate exploring the options available to her. However, she eventually decided not to pursue the matter with the police. Although she clearly had not decided how to address the issue with her mother, Anita told the psychologist that she planned to call the advocate again to discuss with her how to talk to her mother about it.

attendees. Some kissing and "making out" followed. When he told her that he wanted to "do it," she pushed him away, telling him that what they had just done was enough and that she wanted to get back to the party. Kevin, however, was able to overpower her easily, and he restrained her and penetrated her. When he rolled over in exhaustion, someone opened the door to the room looking for a coat and Nicole was able to leave the room and rejoin Cherise downstairs.

Nicole said nothing of the assault until she told Cherise the next morning. The response she received was not what she expected. Cherise pleaded with her not to tell anyone in case the report to the authorities get both of them into trouble for lying to their parents about their whereabouts the night before. Nicole agreed at the time, but a lingering dread about the incident lead her to tell her aunt the next day; her aunt convinced her of the importance of reporting the assault to the police.

Nicole's next step was to tell her parents who then accompanied her to the hospital for a forensic examination. The SANE collected the forensic evidence, and a rape care advocate interviewed Nicole and explained her options available. One of these options, the choice not to proceed with law enforcement, was the one that Nicole

(continued)

CASE PRESENTATION: Nicole, a Case of Date Rape
(continued)

---

chose out of her concerns over publicity for herself and her family. She also expressed some fear that the prosecution of the case would have an adverse impact on her social standing in the high school; Kevin was a popular student, Nicole thought, and pursuing legal charges against him might result in her social ostracism. A discussion with her family over this course of action confirmed her decision not to proceed with the case.

Case Discussion/Crisis Resolution

SANE Eileen Allen sees Nicole's case as not uncommon in her years of experience. "Most of the cases I've seen are victims between the ages of 15 and 25 and are date or acquaintance rapes," she explained. "Many are alcohol-related and involve house parties where there is a lot of drinking." Since the purpose of the collaborative efforts of SART members is to empower the victims of sexual assault to make informed decisions in the aftermath of the attack, individuals have the right to stop the process at any time.

Allen's trained SANE staff averages between 120–140 hospital visits each year to conduct forensic examinations; however, only 100–120 exams are completed. Those calls to the hospital that do not result in exams, she explained, are due either to the fact that the victims "are too drunk and can't give accurate information" or that they "just opt out." As she also has learned, Allen sees the primary reasons for victims opting out of the process as falling into the following categories:

- fear of the medical process
- fear of involvement with law enforcement

CASE PRESENTATION: Courtney, a Case of Date Rape and
Date Rape Drugs

She was 20 years old at the time, attractive, energetic, and popular, and still reeling from the break-up with a long-term boyfriend. Despite numerous offers from other potential suitors, Courtney stayed far from the dating scene, expecting instead that she and her former boyfriend would one day be reunited. Finally, however, she took the advice of family and friends to return to an active social life and accepted the offer of a date from Tom.

Tom was more than just an average guy. "A golden boy," Courtney called him, a young man from a high-profile local family enjoying a successful professional career; he was personable, handsome, and charming. Courtney's later retrospective analysis of some of the events of that night suggested that there may have been some warning signs present early in the evening to which she attributed little meaning until it was too late. For example, the night before the date he requested that she allow him to spend an hour with her parents when he came to pick her up; he asked her specifically not to "rush him out the door." Although an odd request, Courtney thought, for a whole hour to get acquainted, she

- fear of social repercussions, especially for teens
- encouragement by parents to pursue the process, despite the victim's reluctance to do so—in these cases, the victim eventually opts out

Linda Altieri, a registered nurse and coordinator of the Rape Care Program for 180 Turning Lives Around, an agency devoted to providing services and advocacy for women, men, and children affected by domestic violence and sexual assault, described the same reasons why young women decide to forego the process. She added that, like Nicole's case, "Sometimes they're doing something they're not supposed to be doing, like drinking, so they fail to report to avoid trouble at home." Still others, she claimed, don't see themselves as victims, particularly if the assailant was a former or current boyfriend.

One of Altieri's 62 trained rape care advocates are available at all hours, seven days a week, to respond to a reported sexual assault. Their role, as is the role of the entire SART team, is to tell victims what to expect throughout the process of making the report, consenting to the forensic medical examination, and following up with law enforcement. However, she explained, "Our role is to empower them to be able to say 'no' at any step in the process." The victim, whether a child or adult, has the right to consent to these steps, to refuse them altogether, or to withdraw initial consent later in the process. The advocate's role involves obtaining the victim's consent, regardless of age, even if it is contrary to the wishes of a parent.

nevertheless dismissed it as due to his typical friendliness and affability. When he arrived that night, he kissed Courtney's mother on the cheek, shook her father's hand, and sat down at the kitchen table with them. Tom asked her father about his occupation, his long morning commute, and the hours he arose in the morning and returned home in the evening. The entire time, however, Courtney thought that Tom was not much her type and that this date would be a one-time-only encounter.

After close to an hour had passed, Courtney left with Tom. He said that he would take her to a local bar/restaurant, even though Courtney was not old enough to drink, a fact she reminded him of several times that evening. Despite several refusals to accept a drink from the bartender, however, she eventually agreed to take one. The bartender, a personal friend of Tom's, didn't ask Courtney for any identification to verify her drinking age, probably as a favor to Tom, Courtney assumed.

(continued)

C A S E   P R E S E N T A T I O N : Courtney, a Case of Date Rape and
Date Rape Drugs *(continued)*

---

*Within minutes of just a few sips of the drink, Courtney recalled, she felt sick
and lightheaded. She fell off her barstool as she attempted to make her way to the
restroom, but she managed to get there. She knew that she felt very uncomfortable,
both physically and emotionally, so she decided that she would ask Tom to take her
home. Another large frosted drink greeted her at the bar upon her return and Tom
lingered and ignored her request to drive her back home. Courtney just knew that
there was something in that first drink.*

*Tom finally paid the bar bill and as they walked to his car his cell phone rang.
"I'm with her now," he told the caller. "Oh yeah, we'll stop by." Her protests against
this side-trip were silenced as she passed out once she entered the car. "It's the
strangest thing I ever had happen," she said. "I opened my eyes and I was in an entirely different place." The now disoriented and confused Courtney awoke to realize
that Tom had taken her to a go-go bar with exotic dancers to meet up with his
friends.*

*After a few introductions, she overheard Tom say to his friends, "Give me five
minutes and I'll get her into bed." Now an irate Courtney demanded that he take
her home immediately. First he insisted she had to look at the dancers, so he put
his hands on her shoulders and turned her in the direction of the bar area. Then
Courtney once again passed out in the car that, she assumed, was en route to her
home. Instead, she recalled something hitting her on the head, only to realize that
it was the storm door that she banged into as Tom carried her up the steps to his
house. The only other person present was a roommate of Tom's who was inside
the house watching television. Courtney immediately went to the bathroom and
threw up.*

*When she exited the bathroom the roommate was no longer there, and the
only light on in the house was in an empty first-floor bedroom. She entered the
room, fell face-down on the bed, and promptly passed out again. When she
awoke, still disoriented and confused, Courtney realized that the sensation of
paralysis in her right arm was because her arm was stretched behind her and
handcuffed to the bed post; the heaviness on her chest that made it difficult to
breathe was Tom lying on top of her, struggling to remove her pants and under-
wear. Her one-armed struggle was unsuccessful in stopping him from raping her;
within minutes he was inside her. "I remember crying, screaming so that the
roommate would hear me," Courtney reported, but no one came. She also
recalled blacking out several times.*

*When he was finished he just rolled over and slept. In the morning he woke up,
threw Courtney's clothes at her ("like I was yesterday's trash"), and told her that he
would drive her home. He told her at one point that he wanted to keep her like
that so that "he could do that every day after work." The ride home was bizarre,
she thought. Tom apologized for what he did, claiming that he got "carried away."
He also maintained that he wanted to have her as his girlfriend and to take her
shopping that weekend.*

*It was early in the morning, just 15 minutes before her father woke up,
when Tom dropped her off at home. Courtney quickly went upstairs, took off
her clothes, and hopped into bed. Had Tom expressed such an interest the*

night before in her father's working and commuting hours to help him ascertain the best time to have her home without having to run into him? Courtney asked herself this question and others while trying to make sense of the experience.

Case Discussion/Crisis Resolution

Courtney didn't plan to tell her mother about the rape, despite their closeness and openness with each other. She did plan, however, to contact the local women's shelter to speak with a counselor. When her mother arrived home later that day after Courtney awoke, she sensed that something was wrong. Courtney's repeated denials that something was amiss did not stop her mother from probing: *Did something happen last night? What did he do to you?* Finally, Courtney broke down and told her of the ordeal. Unsure of how to proceed, Courtney's mother consulted with her own mother about the best course of action. Courtney ultimately decided not to report the rape to the police, preferring instead to seek out therapy at the women's center.

What eventually changed her mind about pursuing the matter with law enforcement, however, was her discovery that Tom had raped another young woman in the same manner a little more than a week after her assault. This second victim, upon learning Courtney's identity, contacted her and asked her to corroborate her story with the county prosecutor. "Out of pure guilt," Courtney claimed, she visited the prosecutor and told her story, but she still remained ambivalent about pressing charges as the prosecutor suggested until several days later. Finally, she relented and went to trial. A third victim who suffered a similar fate at Tom's hands eventually came forward as well.

The trial was an ordeal for Courtney and for the second victim, but Tom was acquitted of the charges. However, Courtney and the other two victims took their case to an Administrative Law Hearing which, after one unsuccessful try, resulted in Tom's loss of job. Courtney reported that she and the other two women "felt empowered" by exercising their right to pursue the hearing after the courts found him not guilty.

What Courtney did next illustrated one of the core concepts of the meaning of crisis: *danger* and *opportunity* (see Chapter 1). She used her experience as an opportunity to emerge from it stronger than before. Courtney now serves as a speaker during training sessions for rape care advocates sponsored by her local women's crisis center; she speaks to these groups of her rape experience as survivor, not as victim, as well as of the opportunities it afforded her in the aftermath. "It was almost a blessing," she claimed, "because I got angry enough to help other people. I'm a better person for it; I'm one of the lucky ones."

Courtney remains in group therapy with other rape survivors at the same center she called immediately after the rape. In her experience, she claimed, most rape victims don't report it to law enforcement nor follow through with all the steps in the process described above, but they do go to therapy. "I got a different mind frame and moved from the victim to the survivor stage. It changed my life for the better."

CASE PRESENTATION: Kristin, a Case of Rape

NOTE: Like Courtney's story, Kristin tells of her ordeal and of her decision not to file a police report after her rape. And like Courtney, she talks of her response to the assault in a manner which illustrates the *opportunity* offered in the aftermath of her crisis (see Chapter 1).

A medical school student with an intended specialization in oncology, Kristin was a college senior attending a large, prestigious university in the heartland of America at the time of her rape. Bright, popular, and active in one of her campus sororities, Kristin lived off-campus in an apartment with several of her sorority sisters. It was the friend of one of these sisters who visited one weekend and met Kristin. Steve was a senior at another university not far from Kristin's, one that enjoyed a fierce competitive relationship in the sports arena with her school.

Kristin and Steve got to know each other that Saturday night, spending a few hours at a local bar with other friends before parting company. Kristin returned to her apartment; Steve departed to parts unknown. A short while later, however, her phone rang; it was Steve asking her if it was alright for him to come over to see her again. Although second-guessing her decision to allow him this visit now, Kristin agreed to it then.

Steve came to the apartment, which was far from empty; it contained several other friends and sorority sisters, some of them sleeping in the living room. Nevertheless, before long Steve had Kristin in her bedroom and had overpowered and raped her. "I told him to stop, but he told me to 'just hold on'," she remembered. She thought about screaming to awaken her sleeping friends, but in a decision that she considered not to be a conscious one, she thought better of doing so. Perhaps out of embarrassment, she thought, or perhaps for some other reasons she kept quiet; a sense of powerlessness and dread compromised her reasoning during this assault. Instead she maintained her silence and tried to survive the attack by dissociating herself from it, claiming, "I closed my eyes and pretended to be somewhere else."

Soon after the assault, Steve left the apartment. Kristin remained in her bed while several other overnight guests packed up their sleeping bags and left. Unclear as to what to do in the aftermath of her rape, Kristin finally left her room and decided to confide in one of her roommates about her ordeal. Hoping for some solace and support from her friend, Kristin received none. "She tried not to make a big deal out of it." Kristin recalled her friend telling her, "Watch the Gilmore Girls and it'll be fine." Despite feeling rebuffed and minimized by this reaction, Kristin reached out one more time, this time to someone she described as her best friend, Tom, another senior at the university. However, the sense of rejection she experienced at the reaction of her roommate she experienced yet again with Tom. "No offense, Kristin, but you put yourself in that position," he told her. "He made me feel that it was my fault, so I decided not to tell anyone else," Kristin recalled regretfully.

She decided to go about her business and kept quiet about the rape. About two months later, as she became increasingly aware of the possibility of having contracted a sexually transmitted disease (STD) from Steve's attack, she visited the university health center to be tested and treated if she tested positive for disease.

As part of the STD assessment protocol, the attending physician asked Kristin why she was concerned about the disease at that time. Thinking that this question was "another chance for me to tell somebody," Kristin seized the opportunity and said, "Because I was raped." The physician's response, however, was not what Kristin hoped for; instead of being supportive, she maintained, the physician appeared taken aback and simply asked Kristin, "Are you taking care of that?" Feeling "shut down again," Kristin vowed to keep her secret to herself.

When asked about her decision not to report her rape to the police, she replied, "Emotionally I couldn't press charges. The first two people I told as well as the physician at the health center completely shut me down. Besides, stopping the perpetrator by reporting it is not the victim's responsibility."

Case Discussion/Crisis Resolution
As the next few months passed and graduation approached, Kristin began experiencing multiple indicators of RTS (see page 97). "I had nightmares, cold sweats, and even smelling on someone else the same cologne he wore triggered flashbacks. Sometimes while sitting in class, I would just start crying," Kristin remembered.

Finally, the turning point came for Kristin. A university-sponsored Take Back the Night rally was planned on campus. The purpose of these rallies is to empower men and women both to stand up to violence, particularly sexual violence and rape, and to assert the rights of all people to be free from violence. These rallies typically are followed by "speakout sessions" where survivors of violence are offered the opportunity to speak publicly to the rally attendees about their experiences with violence.

Kristin attended the rally and seized the opportunity to ascend to the podium during the follow-up speakout session to tell the story of her rape. She recalled thinking that "telling my story felt good"; a visit to the campus women's center for a social gathering immediately after the speakout session that night also convinced her that she was on the road from victim to survivor. "I was able to spread the word to a lot more people; I wanted to get involved," she stated.

Upon her return home after graduation, Kristin contacted the local women's shelter and eventually completed a training program to become a rape care advocate, a role she continues to this day whenever her medical school studies permit. She not only serves on the local SART, but also speaks to numerous groups of professionals about her experiences and what it takes to become a survivor, rather than a victim. She participates in the training of other rape care advocates as well. "Being an advocate has been my calling; I couldn't imagine my life without it now, it has become an important part of me. I'm in a great position to try to help people," Kristin asserted. As for suggestions she has for other victims of sexual assault, Kristin offered the following: "Get a support system, but you might not find it when you expect to find it; some people just don't know how to respond. Don't be discouraged by people's reactions, just find someone who believes you and supports you."

Guidelines for Treating Victims of Sexual Assault

The National Center for Victims of Crime lists additional suggestions for those who first respond to a sexual assault victim once the disclosure is made, whether to a friend, a family member, or a member of the law enforcement community:

- **Listen without judging**. Sexual assault is a crime that can have staggering consequences for the victim. Coming forward and disclosing the attack to a friend or to a professional is an important, yet difficult step, making it incumbent upon the listener to provide a safe and accepting environment for this disclosure to occur. Communicating a belief that the attack really did happen is one of the most important things to be communicated to the victim. Unconditional acceptance of the victim's story using sound reflective listening techniques is critical.

- **Let them know that the assaults were not their fault**. Many sexual assault victims blame themselves for the assault for a variety of reasons. However, the victim has to hear that what took place was a crime committed by someone else who had no right to do so. Regardless of the victims' thoughts and statements about what they could have done differently to avoid the attack, what should be stressed is that they did nothing wrong and that nothing they did caused the attack.

- **Let them know that they did what was necessary to prevent further harm.** If the victim blames himself or herself for not fighting back enough to avoid or to stop the assault, reassurances should be provided for that such behavior may indeed have resulted in greater harm and that fear often immobilizes people out of a need for survival. Guilt over not doing enough to stop it may linger, so constant reassurances to the contrary are important.

- **Reassure them that they are cared for and loved.** A listener's caring, nonjudgmental demeanor is important to a sexual assault survivor. Steering clear of specific questions about the crime and allowing the individual to choose which details to share are also critical.

- **Encourage them to seek medical attention.** If the victims have not received medical attention or reported it to the authorities, they should be encouraged to do so. Calling 911 or a local or national hotline phone number (see page 99) is the easiest way to do so.

- **Encourage them to talk about the assault with an advocate, mental health professional, or someone else they trust.** Follow-up counseling with a trained professional is essential. Some of the symptoms of PTSD or RTS (see page 97) may not appear until some time after the attack, so it is important that victims seek out a counselor in the community soon after an attack. If the case goes to trial, the victims will have to recount the details of the attack several times, making the need for counseling during this period all the more important. If the victims hesitate to see someone for counseling, they can be encouraged to call one of the hotline numbers to talk with someone experienced in treating sexual assault survivors. These calls also can be made anonymously.

- **Let them know that they do not have to manage the crisis alone.**
  Social support is a powerful mediator of symptoms suffered after a sexual assault. The fact that victims have already disclosed the attack to someone should start the process of engaging others in a helping capacity. Communicating to victims the available network of helping people is important in the recovery process.

RECOMMENDATIONS FOR CHAPTER ENRICHMENT

SUGGESTED FILMS

The Accused **(1988)** Based on a true-life incident, the movie tells the story of Sarah Tobias, a working girl who liked to party with her friends and flirt with the guys. One night after several hours of drinking and flirting, she was brutally gang raped atop a pinball machine in the bar while onlookers cheered on the attack. The film challenges viewers to reassess their own beliefs in rape myths regarding a woman's responsibility in her own rape. Jodie Foster portrays Tobias.

Dead Man Walking **(1995)** This film presents the viewer with difficult choices about capital punishment as an effective or humane punishment for the crime of rape and murder. Sean Penn plays the sexual assailant and murderer on death row.

Casualties of War **(1989)** Set in the jungles of Vietnam during the Vietnam War, the film chronicles the lives of soldiers in combat and their gang rape of a young, innocent Vietnamese girl. Michael J. Fox plays the troop's conscience as he attempts to reason with the assailants about their intended action.

SUGGESTED ACTIVITIES

1. Contact the SART in your own county of residence. Interview a member of the team about the process SART follows in responding to reports of sexual assault. Find out information regarding the numbers and types of calls received annually, and the choices made by victims regarding the services they accept or reject.

2. Interview a rape care advocate in your area. Inquire about what he or she perceives as the most important skills and/or traits required of an advocate for sexual assault victims. What have the experiences been like in the work? What have been the most distressing or frustrating cases?

3. Download a copy of the *National Protocol for Sexual Assault Medical Forensic Examinations (Adolescents/Adults)* from the U.S. Department of Justice's Office on Violence against Women and review it for more details regarding the process of sexual assault response.

7

Alcohol Drug Crises

DISCUSSION QUESTIONS

Have you ever experienced a situation where you had to take care of a friend who was intoxicated or under the influence of drugs? What was the experience like? At any point did you have any concerns for their safety?

Did you ever have a friend who was injured or arrested as a result of being under the influence of alcohol or drugs? How did you react when you first heard about the injury or arrest?

INTRODUCTION

Alcoholism ranks among the top three leading causes of death in the United States (Anthony, Warner, & Kessler, 1997; Substance Abuse & Mental Health Services Administration, 2002); therefore it not uncommon that alcohol and drug abuse will result in many types of crisis situations. Crises that come about as a result of alcohol or drug use are difficult to manage primarily because of the potential for concurrent medical complications. For example, an individual can present under the influence of alcohol or drugs (substance intoxication) and unless that individual is coherent and willing to tell the crisis counselor what chemicals they have ingested, how much, and within what timeframe, the counselor will be left guessing what has contributed to this individual's stupor. Similarly, some individuals will present in crisis because they are in the throes of substance withdrawal. Again, it is known that some drugs of abuse produce complex and potentially fatal withdrawal syndromes (Milzman & Soderstrom, 1994). Alcohol and benzodiazepine withdrawal can result in symptoms such as memory deficits, confusion, delirium, tremor, convulsions, and even visual, auditory, or tactile hallucinations. Thus, a person may experience an alcohol or drug crisis because of either intoxication or withdrawal. It is important that crisis counselors who intervene with people with substance use disorders be familiar with the specific symptoms of intoxication and withdrawal for substances such as alcohol, opiates, ecstasy, methamphetamines, cocaine, benzodiazepines, hallucinogens, and cannabis. Each substance has its own idiosyncratic intoxication and withdrawal syndromes, some of which require hospitalization and medication in order to safely manage the crisis. However, it is important to point out that a crisis may also result from a pattern of substance use that leads to serious problems in daily functioning. An otherwise law-abiding person can be thrown into crisis if arrested for a drunk driving offense or attending a party where drugs are present or if fired from a job due to alcohol- or drug-related tardiness or absenteeism. If this individual lacks a pattern of such problems or they are not psychologically or physically dependent on drugs or alcohol, then a substance abuse diagnosis may be rendered. A diagnosis of substance dependence should be considered if there is a clear loss of control of the individual's use of mood-altering substances, along with physiological or psychological dependence and a definite pattern of problems or unmanageability related to the substance use.

One of the challenges that crisis counselors face is determining whether the immediate crisis (such as intoxication, arrest, forced unemployment, or a break up in a relationship) is evident of a long-standing problem in which alcohol or drug use has played a major role or an isolated instance of substance misuse. An accurate assessment is necessary in prescribing an effective intervention strategy. What makes assessment difficult, however, is that alcoholics and addicts are not always forthcoming in providing background information or they may not be able to recall this information due to alcohol blackouts. To complicate matters further, the issue of comorbidity must also be taken into account (comorbidity refers to individuals who manifest other psychiatric disorders concurrent with substance use disorders). For example, it is estimated that 78% of those with alcohol or drug problems will also experience a psychiatric disorder at some time in their lives (the most common being anxiety disorders, mood disorders, personality disorders, and sexual dysfunctions). Furthermore, it is estimated that 20% of individuals manifesting an anxiety or mood disorder will also manifest a substance use disorder and that 20% of individuals manifesting substance use disorders will also manifest a mood or anxiety disorder (Conway et al., 2006).

In this chapter, we will explore some of the crises that can result from alcohol and drug abuse and how crisis counselors can intervene effectively. In order to best illustrate the different types of crisis, we will present brief cases illustrating substance intoxication, substance withdrawal, and substance dependence.

C A S E   P R E S E N T A T I O N : A Crisis Involving Substance Intoxication

---

Sean is a 19-year-old college sophomore. He is currently on disciplinary probation at the university he attends because in his freshman year, he got into a fight at a party and broke a fellow student's jaw. Sean indicates that in addition to drinking, he has also smoked marijuana since high school and continues to smoke occasionally while at the university. He reports however, that he usually smokes more pot during the summer when he is around his old high school buddies. In the current crisis, Sean was brought to the emergency room (ER) of the university hospital last night after he had passed out on the lawn at a beer party. Fortunately, one of Sean's friends saw that Sean had vomited all over himself and could not be awakened. The friend immediately called 9-1-1 and an ambulance was sent. At the ER, Sean's stomach was pumped and he was given a blood test that revealed an extremely high blood alcohol level along with marijuana (THC) and Oxycontin in his bloodstream. The crisis counselor was called in to see Sean after he regained consciousness the next day.

Sean's crisis starts off as a *medical crisis*. If Sean's friend had just let him "sleep it off" or not tried to wake him, this could have resulted in disastrous consequences. Many individuals will aspirate or vomit while in an intoxicated stupor and will die of asphyxiation (see Trezza & Scheft, 2009). Therefore, most instances of *substance intoxication*, especially when a person is intoxicated to the point of being either unconscious, unable to wake up, or incoherent (for example, being disoriented, not making sense), should be handled as a medical crisis and the person should be brought to an ER or to an immediate health care center where they can be observed and properly treated. The worst thing to do is to leave the person alone. Also, don't assume that because you have rolled the person on their side, that they can't aspirate (regurgitate) food and asphyxiate (suffocate).

Intervention

In Sean's situation, his medical crisis was stabilized and he was evaluated the following day. The crisis counselor approached the situation as follows:

Counselor: Hi Sean, my name is Susan Roberts, I'm a counselor here at the university medical center. The doctor who treated you last night asked that I come in and check on you to see how you're feeling today. I understand you had a rough night. Do you recall being brought to the ER?

Sean: No, the last thing I remember was being at the Sigma house and playing some stupid drinking game, where we were doing jello shots. That was around 10:00 or so, I don't remember much after that.... I feel like shit. My stomach feels like someone jumped on it. Do my parents know I'm here?

Counselor: Your stomach had to be pumped, which is part of why you feel so badly. I don't think Dr. Chung has called your parents though. I'm pretty sure we would need you to sign a release form in order to call them, but I'll check with the ER nurse. You were in a dangerous situation. Sounds like you're pretty worried about your parents knowing you're here?

Sean: If they know, they're going to kill me. They'll probably make me live at home and attend a community college or work. I can't believe I did this again.

Counselor: Has something like this happened before?

Sean: Well, not this bad. In high school I went to one of the school dances and got trashed on some Jack Daniels that a friend and I stole from my parent's liquor cabinet. We thought that no one would be able to tell we were wasted until my friend Kevin started puking all over the gym floor. They figured out that we were drinking together and sent us to see the Student Assistance Counselor, but it was a waste of time. We ended up lying our way out of it. My parents said that if I ever got into trouble for drinking again they wouldn't let me go away to college. They are going to kill me, are you sure my parents weren't called? Could you check now?

COUNSELOR: Sure, I'll check at the Nurse's station and then we'll talk some more. I'd like to get more information about what happened.

SEAN: Okay, who did you say you are? Do you work here at the hospital?

COUNSELOR: Yes, my name is Susan Roberts and I work as a crisis counselor here at the hospital. Dr. Chung asked that I speak with you. I know she is really worried about you.

SEAN: I'll be O.K., as long as my parents don't find out about this.

At this point, the counselor checks to see if Sean's parents have been contacted. Many universities and hospitals have policies that allow for parental contact in the event that their son or daughter are treated in an ER. Although Sean is legally an adult, universities will request that student's sign release forms that allow for contact with parents in cases of emergencies. When the counselor returns she informs Sean that his parents had been notified. Sean decides to call them to let them know he is fine.

COUNSELOR: Sean, besides this incident, have you been having other problems at the university? Any relationship or academic problems?

SEAN: No, not that I can think of. Oh wait, yeah I did have something happen last year during the spring semester of my freshman year. I was at a party at this guy's house who lives off campus, and I got into a fight and broke some kid's jaw. They put me on some kind of disciplinary probation and said that if I didn't have another incident, they would clear my record. Will this get back to them? I didn't get into a fight, did I?

COUNSELOR: Not from what I was told, Sean, but it sound like you don't have much recollection of what happened last night? Has that happened to you before?

SEAN: Not every time I drink but it's happened a bunch of times.

COUNSELOR: Can you tell me what you recall from last night? Did you intend to drink as much as you did?

SEAN: No. I really figured that I would just have a couple of beers and then I was supposed to meet my roommate over at the dorm and go get something to eat.

COUNSELOR: What do you make of the fact that your evening turned out a lot differently from how you planned it?

SEAN: I guess there are just times when I can control my drinking and other times when I can't.

COUNSELOR: Sean, it says on your chart that your blood alcohol level was .34, which is really extreme. The lab also found marijuana and Oxycontin in your bloodstream. You're really lucky you didn't go into a coma. Sean,

(*continued*)

CASE PRESENTATION: **A Crisis Involving Substance**
Intoxication (continued)

---

it's important that you answer this question very truthfully. Were you deliberately trying to harm yourself by drinking and taking drugs? People can overdose by combining alcohol and drugs.

SEAN: You mean like was I suicidal? No, I know that things are pretty screwed up right now, but I'd never do something like that. I just had more to drink than I thought I would, that's all. You don't think I'm a druggie or some kind of psycho, do you?

COUNSELOR: No Sean, it's just important for me to make sure that you weren't trying to intentionally harm yourself because you did take a potentially lethal combination of drugs. Would you tell me more about the marijuana and Oxycontin?

SEAN: Well, I did smoke pot before I went out last night. I sometimes get high. Last year—my freshman year—I was getting high a lot, but once I ended up on Disciplinary Probation, I cut back just in case I was given a drug test.

COUNSELOR: What about the Oxycontin?

SEAN: I was given one of those by a friend of mine who's on the football team. His doctor gave him some for a back injury. They mellow me out even more than pot.

COUNSELOR: Is there any history of drinking or drug problems in your family?

SEAN: My mom and dad almost broke up a few years ago because of my father's drinking. But he started to go to AA and counseling. I don't think he drinks anymore. Not that I know of.

COUNSELOR: Did you feel that your father had a drinking problem?

SEAN: Definitely. He would come home just about every night either drunk and stumbling or buzzed and slurring his words. A couple of times he stayed out all night and my Mom was worried he was in a car accident or thought he might be having an affair or something. I was glad to hear that he quit.

COUNSELOR: Sean, did you know that alcohol and drug problems run in families? Some researchers feel there is pretty convincing evidence that it's a genetic illness.

SEAN: Yeah, I've heard that, but just because I party every once in a while it doesn't mean that I'm like my father or that I have a problem. I'm young and this is what we do to blow off steam.

COUNSELOR: Sure, I see what you mean. I was thinking though that when you set out last night to have a good time, you didn't think you would end up in an ER, right?

SEAN: Right, but this happens to my dormmates all the time, they get wasted and end up in the ER. That alone doesn't mean I have a problem, does it?

COUNSELOR: Right, but Sean it sounds like you've had past problems related to your drinking. I appreciate your being honest with me. Is there anything you might have left out, that would be important for me to know?

SEAN: No, not that I can think of. I'll do anything to stay in school. I don't want to go back home.

COUNSELOR: Since you've already tried the counseling center, why don't we set up an appointment with the outpatient program here at the medical center?

There are a few other students from the university who attend meetings here, and they've been able to help each other out.

SEAN: Like I said, I'll do anything. Would you talk with my parents if they end up hearing about this? I'm afraid of facing them alone.

COUNSELOR: Sure, I'd be happy to meet with them. That sounds like a good idea. Let's see if we can get them to agree with the plan we've discussed.

Case Conceptualization/Crisis Resolution

The crisis session described above attempts to achieve two goals. First, the crisis counselor tries to get needed background information from Sean pertaining to his alcohol and drug use in order to determine the nature of the present crisis and to determine whether this represents an isolated instance of excessive drinking and drug use or a pattern of substance use and consequential problematic behavior, which may suggest a substance use disorder diagnosis. Second, the counselor attempts to determine if the incident may have represented a suicide attempt. There are many instances where people overdose accidentally or use alcohol and drugs with suicidal intentions. According to the Drug Abuse Early Warning Network (DAWN, 2006), which examines emergency department statistics for fifty-one major metropolitan areas, there were 1,742,887 emergency department visits involving alcohol and drugs and approximately 12,500 alcohol- and drug-related deaths and approximately 1,586 alcohol- and drug-related suicide deaths (DAWN, 2006). Furthermore, of the 20 million Americans treated in emergency departments each year, approximately 27% manifest alcohol or drug disorders (Gentilello et al., 2005).

How does one approach the alcoholic or addict in order to effectively work with them and to assist them in resolving the crisis in a professional, competent manner? As in any counseling situation, it is important to first establish rapport. The person in crisis needs to know that you are there to help them, not to criticize nor judge them. Alcoholics and addicts are very attuned to judgmental attitudes. In Sean's case, it was also important for the counselor to **Listen** to his concerns and to his account of what he was able to recall. The next step is to **Assess** the extent and nature of his alcohol and drug use. Some say, "Why bother, most alcoholics or addicts lie anyway." Others suggest that whatever the alcoholic or addict tells you they are using, simply double that amount and you probably have a more accurate picture of their substance use pattern. That is why, whenever possible, it is helpful to get information from significant others such as roommates, friends, family, and coworkers. However, we must caution that with the exception of a life-threatening medical emergency, Federal Confidentiality Laws pertaining to alcohol and drug patients dictate that you must obtain a signed written release from the patient before you can contact anyone. Sean probably would not have allowed the crisis counselor to initiate contact with his parents or friends unless absolutely necessary. It was also noteworthy that Sean disclosed that his father had a problem with alcohol, which suggests a genetic risk factor to Sean's alcohol and drug problems (Hesselbrock & Hesselbrock, 1992; Merikangas, 1990; Schuckit & Smith, 1997).

Prior to Sean's release from the hospital, it is of utmost importance that some definite **Plan** be set up for continued assessment and counseling. Most individuals in situations such as Sean's tend to deny the need for counseling once the crisis has passed. This is why it is important that definite appointment times be set before he is medically cleared to leave and that in the meeting with his parents Sean **Commits** to that plan.

C A S E   P R E S E N T A T I O N : A Crisis Involving Substance
Withdrawal

Ophelia is a 28-year-old retail manager who has been living with her boyfriend Ray
for the past three years. They met while in college and began dating in their senior
year. They have had many "ups and downs" in their relationship and at one point
separated for 10 months, after which they decided to give things one more try. Most
of their problems have revolved around Ophelia's drinking and drug use. Ophelia
explains that she began drinking in high school with friends on weekends. During
the summer, she would rent a house at the beach with these friends and there would
be continuous, wild parties. Ophelia had a DUI last year, but she chalked it up to
"being in the wrong place at the wrong time." Ray was really upset with her. Al-
though he drinks, he feels that he never lets his drinking get out of hand, and that
Ophelia is like "Jekyll and Hyde" after a few drinks. One evening at a dinner party,
after Ophelia consumed several margaritas, Ray caught her in a sexually compromis-
ing situation with one of his best friends. Ophelia has sought crisis counseling today
because Ray has moved out. Ophelia was out drinking with her friends last night and
did not come home until 4:00 in the morning only to find that Raymond had left her.
Ophelia is upset, is crying, and does not know how she can live without Ray. She did
not want to ruin their relationship and feels that her life is out of control. As the
crisis counselor begins to gather more information, Ophelia reveals that in addition
to drinking about a pint of hard liquor per day, she supplements that with a "few
glasses of wine" in the evening and a Valium to "calm" her nerves in the morning.
About 30 minutes into the session, Ophelia's hands are noticeably trembling.

Ophelia has sought crisis counseling with the presenting complaint that her
boyfriend, Ray has left her. (It is not unusual for alcoholics or addicts to present for
help for problems other than their drug or alcohol abuse.) However, as the session
progresses and more information is gathered, it is obvious that Ophelia has a drinking and drug problem. What is significant, although not unique about her pattern of
use, is that she is a functional alcoholic who is also dependent on Valium (another
depressant drug). It is likely that her use of Valium became a means of preventing
the withdrawal symptoms (such as hand tremor and shakiness) that she experienced
in the morning because of her drinking. Very similar to the crisis of substance intoxication, *substance withdrawal* is also a medical emergency. The worst thing a crisis
counselor could do is to let this patient leave an outpatient office unattended or
without being escorted to an ER for a medical evaluation. Also, similarly to the
counselor in Sean's case described earlier, the crisis counselor's approach is to establish rapport with Ophelia and to gather as much information as possible about her
recent use of alcohol and drugs in order to relay this information to the physician
who will assess her in the ER. It is important to gather this information in a sensitive,
nonjudgmental manner, which is the reason to establish rapport and connection first.
With Ophelia, for example, it will be important to hear out her distress about Raymond, and to offer support. Supportive statements might include, "I can see how upset you are about Ray's leaving" or "This separation must be really difficult for you
right now." It is best to steer clear of statements like, "Don't worry, you'll get him
back," or "I know how you feel, it's tough to go through a break up." In making
statements like these, the counselor may be promising something that may not happen ("you'll get him back"), or presuming how Ophelia feels, ("I know how you
feel").

Possibly the most difficult scenario in a substance withdrawal case is when
the person refuses medical attention. Some states have laws that make it per-
missible to hold an intoxicated person in an ER for 48 to 72 hours for observation.

The supposition of these laws is that a person who is intoxicated or in a state of substance withdrawal is not coherent and reasonable enough to make an informed decision regarding their treatment. However, others would argue that keeping a person in an ER against their will is a violation of their civil liberties. Naturally, there are horror stories about intoxicated people leaving the ER against medical advice and being killed as they tried to cross the street. There are no simple solutions to be found. Also, an important point of clarification: The diagnoses of substance intoxication and substance withdrawal refer to the patient's current status at the time they are being seen for crisis intervention. However, once that crisis passes — the person is no longer under the influence of the drug or they have been detoxified from the substance — then the patient still needs to be evaluated to determine if they meet the criteria for a substance use disorder. It is important to remember that a person need not be physically addicted in order to be diagnosed with a substance use disorder. Think, for example, of a binge alcoholic who can often go weeks or months in between binges without drinking, however, once he or she does pick up a drink, their binge can last for days, weeks, or months. If you were to evaluate the person during one of their dry spells, they could still meet the criteria for substance dependence and would still require some type of intensive treatment.

For the crisis counselor, the task is in trying to talk the person into seeking medical attention or staying in the ER. Here's how a crisis counselor might try to convince Ophelia that she needs medical attention:

Intervention

COUNSELOR: Ophelia, from everything you've told me so far, I am really worried about your plan to stop drinking without medical intervention.

OPHELIA: Oh, I've done it before, no big deal. One time, Raymond was angry with me for getting drunk at his father's birthday party and I was completely sober for a few days.

COUNSELOR: I recall your mentioning that, but Ophelia, you mentioned earlier that you were not drinking as much then, plus now you are taking Valium. Taking these two together is a dangerous combination, that's why I'm really worried about what would happen if you were to try to stop on your own.

OPHELIA: I see what you're saying, but I need to get Ray back. I need to talk with him right away. Hell, I don't even know where he is or even if he would talk to me anyway.

COUNSELOR: Right Ophelia, besides you really need to take care of yourself right now. It's important that you let the doctor take a look at you. Would you at least agree to having Dr. Mendez check you over to make sure you'll be O.K.?

OPHELIA: I guess so. I am really shaking and I don't know if I have enough Valium to get me through the day.

COUNSELOR: Sounds like we have an agreement. Let's have Dr. Mendez take a look at you and see what she recommends.

OPHELIA: I'm okay with that, but what if she wants me to stay in the hospital overnight? I'm afraid I won't be able to talk to Ray.

(continued)

CASE PRESENTATION: A Crisis Involving Substance Withdrawal *(continued)*

COUNSELOR: Let's see what Dr. Mendez recommends and if you'd like we can try to call Raymond. Would you like to use the phone while we're waiting? Would you like me to talk with Ray?

OPHELIA: No, but I would like to try and call him again. If he doesn't believe that I'm here, could you talk with him then?

COUNSELOR: Sure, I'd be happy to talk with him.

Case Conceptualization/Crisis Resolution

In the illustration above, the crisis counselor tries to appeal to Ophelia's sense of reason in a nonthreatening way. The counselor also reinforces the idea that for right now, it is appropriate for Ophelia to take care of herself and not focus so much on Ray or on trying to regain the relationship. Naturally, if these strategies are not working, the counselor may need to use more persuasive tactics, such as bringing up

---

CASE PRESENTATION: A Crisis Resulting from Substance Dependence

---

Federico is a 45-year-old attorney with a thriving law practice. Last night he was arrested after getting into an argument with his wife. The argument got very heated and Federico ended up shoving his wife, Claire, to the floor, which resulted in hitting her head. She called the police and Federico was arrested for domestic violence. When asked by the crisis counselor what they were arguing about, Federico admitted that he had been using cocaine that night. He explained to the counselor that he began using cocaine "socially" about six years ago. He described his use as being occasional at first, usually with some of the friends that he plays golf with. However, over the past two years, he had begun using more consistently. He said that on some weekends he would rent a hotel room and would continue to snort lines of cocaine until Monday morning. He states that he would often get paranoid and would be afraid to come out of the hotel room. He would then take Valium to calm down enough to go into his office or court on Monday. Federico explained that Claire does not use drugs and never had any interest in them whatsoever. She resented Federico's use because of the time and money it had taken away from her and their son. Federico felt that Claire was overreacting and was being very prudish. He stated that if Claire would just get off his back, he could work this problem out on his own. He was referred for crisis counseling by the court because of the domestic violence complaint. Federico presently feels he can cut down on using cocaine, especially if he goes back to intranasal (snorting) use and refrains from freebasing, as he has been doing the past two years. He does not feel however, that he can stop using all together, nor does he feel that he needs to. At the time of the crisis counseling session, Federico reports feeling depressed, lethargic and apathetic, which he attributes to his arrest.

This case raises some interesting questions. For example, does Federico have a primary drug problem or is the primary problem with his wife Claire, given her domestic violence complaint? Also, because Federico feels, "depressed, lethargic and apathetic," is this primarily a psychiatric problem? Is Federico really depressed? In this

some of the dangers of trying to detox on her own. Again, while scare tactics are usually to be avoided, some of the realities of withdrawal complications (such as tremor, seizures, hallucinosis) can be brought up in such a way as to try to make a more persuasive argument for treatment. In some instances, there may be a family member or friend present who can also help persuade the patient to stay and get the proper medical attention. It is important that the crisis counselor not lose patience or attempt to force the patient into making a decision too hastily, as this will usually produce resistance or treatment refusal. It is better that the crisis counselor try to help diminish the patients' fears of the detoxification process and assure them that the counselor and other staff will help them through this difficult period with as little distress or pain as possible. A detoxification in a medical setting may take an average of three to seven days depending on the drug of choice. Detoxifications involving opiate drugs (such as heroin, morphine, codeine, oxycontin) usually take longer but can be done on an outpatient basis.

case, Federico's crisis is illustrative of *substance dependence*. In his bravado (many cocaine-dependent individuals often exhibit a sense of invulnerability), Federico declares, "I can cut down." yet, later admits that he probably will not "stop using all together." Federico is cocaine dependent. As was pointed out earlier, although one does not have to use on a daily basis nor experience tolerance or withdrawal in order to be diagnosed as substance dependent, it appears however, that Federico exhibits all of the symptoms of substance dependence. For example, Federico reports a progression to his cocaine use, having started with occasional use then progressing to daily use punctuated with many weekend cocaine binges. His report of feeling "depressed, lethargic, and apathetic" is probably evidence of cocaine withdrawal. One could also make the argument that Federico is experiencing guilt and is feeling depressed over the domestic violence arrest, yet he plans to continue using despite his knowledge that his cocaine use is causing major disruption in his marriage. Yet, it also appears that in order to fend off his guilt, Federico blames Claire as the source of his problems and will not admit that his cocaine addiction is the root cause of his difficulties. This is a common defense among many alcoholics and addicts.

In terms of providing crisis intervention counseling to Federico, it will be necessary to establish rapport or connection with him by hearing him out, listening to his explanations of what happened and the events leading up to the arrest. It will then be helpful to assist Federico to realistically define the current crisis. For example, even though he would like to view Claire as "the problem," it will be necessary to provide feedback to him regarding the events he is describing.

Intervention

COUNSELOR: So, it sounds like if it weren't for Claire, you wouldn't be having all these problems, right? Had you been considering a divorce?

FEDERICO: No, of course not. I could never divorce Claire, besides divorce is frowned upon in my religion.

(continued)

CASE PRESENTATION: **A Crisis Resulting from Substance Dependence** *(continued)*

COUNSELOR: But isn't Claire the source of your problems, the reason why the domestic violence arrest took place? You said before she was "overreacting."

FEDERICO: No, she's not the source of the problem. I just wish she would be O.K. with my doing a few lines of cocaine every once in a while. After all, what's the harm in that? It's the only way I get to relax or have any fun, like a mini-vacation.

COUNSELOR: Federico, you said before that you couldn't use a few lines once in a while. Your use is beyond that, right?

FEDERICO: Yeah, I guess. But I still think I can cut back.

COUNSELOR: Federico, you've spent thousands on cocaine, how much did you tell me your last weekend binge cost you? Also, you now have a domestic violence charge pending. It sounds like things have gone beyond the point where cutting down a little will really work. Besides, do you really think Claire would accept you back under the condition that you've "cut back"?

FEDERICO: No, you're right. No way she would take me back if I was still using.

COUNSELOR: So, I guess the question becomes, "How are you going to stop getting high?"

FEDERICO: Got any ideas?

CASE PRESENTATION: **A Family in Crisis**

Before concluding this section on intervention techniques, it is important to say a few words about family crises. In many crisis intervention settings, it is not unusual for the family to present in crisis, requesting help rather than the substance abuser. Family members often live with an active alcoholic or addict for years, feeling powerless and frustrated in not being able to change their loved one's drinking or drug use (Johnson, 1980). Most families begin to live their lives "around" the alcoholic or addict and their behavior. This works to a point, because sooner or later a crisis will occur. In these instances it is important to encourage the family to "strike while the iron is hot"; in other words, to take advantage of the crisis as an opportunity to intervene with the alcoholic or addict and see to it that they will go for treatment. The other rule of thumb in working with families in crisis is to look for denial in various family members. The dynamics of the chemically dependent family are often unique not just in the various roles of family members, but also in terms of various instances of *triangulation* and *collusion* that may occur. (These terms are used by family therapists to describe family dynamics. In triangulation, for example, an unstable couple, say the husband and wife, will often drag a third party, usually a son or daughter into their conflicts as a means of creating a dysfunctional balance. In collusion, you may have a parent who will collude or confide in a son or daughter who then takes sides with them against the other parent.) Therefore, in dealing with a chemically dependent family in crisis, it is common to find a son or daughter who may defend an alcoholic parent or deny the addiction.

COUNSELOR: As a matter of fact I do, Federico. I strongly feel that the best treatment for you would be an inpatient rehab program. Is that something you would consider?

FEDERICO: I really don't think I need it, but if you think it would help me get my wife back and it would keep the court from disbarring me, I'd consider it.

Case Conceptualization/Crisis Resolution

Naturally, not all crisis sessions go this smoothly. In an actual session, it would probably take some time to get Federico to focus on his cocaine use, as he would most likely be too invested in blaming Claire. The main goal of a crisis session with people who are substance dependent is to get them to question their own faulty addictive logic and accept treatment. As Vernon Johnson states, the approach used in interventions is to "present reality in a receivable way." The reality of Federico's situation is that his cocaine use is out of control and is causing major problems in functioning. The task of the crisis intervention counselor is to present this "reality in a receivable way" with the hope that the alcoholic or addict will commit to treatment, usually in a residential or inpatient setting as a beginning. Other modalities and sequences of treatment will be discussed in the last section of this chapter.

Mr. Brown is a 59-year-old stock broker who has just been transported to the ER by ambulance after getting into a car accident on his way home from the country club, where he had been drinking heavily after playing golf with some friends. Mr. Brown apparently fell asleep at the wheel and crashed into a telephone pole. His blood alcohol level was measured to be .28 which is over twice the legal limit for most states. Mr. Brown is semiconscious, and his wife and two adult daughters have just arrived at the ER. After the Browns are briefed on Mr. Brown's medical condition by the attending physician, the crisis counselor asks to speak with Mrs. Brown and the daughters Erin and Jennifer.

Intervention

The setting of the following case illustration is an ER of a local medical center.

COUNSELOR: Hello Mrs. Brown, my name is Pat Smith, I'm the crisis counselor here at the medical center. I understand that you've been briefed on Mr. Brown's medical condition by Dr. Wilson and that Mr. Brown appears to be stabilized and is resting comfortably at this point. Did Dr. Wilson answer all of your questions?

MRS. BROWN: Yes he did, thank you. These are my daughters, Erin and Jennifer. Erin is a medical student and Jennifer is in her third year in college.

ERIN: Yes, I have some questions. Will my father's blood alcohol level be reported to the police?

(continued)

C A S E   P R E S E N T A T I O N : A Family in Crisis (continued)

COUNSELOR: Yes, since the police were called to the scene, it is a state law that they have access to the blood alcohol results. I believe he will probably be charged with driving under the influence.

MRS. BROWN: I told him not to drive home from the club in this condition. This was bound to happen sooner or later.

ERIN: No, I have never seen Daddy have more than two drinks after playing golf. Was he taking any medications that could have boosted his blood alcohol level? Mom wasn't Daddy taking an anti-anxiety medication that his doctor gave him for his blood pressure? Could that have increased his blood alcohol level?

MRS. BROWN: Yes, he took Xanax occasionally, but I don't think he would take it when he drank because he said it made him too drowsy.

COUNSELOR: Whether he took the Xanax or not, his blood alcohol level was really extreme and usually it would take more than two drinks to have a blood alcohol level that high. Mrs. Brown, you mentioned before that you thought something like this might happen "sooner or later." What did you mean?

MRS. BROWN: Well, I've been after my husband for some time to do something about his drinking. This is not the first time he drove home from the club drunk, Erin.

ERIN: Daddy does not have a drinking problem, he's just been under a lot of stress at work lately. He's a stock broker and the market has had a lot of ups and downs lately. Daddy's been under a lot of stress.

MRS. BROWN: Erin, did you know that Daddy's partner called me about a month ago to tell me that Daddy was coming back from lunch and falling asleep in his office? He also was missing some important documents that his secretary later found in the wastebasket? He even showed up for a sales meeting drunk last month.

ERIN: I don't believe this. Mom, why didn't you tell me all this was going on?

MRS. BROWN: Erin, I didn't want to burden you with all this, you're already under so much pressure with medical school. Besides, I thought it wouldn't do any good. You're always defending your father.

COUNSELOR: Jennifer, you've been listening very patiently, but I can see you're really upset. What are you feeling right now?

JENNIFER: I'm just happy that Daddy didn't kill someone. My mom and dad didn't want me to go away to college, but I am so glad I got out of there. They were always fighting and arguing over Daddy's drinking. I just couldn't stand it.

MRS. BROWN: She's right. Things would get pretty heated at home. I tried to get him to stop drinking, but he just wouldn't listen.

COUNSELOR: Well, in listening to all of you, I think we have an opportunity to try to get him to accept some help for his drinking. But to make this happen, we all need to be on the same page with this. Erin, what do you think?

At this point, the counselor defers to Erin, because she not only has been the most vocal, but she has also been in denial regarding her father's alcoholism. This is also why the counselor has steered clear of using the word alcoholism *in the session, as it would only incite more denial, for example, "Daddy can't be an alcoholic, he goes to work every day."*

ERIN: I'm O.K. with his going to speak with someone, but I think he should see a psychiatrist first to rule out depression over all the work pressure he's been under.

COUNSELOR: We can arrange for a psychiatric consult. I also recommend that we do an intervention while Mr. Brown is here in the hospital and is a "captive audience" so to speak. I want each of you to think of one or two instances where his drinking caused you concern or worry and how you felt about that incident. We will then rehearse what we will say to him and discuss when will be the best time to present this to him. We will also talk about treatment options with him.

JENNIFER: I think he needs to go into a rehab. I can't see him stopping any other way. He has too many "friends" that he hangs out with at the club and gets drunk with. My friend Samantha's dad went to a rehab in Minnesota and he is doing really well now. He even was sober at her graduation party and he's been going to AA meetings and some kind of aftercare program.

ERIN: You think Daddy needs to be in some rehab, Jen?

JENNIFER: You haven't been home for the past six years, except for a few weeks in the summer. Do you know what his drinking is like? Last week, when I brought some friends home after going to the movies, Daddy was passed out half-naked on the couch. He then woke up and started making passes at my friend, Tricia. Or how about the time he was supposed to pick me up at the train station and when he finally did show up about two hours later, he was totally wasted. I had to drive home and I was already exhausted. You don't think he needs a rehab?

COUNSELOR: Jen, that sounds like the kind of thing to include when we meet to do the intervention. So, when do you think should we meet tomorrow to discuss the specifics. We must move quickly though, as I would expect that Mr. Brown will only be kept in the hospital for a few days. If Mr. Brown does go into treatment, it will be helpful if you participate in the family program that the rehab center will offer. They base much of their program on Al-anon, so it will also be helpful to begin going to Al-Anon meetings as soon as possible.

Case Conceptualization/Crisis Resolution

In the crisis illustration above, Erin portrays a daughter who is not only in denial about her father's alcoholism but also someone who has been in collusion perhaps with her father, as she not only seemed to deny or ignore his behavior but also appears to have enabled him by making excuses for him. This type of dynamic is common in alcoholic families (Steinglass, Bennett, Wolin, & Reiss, 1987). Once the immediate crisis has passed, it is often helpful to explore these dynamics further. However, in the initial crisis phase of treatment, it is usually best to focus in on the more important issues at hand, for example, getting Mr. Brown to accept the need for inpatient alcoholism treatment. It is important to mention that referrals to inpatient alcoholism programs do not always go smoothly. Since the advent of managed care, several inpatient treatment programs have closed and treatment options are limited. Also, it is often the case that if an individual is insured through a managed care insurance plan, they may have limited coverage or the managed care case manager may only certify that individual to stay a few days in treatment.

Guidelines for Managing Crises with Alcohol- and/or Drug-Addicted Clients

1. *First determine if the person is in a state of intoxication or withdrawal.* This is not always as easily as it sounds. Some alcoholics and addicts have built up such an extreme tolerance to alcohol or drugs that they may be capable of functioning somewhat "normally" but with a relatively high level of chemicals in their bloodstream. If the person is under the influence or in a state of intoxication or withdrawal, then you may be dealing with a medical crisis and it might be best to have him or her seen in an ER.

2. *Next determine if there is an ongoing alcohol or drug problem.* Crisis counselors who assess individuals with alcohol and/or drug crises are really making two major determinations. First, is the person in a state of medical emergency (as noted above) due to substance intoxication or withdrawal? Second, the counselor must then determine if there is a pattern of substance use resulting in serious life problems in which case a diagnosis of substance abuse or substance dependence may be rendered. Obviously, if a person is in a state of substance withdrawal, it's easier to diagnose the substance dependence. The intoxication and withdrawal diagnosis are important for immediate crisis planning, while the substance abuse or dependence diagnosis is important for longer-range planning beyond the medical crisis.

3. *In the assessment phase it is common for alcoholics and/or addicts to minimize their use.* This is sometimes to be expected and the old "rule of thumb" was to take whatever the alcoholics or addicts said they were using and double it. There are other ways to get a more accurate picture of the addicts' or alcoholics' use but they also have their drawbacks. For example drug screening can sometimes give a counselor a better picture of what the individuals may be using. Unfortunately blood, urine, and breath testing may only give you a qualitative (yes or no) reading instead of a quantitative (a blood alcohol content test tells how much alcohol is in the bloodstream) reading. The problem with testing is that it can sometimes be costly, invasive, and must be done with the client's informed consent.

4. *There is often a thin line between substance abuse and substance dependence.* Although the authors of the *DSM-IV-TR* tried to take into account all the variety of patterns of alcohol and drug use, it is often difficult to make an accurate diagnosis in a crisis situation. Crisis counselors who work as psychiatric screeners in ERs often complain that diagnosing "revolving door" alcoholics and addicts whom they have repeatedly seen and evaluated does not take "rocket science." But it is the first time drunk driver or the young woman who comes in complaining of having had a "panic attack" and who is seeking a benzodiazepine (such as Valium or Xanax) that present diagnostic challenges. Remember, the goal of diagnosis is not to label someone. Diagnosis determines treatment. A good rule of thumb is that if the person's alcohol or drug use is *interfering* in the person's life on a regular basis, then you're probably dealing with substance dependence and a more intensive

level of treatment is probably needed (such as detox and inpatient or at least intensive outpatient treatment).

5. *Treatment planning is often driven by medical insurance coverage.* In many European countries treatment is offered based upon need, so if a person is in need of detoxification or inpatient treatment, they will be referred to a program regardless of insurance coverage. These countries have national medical plans. In the United States today, there are over 40 million Americans that have no medical coverage. What has developed is a two-tiered treatment system for the "haves" and the "have nots." Those individuals with insurance coverage usually have a wider range of treatment options open to them, while those without insurance are usually limited to state-funded programs with often lengthy waiting lists. And not all insurance plans are alike, those who are covered by HMOs will also be limited to certain programs and too often to the length of treatment. Most counselors will tell you that in the "old days" the challenge was trying to convince the addict or alcoholic to enter treatment. Today, the challenge is trying to convince the HMO administrator to let the addict or alcoholic into treatment!

6. *Addicts and alcoholics will often avoid "committing" to treatment.* Most alcoholics and addicts, when offered a menu of treatment choices, will often choose the least intensive treatment. Even though the treatment may not be appropriate for them, addicts and alcoholics will often choose a less intrusive treatment plan or avoid committing to treatment altogether. This too is common. This does not mean that they will fail; it may mean that they are not ready. This is where motivational interviewing approaches are helpful.

7. *Whenever possible, involve family members or significant others in the assessment and crisis planning process.* Here it is important to always include family members and/or significant others in the assessment and treatment planning process. Family members may be an invaluable source of information (as in regarding past treatment attempts) and what resources may be available to their loved one. For example, if a family member indicates that their loved one has tried outpatient several times and has not done well, then it may be time to consider a more intensive form of treatment. Or a family member may be able to provide background information, such as the history of Bipolar Disorder in many other family members, that may impact the crisis counselor's current assessment and treatment planning decisions.

RECOMMENDATIONS FOR CHAPTER ENRICHMENT

SUGGESTED FILMS

Clean and Sober **(1988)** This film portrays the life of a young stockbroker who is addicted to cocaine and alcohol, and whose life spirals out of control as a result of the progression of his addictions. Morgan Freeman plays the role of the counselor. The portrayals of the rehab, the groups, and especially the denial of those in the throes of active addictions are chilling and accurate.

28 Days (2000) This film also portrays the life of an active alcoholic and addict whose life goes into crisis when she gets drunk at her sister's wedding, embarrasses herself and her sister in front of guests, then proceeds to steal the bridal limo and running it through the front porch of someone's home. The remainder of the film takes place in a Hazelden-model, 28-day rehab center. The depiction of this type of rehab is realistic and portrays the many types of individuals who struggle with addictions. This film also does a fairly good job in depicting the denial and anger that other family members of the addict and alcoholic experience.

When a Man Loves a Woman (1994) This film depicts an alcoholic marriage; only this time, it is the wife who is the alcoholic. One unique and important aspect of this film is that it dispels the common stereotype that only husbands or boyfriends become alcoholics. This film is a good portrayal of the impact that alcoholism has on a marriage and family. It also does not give a sanitized version that once the woman enters recovery, everything is wonderful. Far from it, this couple struggles with reorganizing itself in recovery. It helps bring to light why more couples break up or divorce in recovery than they do in active addiction.

Traffic (2000) This film is multilayered in that one theme depicts the life of a drug trafficker, while the other theme depicts the life of a politically appointed Presidential Drug Czar, whose teenage daughter's life is spiraling out of control because of her progressive cocaine addiction. The film is poignantly frightening in its depiction of drug addiction and the dark side of the drug world.

Requiem for a Dream (2000) This film provides a gritty depiction of the impact of drug addiction on three individuals. It provides an interesting contrast of legal prescription addiction with illegal drug addiction, however, in all cases the results are the same. The film also depicts the progression of addiction and how it robs these individuals not only of their life goals and their dreams, but also of their dignity, their values, and their self-worth.

Trainspotting (1996) This film is set in Edinburgh, Scotland, and depicts the impact of heroin on a group of young men who are enslaved to their addiction. The depiction of drug seeking behavior and heroin withdrawal are surrealistic but powerful in its portrayal of the progressive nature of addiction.

Sherrybaby (2006) This film provides a depiction of the life of a woman who has just been released from prison after serving a sentence for drug possession. As Sherry tries to start her life over again there are several problems and stressors she encounters. This film also portrays the impact of child sexual abuse which is common among many woman addicts and alcoholics.

Bill Moyers PBS Series on Addictions **(1998)** This is probably one of the best documentaries made on alcohol and drug addiction. The series is divided into several 30–45-minute segments, each of which deals with a different aspect of addiction. Some of the segments include several chemically dependent individuals who describe how the progression of drug and alcohol use took over their lives. Another segment called "The Hijacked Brain" deals with the neurochemistry of drug use and the similarity that all drugs of abuse have in hijacking the dopamine producing system within the brain. Another segment deals with the societal impact of drugs and alcohol and the government's "War on Drugs."

HBO Series on Addictions **(2007)** This is one of the most up-to-date documentaries on the market. The videos (which can be obtained for a nominal fee through www.hbo.com) contain a 60-minute segment with basic information about various facets of drug and alcohol addiction, its impact on adolescents, families, and adults, and cutting edge treatments for a number of addictions. This lengthy segment is then followed by a number of shorter segments dealing with specific issues, for example, the impact of drug addiction on a parent, new medications to combat drug and alcohol addiction, the impact of drug courts, and so on.

SUGGESTED ACTIVITIES

1. Attend an open Alcoholics Anonymous (AA) or Narcotics Anonymous (NA) meeting. You can find information about when and where meetings take place by calling the number listed in the White Pages of the phone book under "Alcoholics Anonymous" or "Narcotics Anonymous" or on the internet. It is best to attend an *open speakers* meeting, as these meetings are open to anyone and as a student you will be more comfortable with the format. In an open speakers meeting, two speakers will tell the stories of their addictions and how they came to recover in AA and/or NA. Sit and listen, do not take notes. No one will ask you to speak, just sit and listen. Also, remember that the program is anonymous so you cannot reveal to anyone the identities of people you see there that you may know. After the meeting, take note of what stands out the most from what you have heard and observed. Does it match with your impressions of what AA and NA are about? Were the people at the meetings similar or different from what you expected? If so, in what respect?

2. Watch one of the films mentioned above, such as *Clean and Sober, Requiem for a Dream, 28 Days,* or *Traffic.* What are the crisis points in these movies? How did the main characters use denial to convince themselves (and others) that they did not have an alcohol or drug problem?

3. If you had a friend or relative who was in need of alcohol or drug detoxification followed by an inpatient treatment program, where would you send them? Look for alcohol and drug treatment resources in your area. Go online and see what alcohol and drug treatment programs are available

within a 50-mile radius of where you live. How are these programs similar and how do they differ? Does the program require that the person admitted have health insurance or can they accommodate people who cannot afford to pay?

4. What if you had a family member or friend who was just arrested for drug possession? He or she is frantic and reaches out to you for help with the crisis. What would you do to help?

5. Interview someone who is in recovery from drug or alcohol dependence. In your interview, try to find out what brought that individual into recovery. What crises did he or she experience while actively addicted. When did he or she realize there was a problem with drugs and alcohol? Before reaching that realization, how did denial manifest itself to convince himself, herself, or others that there was not a problem?

6. Interview someone from law enforcement (a police officer or a state trooper, or someone from the courts, the prosecutor's office, or the public defender's office) and ask about ways in which alcohol and/or drugs impact the community or state. What types of alcohol or drug problems have he or she seen? What types of alcohol or drug crises have he or she been called to help manage?

8

Psychiatric Crises

DISCUSSION QUESTIONS

Do you feel that depression is the result of chemical imbalances in the brain or can depression be brought on by life events like the loss of a loved one or a break up in a relationship?

In the 1990s there was a major effort to close psychiatric hospitals by discharging mentally ill people into the community, many of whom were assigned to live in boarding homes. What are your opinions and views of the advantages and disadvantages of what has been known as *deinstitutionalization*? How would you feel if a home for the mentally ill was placed in your neighborhood?

People tend to react differently to traumatic events. For example, during the Vietnam War, more enlisted men were found to suffer Posttraumatic Stress Disorder (PTSD) than did officers. Why do you think people react differently to traumatic events?

INTRODUCTION

It is estimated that 44 million Americans suffer from some type of mental illness (U.S. Department of Health & Human Services, 2002). Among these individuals, an estimated 5.4% suffer from severe mental illness (such as Bipolar Disorder, Schizophrenia, or Major Depression). Approximately 20–25% of the nation's 700,000 homeless suffer from mental illness while an estimated 50% suffer from co-occurring mental illness and a substance use disorder. According to estimates from national epidemiological studies, Anxiety Disorders, Mood Disorders and Substance Use Disorders are the three most frequently occurring disorders in the United States (Robins & Reiger, 1991). When conceptualizing various types of mental disorders, as described in the *Diagnostic and Statistical Manual of Mental Disorders*, 4th Edition, Text Revision (*DSM-IV-TR*) (American Psychiatric Association, 2004), it is important to note that there are varying degrees of mental illness. Some severe mental disorders are clearly debilitating while other disorders cause only mild to moderate impairment, which may not interfere with daily functioning. There are, however, particular psychiatric disorders that are associated with crises. This chapter presents various cases to illustrate some of the most prominent types of mental disorders that may result in a psychiatric crisis.

Psychiatric crises are often complex because they may have multiple causal factors. What is also unique to psychiatric crises is that unlike other types of crises in which there is often a clear precipitant (such as a catastrophic or traumatic event), psychiatric crises can occur solely as a result of internal-emotional catalysts. Therefore a psychiatric crisis may be the result of an emotional, psychological, or neurochemical anomaly that then causes impairment or an inability to cope with everyday life. Psychiatric crises can manifest themselves in several ways and will often have a major impact on one's *emotions, thoughts,* or their *behavior and conduct.* Therefore, individuals in psychiatric crisis often present with an array of symptoms that may be difficult to discern from a diagnostic standpoint. For example, if a person reports visual hallucinations, this could be the result of a temporary drug-induced state or it could be symptomatic of Schizophrenia.

Since it is impossible to cover all of the diagnostic categories covered in the *DSM-IV-TR,* we have selected those diagnostic categories that are most prevalent and those that are most likely to result in crises for individuals who suffer from these disorders.

ANXIETY DISORDERS

There are several subtypes of Anxiety Disorders (such as Generalized Anxiety Disorders, Simple Phobias, Agoraphobia, Obsessive-Compulsive Disorder, Panic Disorder, and PTSD), however, what they all share in common is an overwhelming experience of extreme anxiety that interferes with the person's ability to function. Both Panic Disorder and PTSD are two subtypes within Anxiety Disorders that often are associated with crises. It is estimated that approximately 6 million Americans (age 18 and older) suffer from Panic Disorder (Kessler, Chiu, Demler, & Walters, 2005). A person with Panic Disorder will often experience intense anxiety or panic attacks in which they fear they are having a heart attack or other serious physical symptoms. For that reason people with Panic Disorder are often treated in emergency rooms with complaints of chest pains, shortness of breath, and fears that they are going to die. Most often, panic attacks may last for 15–20 minutes. For the person suffering from Panic Disorder, those 15 or 20 minutes may seem like an eternity. Similarly, a person suffering from PTSD may experience acute anxiety when presented with a stimulus similar to those associated with the original traumatic situation. Therefore, soldiers who experience combat-related PTSD may experience intense anxiety and dread as they begin to relive the events surrounding the trauma incident or event. People who have been in a car accident will also find themselves reliving the accident through nightmares or they will avoid driving altogether as a means of coping with the anxiety. It is estimated that approximately 7.7 million Americans suffer from PTSD (Kessler et al., 2005). The following case illustrates a crisis related to Anxiety Disorders.

C A S E   P R E S E N T A T I O N : A Case of Panic Disorder and PTSD

In the following case illustration, Jeff's panic attacks have brought him to the emergency room for treatment:

Jeff is a 37-year-old married father of two children, who is being seen at the local emergency room. He complains of severe chest pains, panicky feelings, and he is hyperventilating. Although he has no history of cardiac problems, he was so frightened about the chest pains that he decided to call an ambulance. After ruling out that there are no cardiac abnormalities, the examining physician asks Jeff what was going on when he began to experience the chest pain and hyperventilation. Jeff explains that the only thing he can recall was how hot he was feeling. He goes on to tell the doctor that he has had two panic attacks since coming home from Iraq approximately four months ago. Jeff states that he is in the National Guard and his unit was deployed to an area near Tikrit. He was not wounded but he states that several of his buddies were injured and two were killed in action. Jeff states that he has nightmares about his friends being killed and wounded. He was reluctant to seek help through the VA because he was told that it might affect future promotions or that they might even discharge him from the National Guard for mental health reasons.

In Jeff's case we note that he first seeks treatment after experiencing a panic attack that mimics a heart attack. Jeff is a good illustration of someone who is experiencing symptoms of Panic Disorder that are directly tied to the trauma he experienced while in combat. The counselor begins by gathering some background information.

Intervention:

Counselor: Jeff, when did you first experience a panic attack?

Jeff: It was about three months ago. I remember that I was driving home from work and I began to feel really hot. I started to get this tightness in my chest, but nothing like I just had. After that first panic attack I began dreading that I was going to have another one. I remember feeling my heart started pounding, It felt like I was going to explode. I couldn't breathe and I think I began to hyperventilate, like I was suffocating. I thought I was having a heart attack or something, but it started to go away, so I didn't go to an emergency room.

Counselor: What do you think triggered this recent panic attack?

Jeff: Well, I was driving and like I said, and I started to feel really hot. I think it reminded me of when I was in Iraq. My National Guard unit was assigned to provide escort to convoys delivering supplies to one of the main bases. I remember on one of these convoys, one of our Humvees was hit by an RPG. There was nothing we could do, just sit there waiting. We didn't know if we were going to be the next to get hit or not. The worst part was when we finally were ordered to move forward we had to drive past the Humvee that was still smoldering. Some of my buddies were still in there but they were trying to get them out. I knew they weren't alive.

(continued)

C A S E   P R E S E N T A T I O N : A Case of Panic Disorder and PTSD
(continued)

COUNSELOR: That must have been a horrible experience for you.

JEFF: It was one of the worst days of my life and probably one of the worst days I had over there. It's funny, most of the time we'd just be sitting around bored, and nothing would happen. Then something like that.

COUNSELOR: So when you had this recent panic attack it was probably brought on by your recollections of your buddies being killed in the convoy attack. Do you experience flashbacks or nightmares very often?

JEFF: Sometimes. I'll get them in waves. Usually it's if I see something on TV that reminds me of being back in combat.

COUNSELOR: Are you receiving any treatment or counseling?

JEFF: No. The guys from my unit keep in touch with one another, that's about it. We were told about PTSD but most of us were reluctant to go for help because we were afraid we might get discharged. One guy did go to the outpatient VA clinic and all they did was put him on medication, which he stopped taking.

COUNSELOR: Jeff, on a scale from 1 to 10, with 1 representing calm and 10 representing panicky feelings, where would you say you are right now?

JEFF: I would put myself at about a 7 right now but if you asked me that question a half hour ago, I was definitely at a 10.

COUNSELOR: Jeff, would you be willing to try something right now that may help calm yourself down without having to use medication?

JEFF: Sure. At this point, I'm willing to try anything.

COUNSELOR: I'd like to begin by having you focus in on your breathing. Just begin to breath in through your nose and exhale through you mouth, at your own pace, not deep breathing. O.K.?

JEFF: Sure. Is it okay to keep my eyes open?

COUNSELOR: Whatever is more comfortable for you. Now as your exhaling, Jeff, imagine that you are exhaling all of the tension and anxiety. Now imagine the muscles of your body becoming more and more relaxed, with each breath that you take. I'd now like you to imagine a safe place. Can you think of a safe place Jeff? Someplace that's totally yours. A place where you can feel total safety and in control?

JEFF: Sure. I think the place I feel the safest is in my garage. I have a work bench there, where I like to tinker on model boats. Is that what you mean?

COUNSELOR: Sounds fine. Now imagine yourself in your garage working on one of your boats, feeling totally relaxed, totally calm with each breath you take. As you're doing this, you begin to feel a cool breeze across your face and feel totally relaxed.

JEFF: I'm feeling a little better, probably about a 3 or 4 right now.

COUNSELOR: That's good Jeff. I'll give you some information on the techniques I've described, but I'm wondering if you'd consider some follow-up at the clinic here. This way it wouldn't be connected to the VA.

JEFF: If it will help me to avoid another panic attack, I'll try anything you say.

Case Conceptualization/Crisis Resolution

In the illustration above, the counselor is focusing on providing Jeff with some immediate tools to manage his anxiety and, in doing so, prevent another panic attack. Some recent research, suggests that Panic Disorder is really a "breathing disorder" in that when a person predisposed to panic attacks begins to feel even slightly anxious, they will often begin to hyperventilate. The escalation of the hyperventilation brings on more anxiety. Some counselors will have their client's breathe into paper bags, which increases the carbon dioxide levels in the bloodstream, thereby decreasing the subjective experience of anxiety. In some instances, techniques like these may not be offered in the context of the initial crisis session, but in longer-term counseling, once more trust has been established. If some of the various techniques did not work and Jeff were to remain in a highly anxious state, then an anti-anxiety medication like Buspar might be used. Benzodiazepines (Valium, Ativan, Xanax, or Klonopin) might be prescribed on only a short-term, interim basis because a disadvantage to these medications is that they can promote dependence; therefore, it is best to try some of the other techniques first. Once the initial crisis has passed, it would be advised to convince Jeff to enter counseling on either an individual or group basis. He may benefit from clinical hypnosis or Eye Movement Desensitization Response treatments (EMDR) (Carlson, Chemtob et al., 1998). Individuals who suffer from PTSD will often have great difficulty in talking about the initial trauma. This usually depends on how intense the trauma they experienced or witnessed was or the level of guilt, shame, or personal responsibility they may feel in connection to the trauma. For example, victims of sexual abuse or childhood molestation will often experience difficulty in discussing their sexual traumatization, usually because of the experience of guilt and shame. People suffering from trauma resulting from combat, like Jeff, may also experience difficulty discussing the traumatic events for different reasons. It is not unusual for PTSD victims to suffer from *suppression* or *repression*. In the former, individuals consciously try to put specific information about the trauma out of their minds. In the latter, the unconscious mind represses the information or puts it out of conscious awareness. When information is repressed, however, it is thought to be "pushed" into the unconscious mind—the part of the mind that we are not aware of but that may be revealed in our dreams. Sometimes however, individuals may be flooded with painful and intrusive recollections of the traumatic incident that plague them throughout the day and disturb their sleep with vivid, frightening nightmares. It is noted that many individuals who suffer from PTSD often go through stages. Initially, they may experience **Outcry**, at which point they are often flooded with many painful emotions related to the trauma. This stage is often followed by **Denial** of the traumatic event, a feeling that "this is not really happening to me," which also may include emotional numbing. This stage is followed by **Intrusiveness**. Here individuals are often bothered by flashbacks or intrusive thoughts or recollections of the traumatic incident. They may also experience nightmares about the incident. In the next stage, **Working Through**, individuals begin the journey of coming to grips with the traumatic event by talking about what they experienced. Often it is necessary to talk about the incident over and over again because each time individuals relive the incident, another piece of the traumatic puzzle is revealed or they are able to express more of the feelings associated with the incident. This is thought to provide some catharsis and relief. It is hoped that individuals will reach the last stage, known as **Completion**, where they can incorporate the trauma into their life experiences, having learned from the trauma and in essence perceiving themselves as survivors of the traumatic incident rather than as victims (Horowitz, 1985).

Practical Guidelines for Crisis Intervention for
Someone with Anxiety

1. In assessing people with an Anxiety Disorder it is helpful to get background information about when they first experienced anxiety, how often thay experience anxiety, how they have coped with their anxiety to date. If they experience anxiety attacks, how long do they last and have they received any prior treatment for anxiety— whether it be emergency room treatment, medication, or psychotherapeutic efforts.

2. Find out whether there have been any periods of remission, such as times without anxiety experiences, If so, it is helpful to find out what may have accounted for these symptom-free periods. What worked for patients during this period? Also what may bring on their symptoms?

3. In order to get an idea as to how intense anxiety has been, it is helpful to use a rating scale or subjective units of distress (SUD) as a means of assessing the anxiety level (Wolpe, 1982). Patients are asked to rate their anxiety on scale of 0 to 10, with 0 indicating total calm and 10 indicating panic or extremely intense anxiety.

4. Determine what coping strategies have been attempted. Usually before seeking treatment, most people try to cope with anxiety on their own. Here it is important to assess what patients have done to try and cope with anxiety or panic attacks. It is not unusual for people to self-medicate, so alcohol or drug abuse should be assessed at each session.

5. Help develop some immediate strategies that will help to alleviate patients' anxiety, such as relaxation techniques, diaphragmatic breathing, or guided imagery.

6. In cases of PTSD, allow the patients to discuss the traumatic incident in a way that they are comfortable with. Do not try to push for information that they are not ready to discuss. Ascertain if they might be willing to continue with ongoing counseling or help through a support group specific to that type of trauma, such as a rape survivors group or combat veterans group.

MOOD DISORDERS

There are two major subtypes of mood disorder, Unipolar Depression and Bipolar Depression, and both may result in a state of crises. Unipolar Depression refers to individuals who experience depressive moods that permeate their daily lives to such an extent that they have difficulty in functioning. The subtypes of Unipolar Depression (Major Depression and Dysthymia) differ in terms of degree or intensity. Approximately 14.8 million Americans are affected by Major Depressive Disorder, which is the leading cause of disability in the United States (Kessler et al., 2005; World Health Organization, 2004). Symptoms of Major Depression include physical symptoms such as low energy level, difficulty staying asleep, and poor appetite. Cognitive symptoms include anger outbursts, negative thinking, pessimism, and difficulty concentrating. Individuals who are depressed usually tend to isolate from others and have difficulty being around other people. In the following case vignette, Jill suffers from Major Depression.

CASE PRESENTATION: A Case of Major Depression

Jill is a married mother of two sons aged 16 and 12. Her husband Tim had called the crisis hotline explaining that Jill has been feeling increasingly "lethargic and depressed for the past eight months or so. She doesn't want to go out—not even to her sister's home, which she always enjoyed doing. She won't take calls from her friends or coworkers. Jill had worked as a receptionist at a local car dealership, but has been unable to go to work for the past two weeks because she just doesn't have the energy to make it through the day. She refuses to go to a movie or, even to leave the house for that matter. All she does is sit around and cry all day."

Jill has been feeling hopeless and helpless, although she claims that she is not suicidal because of her "religious beliefs." Jill's medical doctor suggested that Tim should bring Jill to the mental health clinic for an evaluation. After some persuasion on Tim's part, Jill agreed to speak with a counselor. The background information that Jill provided indicates that Jill's father had gone through several bouts of depression in his late 30s and had been hospitalized briefly for "a nervous breakdown." Jill is unable to explain exactly when or why she began to feel depressed. In exploring possible explanations, Jill explains that prior to her sons being born she had given birth to a baby girl who died from Sudden Infant Death Syndrome (SIDS). Jill admits that she never really forgave herself for this and now she feels that she doesn't deserve to be happy.

In the following excerpt, the crisis counselor first tries to establish rapport with Jill and then moves into talking about her depression:

Intervention:

COUNSELOR: Hello Jill, my name is Sandra Mackey, is it O.K. if Tim waits outside and fills out some paperwork while we talk?

JILL: Sure.

COUNSELOR: It took a lot of courage for you to come in today. From what Tim shared over the phone, it sounds like you've been feeling down for some time now.

JILL: It seems like forever.

COUNSELOR: Could you tell me more about what you've been feeling?

JILL: I just feel depressed and sad all the time. I cry at the drop of a hat. I can't get out of bed in the morning; I just want to lay there with the covers over my head.

COUNSELOR: Do you know how long you've felt this way?

JILL: My husband says it has been the past 8 or 9 months, I think it began way before that. Maybe I just hid it better then.

COUNSELOR: What's a typical day like?

JILL: I usually get Tim off to work, the boys off to school, and then I go back to bed until the kids get home from football practice. I make dinner then I fall asleep on the couch until bedtime. I've not been able to even think about going back to work. I just don't have the energy.

COUNSELOR: What type of work do you do?

JILL: I work as a receptionist at a car dealership. I answer the phones and make appointments with the sales people. I like the work and the people I work with, but I just can't stand to be around anyone right now.

(continued)

C A S E   P R E S E N T A T I O N :   A Case of Major Depression
(*continued*)

COUNSELOR: Do you go out at all or visit any friends or relatives?

JILL: No, not really. I used to like to visit my sister. She has a beautiful home over in Mount Royal, but I haven't had the energy to go and see her.

COUNSELOR: When you sleep, do you feel rested when you wake up?

JILL: No, I could sleep for days and still wake up feeling tired. I'll often get up at 4 or 5 a.m. and then I can't get back to sleep. That's the worst part. Things seem pretty bleak at 4 a.m.

COUNSELOR: How so?

JILL: I just begin to dwell on all the things I've done wrong in my life. I wish I could go back and undo all the wrongs I've done.

COUNSELOR: Sounds like you feel a lot of guilt.

JILL: Some days I just feel guilty for being alive, like I don't deserve to live.

COUNSELOR: Have you had suicidal thoughts?

JILL: No, I couldn't do that to Tim and the boys.

COUNSELOR: Jill, what you've been describing is common among people who are going through major depression. But the good news is that there are ways to treat depression so that you can begin to function again. Is that something you'd be willing to explore with me?

JILL: Yes, I would. I know I can't go on feeling like this.

Case Conceptualization/Crisis Resolution

Jill is experiencing a crisis related to Major Depression. The crisis counselor first tries to establish a rapport or connection with her, and to convey that she is there to help Jill with the difficulties she is experiencing. Once Jill has established trust in the counselor, the first step is to explore the nature and details of Jill's depressive symptoms before discussing ways to begin to lessen these symptoms. This might involve an exploration of whether Jill would be a candidate for antidepressant medication. Once this is established, the counselor would also need to gain a commitment from Jill that she will participate in counseling beyond the crisis intervention phase. Given that Jill's depression seems to be of a long-standing nature, it is probable that her issues will not be resolved within six to eight weeks. It is possible that there could be genetic influences to Jill's depression, since her father was apparently depressed and needed to be hospitalized, while there are also clearly environmental factors as well as Jill's feelings of guilt, which will need to be explored in more depth. The focus of this crisis intervention session, however, would *not* be to uncover these causal factors, but rather to deal with the immediate crisis—Jill is depressed and has been unable to function in everyday life.

In the initial crisis session, the counselor would continue to explore other aspects of Jill's depression and the symptoms she is experiencing. Once enough background information has been gathered and it has been determined that Jill is not in danger of harming herself, a crisis plan would begin to be developed. At that point, it would be helpful to involve Tim in the planning process and to elicit his support in helping Jill implement the plan. For example, given Jill's history, it may be helpful to have her evaluated by a psychiatrist for antidepressant medication. She will also need ongoing counseling to help her work on the issues that are contributing to her feelings of guilt and self-doubt.

CASE PRESENTATION: A Crisis Involving Bipolar Disorder

With Bipolar Disorders there are often two phases: The manic phase is characterized by extremely high levels of energy, talking incessantly, expression of grandiose ideas or plans, inflated self-esteem, racing thoughts, easily distracted, and excessive activity in pleasurable, often risky activities (including gambling sprees, spending sprees, or sexual promiscuity). When individuals are in the midst of a manic phase, they are usually unaware of their condition or may be so energized that they don't want the feeling to stop. This becomes a problem for people with Bipolar Disorder who go off of their medication (usually Depakote, Lithium, or some other mood stabilizer) because they "miss" the high of the manic phase. Unfortunately, when people with Bipolar Disorder crash into depression, they often crash hard into the depressive phase, which is one of the reasons why they are considered at higher risk for suicide. It is also not unusual for Bipolar individuals to abuse alcohol or drugs, which only exacerbates their problems and can even further increase their risk for suicidal action or other dangerous risk-taking behavior.

Glen is a 42-year-old district manager for a computer manufacturing company. He was brought to the crisis counseling center today accompanied by his wife, Barbara. When interviewed by the crisis counselor, Glen states that he has "never felt better in his life" and can't understand why his wife insisted that he come to speak with someone. She tells the crisis counselor that Glen has been "on a high for the past week." Barbara explains that Glen had disappeared last Tuesday and did not show up until four days later. She did not know where he went, although he claims he just went to Atlantic City, "to have a little fun." Barbara then got a call from a casino in Atlantic City claiming that he had run up a $20,000 tab at the roulette table and that security had to kick him out of his room because of the wild party he was having at 4:00 a.m., which was disturbing other guests. Glen continues to tell the crisis counselor that he was "just having a little fun—what's the harm in that?" The crisis counselor orders a toxicology screen and Glen has a small amount of alcohol in his system but no other drugs are detected. Barbara goes on to explain that Glen has "disappeared" like this in the past over their 15 years of marriage. At one point, she did get Glen to see a psychiatrist and he was prescribed Lithium, however, Glen stopped taking the medication claiming that it gave him a hand tremor and he also didn't like feeling "like a dishrag" all the time. Since that time, about two to three times a year, Glen will go on sprees like this. Barbara is fed up and threatened to leave Glen if he didn't get help. Glen begins crying at this point and agrees that he "will do anything" in order to keep the family together. The crisis counselor, Glen, and Barbara begin to formulate a plan.

Glen presents with many of the signs of Bipolar Disorder. His presentation in the crisis interview is one of non-stop talking and boundless energy. Individuals with Bipolar Disorder can often go days without sleep or rest. It is also common that they will lack awareness or insight into how outlandish their behavior has become when they are in the throes of a manic phase, or they will deny the seriousness of their symptoms. Nothing seems to phase them … until the depressive phase sets in, at least. At that point, usually everything begins to crash in and there is often a realization of the problematic behavior that occurred during the manic phase. This is when a person with Bipolar Disorder may be at a greatest risk for suicide. Their suicidal risk can be further exacerbated by alcohol or drug abuse. Ernest Hemingway, the Pulitzer Prize winning author, was thought to have suffered with Bipolar Disorder. He was also known as being a heavy drinker. Sadly, Hemingway committed suicide by shooting himself.

The role of the crisis counselor is to ensure the patient's safety by making certain the person's emotional condition at the time can be managed. Fortunately, mood stabilizing medications are effective in treating Bipolar Disorder. As indicated earlier, however, the problem with many individuals with Bipolar Disorder is that they will

(continued)

CASE PRESENTATION: A Crisis Involving Bipolar Disorder
(continued)

---

often stop taking the medication, either because of side effects or because they "miss" the manic high. The crisis counselor must, therefore, impress upon the patient and family the importance of taking the medication regularly, not going off of it impulsively, and to follow the psychiatrist's orders regarding having their Lithium blood levels checked. As was indicated in the case of Glen, sometimes it is difficult to convince a person who is in the midst of a manic phase that they need medication and ongoing counseling. In the following case excerpt, the crisis counselor is trying to convince Glen that he will need to go back on his medication as part of the **Planning** phase of the intervention.

Intervention:
COUNSELOR: Glen, I can see how upset you are at the thought that Barbara might leave you. Do you think she would carry through with a divorce?

GLEN: Yes, I know she is serious, you heard her. There are times, though, when I think maybe we would be better off apart.

BARBARA: Glen, I don't want us to split up, I want to stay together, I know we can be happy. I don't want to break up our marriage, you know that.

GLEN: Yes, I know that, you want me to get help, stay on my medication right?

BARBARA: Yes, of course I do. When you're on the medication, we have a good life together. When you go off it, we don't know what's going to happen.

COUNSELOR: Glen, honestly, what are you thinking about the medication at this point?

GLEN: You know, as nuts as it seems, there is a part of me that likes these crazy manic phases I go through. I think I would miss them. But the other part of me knows I can't keep putting Barbara through this.

COUNSELOR: Are there things that you don't like about the manic phases?

GLEN: Well, ending up $20,000 in debt, for one. Plus, the guilt I feel afterward … and then there's the months of depressive hell that I go through. I see where you're going with this.

COUNSELOR: The things you mention are very common among people who suffer with Bipolar Disorder. The thing is Glen, you don't have to suffer as you have been. Even though no medication is perfect, it does work, right?

GLEN: It does work, but you're right, I don't feel perfect on it.

BARBARA: I know that you were much better off when you were taking the medicine.

COUNSELOR: Glen, would you be agreeable to seeing Dr. Jones again, since he is familiar with your medication history?

Case Conceptualization/Crisis Resolution
Glen agrees to see Dr. Jones. The medication issue is discussed in the subsequent crisis sessions along with a plan of how Glen will manage the gambling debt. Ongoing counseling will be helpful in this case in order to make certain that Glen's moods remain stable and that he is not reconsidering going off his medication. Ongoing therapy is also helpful in anticipating and avoiding triggers that may result in changes in mood. Some recent studies have pointed to the role of environmental "triggers" that may serve as a catalyst to manic or depressive phases. Therapy may be useful in helping individuals with Bipolar Disorder to identify and manage these triggers.

Practical Guidelines for Crisis Intervention with Mood Disorders

1. Given the correlation between Major Depression and Bipolar Disorder with suicidality, it is important to make certain that the person in crisis is not experiencing suicidal thoughts or ideation. If they are, it is then important to ascertain whether or not they have a plan for suicide. If so, then hospitalization for safety will need to be considered.

2. Some mood disorders may have a more reactive nature—as a result of suffering a major loss, for example—so it is important to explore whether or not the person has experienced recent losses. However, many Mood Disorders result from internal factors such as serotonin imbalances. In those instances it is important to explore whether the person in crisis might be a candidate for antidepressant medication (as in the case of someone suffering from Major Depression) or a mood stabilizer (as in the case of someone suffering from Bipolar Disorder).

3. In assessing someone who is experiencing depression it is often helpful to ask about "biological symptoms" such as sleep, appetite, and energy disturbances. In many instances, depressed individuals will often lack appetite or sometimes will binge eat. Similarly some will sleep excessive hours, while others will experience early morning awakening and disrupted sleep patterns. Energy levels also tend to be low and sometimes just getting through the day is a major chore, whereas with Bipolar Disorder sudden shifts in energy level are common.

4. It is important to determine if the person in crisis has a good support system. If so, have they pulled away from those who may be sources of support? It is common for people experiencing Mood Disorders to withdraw from others, or to report that just being around others is difficult.

SCHIZOPHRENIA

It is estimated that approximately 2.4 million American adults are diagnosed with Schizophrenia (Reiger, Narrow, Rae, Maderschied, Locke, & Goodwin, 1993). Schizophrenia is commonly known as a "thought disorder" because people with Schizophrenia often experience perceptual disturbances such as auditory, visual, tactile (touch), or olfactory (smell) hallucinations, or delusional thinking (which is a false personal belief based upon an incorrect inference about external reality, even when evidence to the contrary is presented). Although psychoses can come about as a result of a toxic reaction to certain drugs, alcohol, or medications, the majority of psychotic reactions are thought to represent a class of mental disorders known as Schizophrenia. The symptoms of Schizophrenia can be grouped into two major categories: *positive symptoms* which included hallucinations, delusions, difficulty communicating thoughts logically, abnormal movements such as rocking or head banging, and paranoia or anxiety, and *negative symptoms* such as anhedonia (inability to experience pleasure in day-to-day life), lack of ability to socialize or connect with others, lack of energy, and difficulty

---

C A S E   P R E S E N T A T I O N :   A Crisis Involving Schizophrenia

---

Robert is 25 years old. He has come to the local mental health clinic today, complaining that he is "hearing voices." Robert lives in one of the group boarding homes in the area; unfortunately, it is not one of the better ones. He will often go without his medication because no one is there to supervise that he actually takes it. He states that it has been about three weeks since he last took his Risperdal and he is now beginning to feel "edgy." Robert says he will usually start to feel restless and will then hear voices telling him that someone is trying to poison his food and steal his brain. When he felt this way once before, the examining psychiatrist had Robert admitted to a state psychiatric hospital for observation. When asked about the voices, Robert explains that the voices he hears are "from Satan" and that they also tell him to do "bad things." Fortunately, Robert has not been in trouble with the law before and he usually knows that when he begins to feel this way, it is time to go back on his medication.

The two most essential components for successfully intervening with people suffering with Schizophrenia are *safety* and *stabilization*. The safety factor comes into play both in terms of ensuring the safety of the Schizophrenic, and of those around the Schizophrenic. It appears that approximately 50% of those with Schizophrenia are somewhat oblivious to their symptoms, or they are convinced that the distortions of thought and perception are accurate. The other 50% are painfully aware of their symptoms and the devastating effects of this disorder on their ability to function in everyday life; therefore, they are in more turmoil over these symptoms. It is not unusual, then, to find that about 50% of Schizophrenics also experience depression. It is estimated that about 10% of Schizophrenics commit suicide and that 20% attempt it (Maxmen & Ward, 1995). Interestingly, most Schizophrenics do not commit suicide in the midst of the psychosis, but rather as they become more painfully aware of their illness in the aftermath of psychosis. Those with better premorbid adjustment and higher education levels are more at risk for suicide. This seems paradoxical, however, considering that these individuals probably have higher expectations of themselves, it is not unusual to find that they are harder hit by depression in the aftermath of a psychotic episode. Therefore, safety concerns cannot be too highly emphasized, whether it be in the active psychotic phases of the illness when the person is unable to make sound decisions or in the aftermath of the psychosis, risk for harming oneself or being harmed certainly exists.

With regards to stabilization, often antipsychotic medications are utilized to control delusional and hallucinatory symptoms. Antipsychotic medications are often quite effective in ameliorating psychotic symptoms. Unfortunately, as effective as the antipsychotic medications have been in controlling psychotic symptoms, they also produce major side effects, some of which mimic Parkinson's Disease (such as hand tremors, lip smacking, and facial grimacing). These side effects are sometimes referred to as Tardive Dyskinesias. Some of the newer antipsychotic medications have fewer of these Parkinson's-like side effects, such as Clozaril, Zyprexa, and Risperdal.

In the case of Robert, we see someone who most likely manifests Paranoid Schizophrenia. He fears that someone is trying to poison his food and steal his brain. He also alludes to hearing voices from Satan that are telling him to "do bad things," although he does not explain what these "bad things" are. He also tells the crisis counselor that he had been in a state hospital and that he also had been taking Risperdal, all of which are indicators that Robert can most likely be diagnosed with Schizophrenia. When a person, who is diagnosed with Schizophrenia and whose symptoms have been successfully controlled by medication, begins to re-experience psychotic symptoms, we refer to them as *decompensating*. Decompensation can occur rather abruptly or they can take place over the course of several weeks.

Naturally, in making a thorough assessment, other corroborating information is needed. Here, it would be helpful to talk with a reliable family member, get permission to look at Robert's prior medical records, or talk with the psychiatrist who had been prescribing his medication. What is difficult, however, in working with individuals with Paranoid Schizophrenia is that they will be suspicious of any attempts to help them and may therefore be unlikely to sign a release for prior treatment records.

It is likely that Robert may not be willing to sign any releases. It does seem that he has some insight into his condition, as he states that when he begins to feel out of touch with reality, he realizes that it is time for him to go back on his medication. In such a case, stabilization then entails making certain that Robert receives the correct medication at the proper dose. As with Bipolar Disorder, where a person may go off the medication against medical advice, it is common that Schizophrenics will go off medication in order to lessen the side effects. Another complicating factor toward stabilization is that many schizophrenics will sometimes stop taking their medication because of poor supervision in their living situation (such as at a boarding home), or because they are abusing alcohol or other drugs and do not like the effect that is produced by combining the medication with drinking or illicit drug abuse. Alcohol and drug abuse is a common factor in psychotic decompensation. Once rapport has been established, the crisis counselor interviewing Robert will try to explore many aspects of his decompensation in order to determine what level of treatment is needed:

Intervention:

COUNSELOR: Robert, you mentioned earlier that the voices you hear tell you to do "bad things." Could you tell me what kinds of "bad things"?

ROBERT: If I tell you, you're not going to lock me up in the state hospital, are you?

COUNSELOR: Robert it is important that we talk about this, I don't want to lock you up, I just need to get a sense for what types of "bad things" you've been hearing.

ROBERT: (hesitates) Well, the voices tell me to hurt people. People that are bad.

COUNSELOR: Do the voices tell you how to hurt them or who to hurt?

ROBERT: No, just that I should hurt bad people and that I'm bad too. I think the voice is the devil's voice.

COUNSELOR: Robert, you don't seem to be a bad person though. Are there any other things that you've done or think about that make you bad?

ROBERT: No, nothing that I can remember. I just want the voices to go away. I know I should take my medicine but I hate how it makes me feel.

COUNSELOR: What do you dislike about it?

ROBERT: It makes me feel numb and spaced out. My face starts to twitch when I take it, and I'm afraid people are going to know I'm crazy and make fun of me.

COUNSELOR: So, you stop taking your medication when you feel that people know about it?

ROBERT: Yeah, but that's when the thoughts about being poisoned or about the CIA trying to steal my brain come back really bad.

(continued)

CASE PRESENTATION: **A Crisis Involving Schizophrenia**
(continued)

COUNSELOR: It sounds like you usually feel and think better when you're taking the medication, except for the twitches, right?

ROBERT: Yeah, I guess I should start taking it again.

COUNSELOR: What do you do during the day?

ROBERT: Well, I wake up and then have coffee in the dayroom of the boarding home where I live. Then I walk around town until it's time for lunch. Then after lunch I walk around some more until dinner time. Is that what you mean?

COUNSELOR: Yes, Robert. Were you in some kind of day program at one time? I thought I saw that in your chart?

ROBERT: I was in a program at Central Medical Center, but I was getting up late and the bus stopped picking me up.

COUNSELOR: How did you like the program?

ROBERT: It was good when I went. They gave us lunch, we had groups to work on different skills, and we got to go bowling twice a week in the winter.

COUNSELOR: Here's what I'd like to do. Why don't you come into the hospital for a couple of days so we can get you started back on the medication and make sure the twitches don't come back and in the meantime, I can call over to Central and arrange for you to begin the program again.

ROBERT: What about my not getting up on time.

COUNSELOR: We can work on that. We'll get you an alarm clock and I'll talk with the boarding home manager about making sure they wake you up until you get used to waking up on your own again. What do you think?

ROBERT: That sounds good. You're not going to ship me off to the state hospital are you?

COUNSELOR: No, Robert, I think we can get you feeling better again. Would you consider moving to a different boarding home?

ROBERT: I would but you're not going to put me back in the state hospital?

COUNSELOR: No, just a different boarding home. A better one than the one you're living in.

---

with maintaining concentration. Usually when individuals with Schizophrenia present in crisis, it is when they are experiencing active and acute *positive symptoms* (as in the case of Robert starting on page 142) as opposed to negative symptoms. Positive symptoms are often more serious and more distressing to the individual and their family. At this point they are more likely to act out or be referred for psychiatric evaluation. Schizophrenia often makes its first appearance in the late teens or early 20s and, interestingly, those individuals with acute positive symptoms are considered to have a better prognosis than individuals with chronic, long-term, negative symptoms. It should be noted that Schizophrenics are also at a high risk for suicide.

Case Conceptualization/Crisis Resolution

In this case example there are several noteworthy issues. First, regarding safety, when Robert refers to hearing voices that tell him to do "bad things," the counselor makes certain that Robert is not harboring plans to hurt someone else or himself. If that were the case, Robert would need to be hospitalized immediately. The goal of this crisis session is to make certain that Robert will be safe, that he will go back on his medication, and that he will begin to go to the day program again in order to avoid a future decompensation. The other issue regarding stabilization is brought out in the discussion regarding Robert's going back on his medication. Fortunately, Robert is able to see more advantages than disadvantages to resuming his medication at this time. This is not always the case, and it may take some persuading and convincing before some patients will go back on their medication. There are some medications (such as Artane, Benadryl, or Cogentin) that are designed to control some of the side effects that Robert complains of. Often, stabilization is rather difficult because a particular antipsychotic medication may work well with some patients and not with others. Also, certain doses will work well, while other doses will produce a stuporous or drugged appearance. The role of the psychiatrist is to adjust the medications to produce the greatest benefits with the least amount of side effects.

Stabilization concerns are also addressed when the counselor brings up the issue of Robert going back to the day program. Day hospitals or day programs have been quite effective in providing Schizophrenic patients with very much needed social support and social interaction, along with social- and occupational-skills training. Day program staff can also monitor each patient's overall physical and psychological condition. In many instances, astute counselors can head off a full-blown psychotic decompensation by recognizing the telltale symptoms of a pending break. What is problematic, however, is that Schizophrenic patients will often drop out of these day programs due to lack of transportation or motivation, because they stop taking their medication, or because of alcohol and drug abuse. These patients then often become revolving-door patients who police will bring to emergency rooms time-and-time again or they will be arrested for vagrancy.

Guidelines for Crisis Intervention for Those with Schizophrenia

Murphy and Moller (1997) offer some helpful strategies for counselors working with individuals with hallucinations and/or delusions. These recommendations include:

1. Establish a trusting interpersonal relationship. In doing so, express your feelings in an open, honest, and direct manner.
2. Assess the hallucination and/or delusion including duration, intensity, and frequency. Be patient and listen when the patient is ready to talk.

3. Focus on the symptoms and ask the person to describe what is happening. The goal is to understand the symptoms experienced or demonstrated. Pay attention to the content of the hallucination or delusion, for example, some delusions are nihilistic involving themes of nonexistence or annihilation, some are grandiose involving an exaggerated sense of self-importance, and some are persecutory involving themes of being attacked or persecuted, conspired against, or cheated.

4. Identify if drugs and alcohol have been used, including prescription drugs. Morphine and Codeine induce hallucinations in some people.

5. If asked, point out simply that you are not experiencing the same stimuli. The goal is to let the person know what is actually happening in the environment. Do not argue about what is not occurring. When a hallucination occurs, do not leave the person alone.

6. Help the person to describe and compare present and recently past hallucinations.

7. Encourage the person to observe and describe the thoughts, feelings, and actions, both present and past, as they relate to the hallucinations.

8. Help the person describe needs that may be reflected in the content of the hallucination.

9. Help the person identify triggers of the hallucination.

10. Suggest and reinforce the use of interpersonal relationships as a means of helping them manage their symptoms, such as talking with someone they trust who can give them corrective feedback.

11. Identify how symptoms of psychosis have affected the person's ability to carry out activities of daily living. It is also helpful not to push the person to disclose too quickly and to let them know that they have a right to say, "I don't want to answer that question at this time." Also, don't play "analyst" by trying to interpret the hallucination or delusion, it is better to listen and try to gain an understanding of what the person is experiencing (Bohen, 2002).

PERSONALITY DISORDERS

When certain personality traits become inflexible and maladaptive, or if they cause significant impairment in everyday functioning or emotional distress; they may constitute a Personality Disorder. According to the DSM-IV-TR, (American Psychiatric Association, 2000), there are currently ten subtypes of Personality Disorders. There are a few, however, that are most likely to experience crises. Cluster B—or dramatic, erratic subtypes—are those most likely to present in crisis. Cluster B is composed of the following Personality Disorder subtypes: 1) the Narcissistic Personality (individuals with Narcissistic Personality Disorders are characterized by their incredible self-centeredness, their grandiose sense of self-importance, their preoccupations with unlimited success, power, wealth, and their drive to be admired), 2) the Borderline Personality (who often present in a state of crisis because they often experience tremendous difficulty in modulating or regulating their emotions, especially when it comes to tolerating boredom, loneliness or feelings of rejection), 3) the Histrionic Personality (noted for their need for attention from others and drama in their lives; they are the "life of the party" and can be quite seductive and charming, but they are also very prone to experiencing crisis), and 4) the Antisocial Personality (known for their lack of conscience and a lack of remorse—known for their criminal behavior, their manipulativeness, ability to con people, and their total lack of concern for the well-being of others).

Of all the Personality Disorders, individuals with Borderline Personality Disorder (BPD) are most likely to present in crisis. Individuals with BPD are among the most difficult and most demanding individuals to work with. One of the commonalties shared by Borderline and Histrionic Personality Disorders is that these individuals seem to live from crisis to crisis. A colleague once remarked that he could never get an adequate history from a particular BPD patient, because she was *always* in crisis. Each session with this patient was a crisis session in which she would rant and rave, cry and scream, and she would usually end the session with "Why aren't you doing anything to help me?" as she would storm out of the office. According to Linehan (1995), BPD is marked by "emotional dysregulation," which means that BPD patients have difficulty coping with the daily ups and downs or emotional upsets that most people experience. BPD patients seem to lack the ability to self-soothe or comfort themselves during times of disappointment or apprehension. Because of this emotional instability, BPD patients are often prone to suicidal acting out and self-mutilation (such as cutting arms or legs with razor blades). According to Maxmen and Ward (1995), "Many slash their wrists or douse lit cigarettes on their arms, not to kill or hurt themselves, but to *feel* something ('I feel so dead, cutting myself is the only way I know I'm alive') or to relieve tension." (pp. 407–408)

BPD is also characterized by impulsivity, by unstable and intense interpersonal relationships, by inappropriate and intense anger, identity confusion, problems with being alone, and chronic feelings of emptiness and boredom (Maxmen & Ward, 1995). Borderlines are sometimes difficult to diagnose, especially in a crisis situation, because they can often present with so many other problems. They may seek crisis services because of a relationship loss, sexual acting out, alcohol or drug abuse, a fight or argument, suicidal behavior, or some other impulsive act. They may also complain of anxiety or panic. Borderlines also tend to be involved in very intense "all or nothing" types of relationships—anything less than total love and devotion is considered rejection or hate.

Guidelines for Crisis Intervention for Someone with Borderline Personality Disorder

Linehan's work with BPD individuals is considered to be some of the highly regarded work in the field. Her Dialectical Behavior Therapy (DBT) provides counselors with effective strategies for both short-term and long-term case management of BPD. The following guidelines are derived from some of Linehan's (1995) recommendations that would occur at the time of crisis and pertain to

---

**C A S E   P R E S E N T A T I O N :   A Crisis Involving Borderline
Personality Disorder**

---

*Sara is 23 years old and presently lives with her parents and her younger brother.
She called the hotline stating that she had cut her arms and did not want to
"live anymore." Her parents agreed to bring her to the emergency room for an
evaluation, and to talk with the crisis counselor. Sara explains that when her
boyfriend Sean broke up with her, she felt "empty" and could not stand living
without him. She states that she has a difficult time being alone and that she cannot
tolerate boredom. Sara admits that sometimes she will make superficial cuts on her
arms and thighs with a razor blade when she feels "empty." She will also engage in a
lot of risky behaviors such as getting drunk and racing down the highway or going
out to bars and getting picked up by strange guys.*

Sara has many classic symptoms of BPD. She reports having an intense and stormy
relationship with her boyfriend, Sean. She also talks about feeling empty and bored
since the relationship ended. Sara also reports suicidal ideation and self-mutilative
behavior. One of the first rules in working with BPD patients is to establish a contract to
stop any and all acting out behavior. Unfortunately, Borderlines often relate to others
by way of acting out their feelings impulsively, so to expect that all Borderlines will
respond to behavioral contracting is unrealistic. In many instances, any therapeutic
contract is developed with the understanding that BPD patients have certain goals and
the counselor can help them attain those goals. However, the crisis counselor would
need to examine whether Sara's goals are attainable (for example, to reunite with Sean
or make him into the kind of boyfriend she wants may not be realistic). Obviously these
things are not going to happen. In the intervention below, the crisis counselor tries to
offer encouraging support to Sara while setting boundaries, and yet making certain
that she does not interpret these remarks as abandonment.

Intervention:

COUNSELOR: Sara, from what you've told me so far, it sounds like the break up with
Sean was really tough for you, but now you're saying he was a loser. How
long did you and Sean date?

SARA: Only about two months or so. We met in the Roadside Bar down on Route 7.
He was really cute. We slept together the first night, although that's nothing
new I guess. I remember I was pretty drunk that night. I had just broken up
with Doug ... I found out he was married and had a kid, the rat bastard.

COUNSELOR: Sounds like you've been having a rough time with relationships.

SARA: I keep meeting up with losers. Maybe I should stop hanging out at the
Roadside.

COUNSELOR: That may help. Sara, before you mentioned cutting yourself. Have you
done that recently?

SARA: Last night I did, after getting off the phone with Sean. He was being such
a pain in the neck. After I got off the phone with him, I was feeling really
upset, like I was going to explode or something, so I cut my thighs with a
razor blade—not deep though, I didn't want to kill myself. Do you want
to see the cuts?

COUNSELOR: Maybe we can have our medical doctor check the cuts out later. Were you
also drinking last night?

SARA: Yes, I had about three vodka and cranberry juices. Or maybe it was four,
I lost count after a while.

COUNSELOR: Sara, I'd like to suggest something and see if you would be willing to make an agreement with me. Would you hear me out?

SARA: Sure

COUNSELOR: Well, it sounds like there is a pattern to the types of problems you've been having. You get involved with guys who probably are not good for you, then you end up breaking up and feeling suicidal or cutting yourself because you feel empty or abandoned, right? Then when you add alcohol to the mix, things get even more out of hand. What I'd like to recommend is that we write up an agreement that you will stop these things that seem to be hurting you in the long run. What do you think?

SARA: What do you mean, stop hanging out at the Roadside? What would I do?

COUNSELOR: We would have to come up with other things you could do that would be enjoyable or other ways to be social.

SARA: But you mean stop having sex with strangers, stop drinking and stuff, right?

COUNSELOR: Yes, exactly. Would you agree to that and also agree to continue with counseling?

SARA: What if I do stop, does that mean you'll dump me or stop the counseling?

COUNSELOR: No, there is still a lot of work for us to do, but if you stop these dangerous behaviors, then at least that would be a beginning. Would you agree to put some of these things on paper?

Case Conceptualization/Crisis Resolution

In this crisis session, the counselor is focused on trying to set some realistic limits to Sara's behavior. He also is trying to support her emotionally, while at the same time to convey a sense of reassurance that Sara will not be "dumped" if she is making progress. The counselor would also need to come up with a crisis prevention plan with Sara. In other words, if she were to feel anger, rage, suicidal feelings, or self-mutilative, then she would also agree to call the crisis hotline and talk with the counselor on-call. There are naturally advantages and disadvantages to this type of a plan. The advantage is that it does not promote dependency on just one counselor and allows Sara to get other points of view when she is feeling upset. The disadvantage is that BPD patients will often engage in other splitting maneuvers, like playing one staff member against the other or manipulating a staff member who may not be familiar with the importance of boundary setting with BPD patients. The other disadvantage is that Borderlines can often be demanding of time and resources, therefore, they may call many times and for the least little thing. One Borderline patient would often page her therapist on Sunday mornings. Weekends tend to be particularly difficult for BPD patients because they may be more prone to feeling lonely and bored. Eventually, the therapist had this patient plan her weekends during their sessions and encouraged her to call to report how the weekend plans went. Eventually, the patient stopped calling once she realized that she was capable of adequately planning her weekend independently of her therapist.

In some instances psychotropic medication may be of some use in helping to stabilize the extreme mood fluctuations of the Borderline. According to research literature, MAO inhibitors—a subclass of antidepressant drugs and antipsychotic drugs—in low doses for irritability have been found to be effective in treating the transient emotional lability of some BPD patients (Cornelius, Soloff, Perel, & Ulrich, 1993).

(continued)

**CASE PRESENTATION: A Crisis Involving Borderline
Personality Disorder** (*continued*)

Unfortunately, benzodiazepines like Valium, Librium, or Tranxene can disinhibit BPD patients and may create more impulsivity and possible substance dependence. Tricyclic antidepressants such as Elavil and Triavil have not been found to be very effective. Some anticonvulsant drugs such as carbamazepine (Tegretol) have been found to reduce self-destructive behavior in BPD patients.

The aforementioned Personality Disorders that have been discussed thus far raise the issue of whether there exists a *crisis-prone patient*. According to Freeman and Fusco (2000), crisis-prone patients may become easily overwhelmed by emotions and will therefore tend to have a reactive style and little ability to assess the crisis situation and appropriately utilize strengths, supports, and resources. They appear to lack coping resources and, as a result, will often resort to impulsive or dramatic gestures in order to decrease the anxiety brought on by the crisis. Crisis-prone patients are also likely to misinterpret statements made by others, or will tend to exaggerate the events they have experienced. As Freeman and Fusco (2000) so aptly state, "The high arousal individuals are either in crisis, about to go into crisis, or live their lives with crisis always on the horizon." (p. 28)

---

engaging the patient in ongoing treatment. The major goal is to encourage the patient to commit to ongoing therapy.

1. Encourage the patient to enter and stay in treatment for a specified period of time.
2. Encourage the patient to commit to attending all scheduled therapy sessions.
3. Work on reducing suicidal and self-injurious behavior.
4. Engage the client in skills training that focuses on regulation of mood, and that increases problem solving.

MEDICAL CONDITIONS & MEDICATIONS THAT CAN CAUSE PSYCHIATRIC SYMPTOMS

Earlier, it was mentioned that psychiatric crises are often complex and often there are a multitude of symptoms and problems, which often converge to exacerbate a particular crisis. These crises can also be either created or exacerbated by certain medical conditions. For example, there are many medical conditions that can often look like psychiatric conditions. Such would be the case with Hyperthyroidism (overactive thyroid hormone), which can produce symptoms such as anxiety, irritability, grandiosity and manic-like symptoms. Conversely, Hypothyroidism will often produce symptoms that are depressive in nature and include impaired cognition, social withdrawal, and sleepiness or drowsiness. The following table contains some other medical conditions that can cause psychiatric symptoms.

T A B L E   8.1   Medical conditions that may cause psychiatric symptoms*

Endocrine/Metabolic Disease	Psychiatric Symptoms
Hyperadrenalism (Cushing's Syndrome)	depression, mood lability
Adrenal cortical insufficiency (Addison's Disease)	apathy, depression
Hyperparathyroidism	depression, anxiety, confusion, irritability, psychosis
Hypoglycemia	anxiety, irritability, confusion
Hyperthyroidism	anxiety, irritability, grandiosity
Hypothyroidism	depression, sleepiness, social withdrawal
Hypernatremia (excessive sodium)	sleepiness, drowsiness, confusion, lack of emotion, dullness

Gastrointestinal Disease	Psychiatric Symptoms
Wilson's Disease	personality changes, Schizophrenia-like symptoms dementia
Anemia	Decreased concentration, mood disturbance
Porphyria	anxiety, insomnia, depression, hallucinations, paranoia, delirium

Infectious Diseases	Psychiatric Symptoms
AIDS	early: decreased attention & concentration late: dementia, personality change, apathy, agitation
Meningitis	confusion, coma
Creutzfeldt-Jakob Disease (Mad Cow Disease)	rapidly progressive dementia

Neurologic Symptoms	Psychiatric Symptoms
Intracranial tumors	personality changes, dementia, depression, anxiety
Subdural Hematoma	irritability, confusion, extreme sleepiness

Nutritional Syndromes	Psychiatric Symptoms
Pernicious anemia	anxiety, depression, mania, confusion
Wernicke's Encephalopathy (thiamine deficiency)	amnesia, apathy, delirium, coma
Korsakoff's Psychosis (thiamine deficiency)	amnesia, confabulation, disorientation

*Adapted from Asaad (1995)

There are also particular medications that can create, exacerbate, or mimic certain psychiatric conditions. For example, there are certain medications prescribed for hypertension or high blood pressure that will cause depressive symptoms. This does not mean, however, that crisis counselors will recommend that an individual stop taking their high blood pressure medication. Instead, the counselor will usually consult with the physician or cardiologist who is prescribing this medication in order to determine if they may be able to prescribe an antihypertensive medicine that has less of an impact on the patient's emotional state. Table 8.2 provides a partial list of some other medications that can produce various emotional reactions. It is always important when assessing any individual who is in crisis to ask questions about their medical history and what medications they are currently taking.

T A B L E 8.2   Medications that may cause depressive symptoms

Analgesics and Anti-inflammatory medicine

> Ibuprofen
>
> Indomethacin (can also create mental confusion, acute psychosis, or depression with suicide attempts)

Opioids

> Percodan
>
> Percocet
>
> Darvon
>
> Darvocet
>
> Demerol
>
> Methadone

Antibacterial and antifungals

> Ampicillin
>
> Clycloserine
>
> Ethionamide
>
> Streptomycin
>
> Sulfamethoxazole
>
> Sulfonamides
>
> Tetracylcine

Antihypertensive and cardiac medications

> Alphamethyldopa
>
> Bethanidine
>
> Beta Blockers (such as propranolol)
>
> Clonidine
>
> Digitalis
>
> Hydralazine
>
> Lidocaine
>
> Procainamide
>
> Reserpine
>
> Rescinnamine
>
> Veratrum

Hypoglycemic medications

    Oral insulin

    Injectable insulin

Prostate enlargement medications

    Flomax

A FINAL WORD ABOUT PSYCHIATRIC CRISES

In talking with a colleague who works as a mobile psychiatric screener, he happened to mention that he has been called out on a number of cases involving older adults with Dementia. Many of these individuals live alone in the community and are often isolated from family and friends. Often, Dementia has its greatest impact on short-term memory, however, other cognitive deficits soon appear, such as the inability to express oneself (aphasia), to engage in purposeful activity (apraxia), or to properly name objects (agnosia). These older Americans are often unable to care for themselves, their homes, or their pets, which sometimes brings them to the attention of their neighbors or police. With the aging of the vast numbers of baby boomers, crisis counselors will probably be called in to intervene in this type of case with greater frequency in the future.

RECOMMENDATIONS FOR CHAPTER ENRICHMENT

SUGGESTED FILMS

Born on the Fourth of July (**1989**) This film provides an accurate depiction of a disabled Vietnam veteran who suffers from PTSD-related symptoms.

The Deer Hunter (**1978**) This film also provides an accurate depiction of Vietnam veterans who suffer from PTSD-related symptoms.

Girl Interrupted (**1999**) This film is set in an exclusive Northeastern psychiatric hospital, and focuses on young women who are battling Major Depression and BPD. The film is based on the novel by Susanna Kayson, which provides a chilling and accurate description of women whose lives are in various states of crisis.

A Beautiful Mind (**2001**) This film is based on the true story of Dr. John Nash, a mathematics professor at Princeton University and a Nobel prize winner. This film depicts Dr. Nash's struggle with Schizophrenia, and portrays the crises that he and his wife had experienced when the disease would take hold of him.

Fatal Attraction (**1987**) In this film, Glenn Close portrays a woman who has many characteristics of BPD.

SUGGESTED ACTIVITIES

1. Imagine that a friend or family member is suffering from Major Depression and needs psychiatric hospitalization. What resources can you find in your community or within a 25-mile radius that might be of help? Would your friend or family member need medical insurance in order to obtain treatment at these facilities? What about for follow-up treatment at an outpatient treatment clinic?

2. The following is a list of medications that are used to treat psychiatric problems. Find out what the medication is used for, as well as the benefits and side effects:

   Librium

   Depakote

   Topamax

   Seroquel

   Cymbalta

   Luvox

3. The National Alliance for the Mentally Ill (NAMI) is an organization that does a lot of advocacy work for people with mental disorders. See what you can find out about NAMI and the type of work they do.

9

Health Crisis

DISCUSSION QUESTIONS

Imagine you go to your family doctor for a routine medical checkup, and when your lab results come back, your doctor informs you that you may have a "serious medical condition." What would your reaction be? What would you do?

How do you think healthcare has changed since your grandparents were your age? What changes do you expect will happen in the future? For example, will there be a cure for cancer be discovered in your lifetime? a cure for AIDS?

INTRODUCTION

Despite all of the technological advances in medicine and the increase in life expectancy, the mortality rate and incidence/prevalence rates of particular diseases are alarmingly high in the United States. Interestingly, cardiovascular diseases (like heart disease and stroke) remain among the leading causes of death, along with cancer and chronic respiratory disease (Centers for Disease Control and Prevention, 2009). Other lifestyle-related illnesses have made their way onto the Leading Causes of Death list, and explain the need for crisis counselors in our emergency care system.

The World Health Organization (WHO) ranks the United States as 37th of 191 countries surveyed in healthcare delivery (Landers, 2000). What is disturbing is that one of the reasons the U.S. ranks as high as 37th is because of our specialized heroic lifesaving treatment (such as emergency medical care and emergency room treatment) and because the United States spends more on healthcare than the other 191 countries in the WHO survey. Why, then, does the U.S. rank so low? The answer to this lies, in part, to the estimated 48 million Americans who have no access to routine or preventative healthcare due to a lack of health insurance. It appears that not only are many Americans experiencing medical crises,

TABLE 9.1   The Leading Causes of Death in the United States in 1900 and in 2006 (rates in 100,000)

1900	Rate	2006	Rate
1. Cardiovascular disease (heart disease, stroke)	345	1. Cardiovascular disease (heart disease, CVA)	631
2. Influenza and pneumonia	202	2. Cancer	559
3. Tuberculosis	194	3. Stroke	137
4. Gastritis, duodenitis, enteritis, and colitis	143	4. Chronic pulmonary disease	124
5. Accidents	72	5. Accidents	121
6. Cancer	64	6. Diabetes	72
7. Diphtheria	40	7. Alzheimers	72
8. Typhoid fever	31	8. Influenza/Pneumonia	56
9. Measles	13	9. Nephritis, Nephosis	45
10. Chronic liver disease and cirrhosis	*	10. Septicemia	34

*data unavailable

Source: Figures from 1990 from *Historical Statistics of the United States: Colonial Times to 1970,* U.S. Bureau of the Census, 1975, Washington, D.C.: U.S. Government Printing Office. Figures for 2006 from Center for Disease Control and Prevention (2009). National Vital Statistics Report, 57, (14), 1-98. Washington, D.C.: U.S. Government Printing Office.

but the United States healthcare system is also in a state of crisis. Naturally, the fear of being denied medical treatment, being given less than adequate medical treatment, or facing financial ruin, can only exacerbate any personal medical crisis.

Medical crises differ in their origin or etiology and chronicity. For example, a medical condition that is brought on by one's behavior (such as emphysema brought on by smoking, liver inflammation brought on by excessive alcohol intake, or a cardiovascular incident brought on by obesity) may be perceived differently by individuals (and their families), and may have a different impact than does a condition where the person bears no personal responsibility (such as certain types of cancer, which may be genetic in origin). Naturally, whether the condition is *acute* (influenza or ear infections) versus *chronic* (diabetes or Lupus) will also have tremendous bearing on whether or not the individual experiences a medical crisis. What all medical conditions have in common, however, regardless of etiology or chronicity, is that there is a psychological or emotional component. Again, not all psychological or emotional responses to illness will constitute a "medical crisis," however, the intensity of one's reaction will usually be equal to the amount of disequilibrium the illness will cause in the person's life and the lasting effects of the disruption of functioning.

Crises often arise not only at the time of the diagnosis, but also at the time when treatment decisions need to be made. There are a variety of situations where treatment decisions could result in crises. For example, with a woman diagnosed with breast cancer, treatment decisions may pertain to whether a radical mastectomy should be performed or whether a lumpectomy followed by radiation or chemotherapy treatment can save her. Another example of treatment decision crisis can arise with a diabetic male in his late 50s, who because of extremely poor circulation, is advised to have his leg amputated. With an elderly woman who is living alone with advanced arthritis, a treatment decision crisis may arise when her physician recommends an assisted living facility in order to prevent injuries and to provide proper nutritional care.

EMOTIONAL-PSYCHOLOGICAL RESPONSE
TO MEDICAL CRISES

DiTomasso, Martin, and Kovnat (2000) have determined that a medical crisis is comprised of the following elements: *a triggering event, cognitive factors, behavioral factors,* and *physical factors.* They point out that the triggering event alone (for example, a medical illness) may not necessarily account for whether or not the individual is in crisis, but rather whether or not that event takes place in combination with other stressors and how the person perceives the triggering event. This leads to the notion that the *triggering event* leads to an interpretation by the person that brings into play *cognitive factors.* In other words, the person's response to the event is influenced by "unrealistic beliefs, attitudes, and assumptions; cognitive distortions; biased recall and perception; negative view of self, world, and future; decreased self-efficacy; and lack of accurate information" (DiTomasso, Martin, & Kovat, 2000, p. 413). So, for example, patients who unrealistically expect to make a full recovery after a surgical procedure may find themselves in a depressive crisis when they realize they may not have the same freedom of mobility they once had. Cognitive distortions will also bring about a state of crisis when the medical condition brings about a change in self-perception and self-efficacy. Such as a young man with ulcerative colitis that results in a colostomy. He may feel that he would never be able to date or marry, as no woman would ever want him as long as he had a colostomy bag. In biased recall and perception, DiTomasso, Martin, and Kovnat (2000) point out that it is more likely that people in general will recall negative events when they are in a negative mood. A negative mood state brought on by medical illness is no exception. Anyone who has been immobilized by the flu, even for a week, knows how difficult it is to have a cheerful, optimistic attitude. A negative view of oneself, the world, and the future, according to Beck (1976), is a recipe for a depressive response, which can lead to or exacerbate a medical crisis. The patients who feel that they will never fully recover or those who are forever scarred physically and emotionally by an illness or accident will naturally experience depressive emotional reactions, which become an integral part of their medical crisis. Finally, a lack of accurate information will also exacerbate the crisis.

Misinformation or a lack of accurate information will foster cognitive distortions and misperceptions, which will only serve to further exacerbate the crisis.

Behavioral factors can also play a role in whether or not one experiences a crisis and the extent or severity of the crisis. For example, DiTomasso, Martin, and Kovnat (2000) indicate that a *lack of coping strategies*, *negative means of coping*, *lack of available social supports*, and *inability to request support* all become part of the behavioral factors that will influence the course of a medical crisis. A person who has been able to handle other crises in their lives will usually have a better prognosis in being able to cope with the medical crisis.

Finally, the physical factors are the most obvious and important aspects in determining a medical crisis. Here the nature and extent of the physical illness is taken into account. An acute physical condition, such as an acute childhood ear infection, is easily treated with antibiotics and may result in an immediate medical crisis because of the child's pain. However, when the child's hearing loss is permanent because of repeated ear infections, which has also resulted in several surgical procedures, then another ear infection can represent a more enduring major medical crisis. Similarly, those physical disorders which are life-threatening, such as cancer, leukemia, tuberculosis, coronary artery blockage, will also result in a medical crisis. Illnesses or accidents that result in permanent physical or bodily change will also create an intense medical crisis. Such would be the case with the young teenager or college athlete who has an arm or leg disabled or amputated after a near-fatal car collision.

THE CRISIS RESPONSE OF THE FAMILY AND CULTURAL CONSIDERATIONS

Just as the person who suffers the medical crisis will experience a variety of reactions to a medical crisis, so too will the family. The family's reactions will play a major role in how the crisis is experienced and how the crisis evolves over time. A warm, loving, supportive family who pull together in times of crisis will naturally have a much different impact on the person suffering the medical crisis. In general, medical crises tend to bring out the best or worst in families.

Children also react to medical crises, although their reactions and the expression of the concomitant feelings about the crisis may be quite different from that of adults. A child, for example, may develop symptoms when a parent or sibling is diagnosed with a medical illness. Or the child may regress (by bedwetting or thumb sucking) or begin to act out in some way (fighting in school). Children may also adopt certain roles within the family as a means of trying to manage the stress brought on by the illness. It is noteworthy that the roles that are often associated with growing up in an alcoholic home—the hero, the scapegoat, the lost child, the mascot (Wegscheider, 1981)—were first discovered by Virginia Satir, a pioneer in the field of family therapy who was working with families in which a parent had been diagnosed with cancer.

There are several factors that also come into play when considering how culture may influence how a medical crisis will impact a family. Just as culture will play a role in determining the acceptable norms for emotional expression, so too will families of various cultures differ in how they respond to a medical crisis. For example, some cultures tend to be more stoic in response to crisis, while others are more openly expressive and do not hold back their tears or rage.

In some cultures, illnesses may be perceived as originating from "bad luck," personal behavior, evil spirits, or through the ill-will of others. For example, in countries with strong Christian values, a medical illness may be viewed as resulting from sinful behavior or it may be perceived that God has given this person the illness or injury to test his or her faith. Irish Americans find "virtue and sanctity in silent suffering" or in "offering up" their pain to God "as an imitation of Christ" (McGoldrick, 1982). In Italian culture, some believe in the notion of the "the evil eye" or *malocchio*, which suggests that others who wish harm or bad luck on a person can so do intentionally or unintentionally by casting the "evil eye" on this individual or their relatives. Prior to seeking formal medical consultation, many first generation Italian Americans may seek help from a "therapeutic woman" who is usually first generation Italian and is consulted in cases of anxiety, depression, or stress (Ragucci, 1982). Similarly, in Puerto Rican culture, a variation of the "evil eye" exists known as *mal de ojo*. This concept is often used to explain the sudden illness of children (ranging from mild discomfort to severe pain and even death).

Culture may also influence the types of treatment (mainstream or nonmainstream) that may be sought for particular illnesses. For example, many individuals of Puerto Rican and Cuban ancestry endorse faith-healing beliefs and may be as likely to consult a spiritist as they would a medical doctor. A spiritist acts as a medium, counselor, or healer in order to exorcize the spirits, which are believed to cause illness. *Santeros* and *espiritistas* are found throughout many Latino communities in the United States (Bernal, 1982). *Curanderos* are common among Mexican Americans, *bonesetters* are common treatment providers among the French Canadians, *remede-mans* are common among the Louisiana Cajuns, *singers* are found among the Navajo and *herbalists* are common healers among the Chinese (Harwood, 1982). Many of the aforementioned beliefs regarding causes of illness and nonmainstream treatments have waned somewhat among those second- and third-generation people of immigrant ancestry, as these individuals have often become more acculturated and English is spoken as the primary language in their homes, thereby making for easier communication in accessing healthcare. As second- and third-generation sons and daughters have become more sophisticated and educated, there is less of a tendency to hold onto old world beliefs and customs, and this had resulted in a greater likelihood of accessing more traditional healthcare treatment. In the section that follows, intervention strategies for various medical crises will be discussed in greater detail.

C A S E   P R E S E N T A T I O N : A Crisis at the Time of Diagnosis

---

Helen is a 36-year-old divorced woman. She was referred for crisis counseling by the Women's Health Center of her local medical center following her being notified of having received a positive breast biopsy. Helen has been attending the Women's Health Center regularly after her sister died of breast cancer about nine years ago. Because breast cancer runs in her family, Helen had begun to receive regular mammograms and checkups.

Helen's medical crises began at the point when she received a phone call to return to the office. She knew the news was not good. Given the history of breast cancer in her family, she had dreaded such a call since her sister's death. After meeting with the doctor, but before making any decisions regarding what steps to take medically, Helen was agreeable to speaking with a counselor at the Women's Health Center. The counselor introduced herself to Helen and meeting went as follows:

Intervention

COUNSELOR: Hello Helen, I'm Jennifer Smith. Your medical doctor asked that I speak with you. She told me about your biopsy results and that you were willing to come in today. Did you find the office O.K.?

HELEN: Yes, the directions the receptionist gave me were fine. I was just so upset when I got the call and they said I had to come in to speak with Dr. Johnston, I knew something had to be wrong. Usually they would just tell me my mammogram was negative and to reschedule in a year.

COUNSELOR: What was your initial reaction or feeling when you received the call?

HELEN: At first I was in shock or disbelief, like they must have the wrong lab results or something. Then I got really upset, like afraid mostly. It's hard to describe. I kept thinking about what my sister went through and I kept flashing back to when she was diagnosed with cancer.

COUNSELOR: How long ago was that?

HELEN: She was diagnosed in April of 1997, and by that Christmas she was dead.

COUNSELOR: I'm so sorry to hear about your sister. Were you and she close?

HELEN: I guess you can say we were. We were always competing against one another, probably because we were only a couple of years apart. So whether it was sports, or grades, or boys in high school, we always trying to see who would come out ahead. When she died, I felt like a part of me died along with her. She made me promise to get regular checkups though. Something I'd always avoided. I guess you can see why.

COUNSELOR: So you kept up with yearly checkups like you promised your sister?

HELEN: Yeah, I've been coming to the Women's Health Center since she died. I've always dreaded this day though. I knew that one day I'd get a call like this. Part of me wants to know every detail of what to expect and what the treatments will be like, while the other part of me just wants to run away and never come back.

COUNSELOR: Did your sister go through a lot of treatments?

HELEN: Yes, but I guess the cancer was so far advanced by then that it really didn't do her any good. I think it just made her worse. It probably would have been better to have left her alone and let her live out her last months in dignity.

COUNSELOR: It sounds like you've given a lot of thought to what you would do?

HELEN: I guess I have. Since getting divorced a couple of years ago, I thought about what I'd do if I was ever diagnosed with breast cancer.

COUNSELOR: When will you meet with Dr. Johnston?

HELEN: I'm scheduled to meet with her next Wednesday.

COUNSELOR: What steps are you willing or not willing to take?

HELEN: If she recommends removing a lump or mass, I would do it, but I just don't know if I'd do all that radiation or chemotherapy. My sister went through all that and she was weak and throwing up all the time. Plus it really didn't help her. And I would only do a radical mastectomy if they were certain that it hasn't spread. I don't think I'll ever get remarried anyway so I figure it doesn't matter if I have one breast or two.

COUNSELOR: It does sound like you've given a lot of thought to this in terms of what you're willing and not willing to do.

HELEN: I have. What would you do if you were in my shoes?

COUNSELOR: I would probably do exactly what you're doing. I'd talk with someone, get some help, get support, and then I'd find out the facts and make a decision from there. Do you have other help or support? Other friends or family you can talk to?

HELEN: No, I mean other than a couple of friends I have at work. I have no other family living in the area and I don't have children. I do have a brother that lives outside of Seattle, but I don't get to see much of him. Plus I don't know if I could talk with him about this kind of issue. If my sister were alive, I could talk with her.

COUNSELOR: What do you think your sister would recommend?

HELEN: I think she would tell me to go out and enjoy life. She always wanted to go to Paris but never went. I know she always regretted not having done that when she was alive and healthy.

COUNSELOR: Where would you want to go or what would you want to do?

HELEN: I've always wanted to go to Italy.

COUNSELOR: Tell me more about your plan? Where would you want to go in Italy?

Case Conceptualization/Crisis Resolution

One of the first tasks of intervening in a crisis situation is to try and establish a rapport with the individual, making him or her feel comfortable enough to talk.

This counselor also empowered Helen by asking her what she wants to do regarding treatment rather than to impose any expectations on her. Plus, at the time of the initial crisis session, Helen has not yet met with her doctor and does not know what recommendations will be made regarding treatment. What Helen knows is that she does not want to go through the suffering her sister went through, and this becomes a source of fear and apprehension regarding the diagnosis. By talking with the crisis counselor, Helen is able to gain support from someone that she can talk to, who will help her weigh out decisions. Helen has few friends and, although it would have been helpful to gain more information about her divorce and other past

(continued)

CASE PRESENTATION: A Crisis at the Time of Diagnosis
(continued)

---

history, it was not relevant to the crisis at hand and therefore could be discussed at a later date.

In the vignette presented here, the counselor is intent on gathering information about the nature of the crisis, factors that are contributing to, and maintaining it. This is all part of the **Listening** stage as described in the LAPC Model. In discussing her present reactions, the counselor is trying to gain a sense as to Helen's state of mind, her feeling and other reactions, as well as what other support systems she may have. This is all part of the **Assessment** stage. In the **Planning** stage, the counselor will conclude this initial session by getting Helen to come back after her meeting with Dr. Johnston in order to discuss her reactions to the new information she is given. Helen is willing to **Commit** to returning later in the day after her meeting with Dr. Johnston. The following describes some of the next session:

COUNSELOR: I'm glad you were able to come in today Helen. How did the meeting with Dr. Johnston go?

HELEN: I'm not totally sure, to tell you the truth. It was much different than what I was expecting?

COUNSELOR: In what way was it different?

HELEN: I was really expecting the worst, like I'd have to undergo radical surgery followed by a year or so of chemo; but that's not what happened. Dr. Johnston told me that she could do a lumpectomy and that they could then do chemo for a few months. I could keep working during this time. I was expecting that I'd have to go on disability.

COUNSELOR: It sounds like you're agreeable to what Dr. Johnston was proposing?

HELEN: Yes, I think it's something I could do, something I could get through.

COUNSELOR: You sound much more optimistic.

HELEN: I am, but I don't want to be overly optimistic. I feel I have to always be on guard. Like they say, I'm "hoping for the best, but preparing for the worst."

COUNSELOR: I see what you mean.

HELEN: But I'm going to take that trip to Italy. I don't want to wait until things are worse before I do some things for myself.

In Helen's medical crisis, it appears that she is trying not to be overly optimistic, and she has been cautious up to this point, especially because her sister has died of breast cancer. Yet, Helen has decided not to postpone things she wants to do in life. Her wanting to go to Italy is an example of this. It may be helpful for the crisis counselor to meet with Helen a few more times, especially around the time of her lumpectomy and while she is undergoing chemotherapy. Although Helen has made a good connection to the counselor, it remains to be seen whether she will be willing to attend a support group for breast cancer survivors. This may be explored as a possibility in future sessions with the crisis counselor.

CASE PRESENTATION: A Crisis Involving Chronic
Back Pain

Antonio is a 47-year-old married father of three. After graduating high school, Antonio had enlisted in the Navy where he served for six years. Upon receiving his discharge, he then went to work for his uncle in the family masonry business. He had been working successfully and had become a foreman when he was injured on the job while lifting a cinder block. This resulted in three herniated lumbar discs. Antonio had received physical therapy. however, the therapy was not helpful. Finally, his orthopedic surgeon recommended that metal plates be screwed into his spine to support the weight that the discs could no longer support. Antonio has received several other surgeries since that time, including a spinal fusion using cadaver bone and more recently a titanium cage, which is wired to his spine. All of these surgeries have provided only minor relief and Antonio finds that he is unable to work and unable to do much of anything in the way of physical work or exercise. Even driving a car is painful. Antonio had sought crisis counseling at the advice of his pain management physician who felt that Antonio was slipping into a deep depression.

The case of Antonio represents a medical crisis that involves both chronic pain, brought on by a chronic back condition, and depression, which has resulted from a combination of factors including the pain medication, the lack of mobility, and the loss of his occupational identity. These factors have created a synergistic effect, which had resulted in the current crisis. Antonio had prided himself on being a hard worker and a good provider for his wife and children. Now he found that even driving a car had become painful and he felt that he was "useless" around the house. Antonio also had once hoped that he would be able to return to work and get off of medical disability, however, he was now coming to the realization that this probably will not happen. Each time he had surgery, he would muster hope that this would be the one that would restore him to full functioning, however, in each instance the gains were minor and in some instances were also short-lived.

In this initial session with Antonio, the crisis counselor was intent on listening to the reasons why he was seeking counseling at this particular point in time. (Why now, as opposed to a month or a year ago?). The counselor was also intent on establishing some rapport with Antonio so that he might avail himself of future counseling to help him cope with his present dilemma.

Intervention

COUNSELOR: Antonio, I understand that your pain management doctor referred you here?

ANTONIO: Yeah, he sent me here when I told him how depressed I had been feeling lately. I didn't say that I was going to kill myself or anything, but he felt it was serious enough to suggest I come here.

COUNSELOR: Could you tell me how depressed you have been feeling lately?

ANTONIO: Doc, I've just been miserable. I can't sleep, and when I do sleep, I wake up in the middle of the night in a sweat. I don't want to eat or go out. People annoy the hell out of me, I guess I would rather be left alone.

(continued)

CASE PRESENTATION: A Crisis Involving Chronic Back Pain (*continued*)

COUNSELOR: How long have you been feeling this way?

ANTONIO: I guess it started about four months ago. I noticed that I was feeling more and more hopeless about my back, about all the surgeries, all the medication.

COUNSELOR: What was going on four months ago that was different from before?

ANTONIO: Well, for one thing, I had just finished physical therapy after my most recent surgery, which was six months ago. I had the titanium cage operation. That's the one where they go in through your stomach and push all of your intestines out of the way so they can get to your spine, and then attach this cage-like thing into your spine to support the weight that the discs can't support.

COUNSELOR: It sounds like a really involved surgery. How long were you under anesthesia?

ANTONIO: I was under for about eight hours. The recuperation was even worse though. Then, once I was discharged from the hospital, I couldn't get out of bed for weeks.

COUNSELOR: Was this recuperation different from the other surgeries you had?

ANTONIO: It really took much longer for me to get to where I could even attempt to get out of bed.

COUNSELOR: Then you began physical therapy, right?

ANTONIO: I did that religiously, but when I was done with it, I felt I was no better off than before I had the surgery. I guess that's when I went into a tailspin.

COUNSELOR: That must have been really tough for you, having gone through all that and then not feeling much better than you had before the surgery.

Here the counselor is providing some validation of how difficult it must have been for Antonio to have gone through such a difficult procedure and not to have derived some benefit from it.

ANTONIO: Exactly. I felt like I had wasted all that time for nothing.

COUNSELOR: What has your orthopedic surgeon had to say about the operation?

ANTONIO: Well, he said it was successful and that I just need to give it more time.

COUNSELOR: Do you feel you've given the recuperation enough time?

ANTONIO: Well, I guess it may get better. I spoke with someone online who had this same procedure and he said it took many months before he began to feel some relief. I just feel like I'm running out of time.

Guidelines for Counselors Working With Medical Crises

Medical crises can be very difficult to manage because of the often serious implications of various medical illnesses or medical trauma. This is certainly the case with terminal conditions such as many types of cancer, leukemia, and advanced

COUNSELOR: Are there options other than waiting?

ANTONIO: Well, not surgery that's for sure! I can't go under the knife again. But I did hear of about some kind of morphine pump that delivers the painkiller right to the back rather than taking the pills that space me out and make me even more depressed.

COUNSELOR: Maybe that is an option for you. Have you discussed that with your doctor or pain management specialist yet?

ANTONIO: No, I just heard about it, but I think I will the next time I meet with them. I can't take this anymore. I'm either in constant pain or I'm spaced out on the medication.

COUNSELOR: Antonio, are you going to be safe in the meantime?

ANTONIO: I wouldn't do anything to myself. I couldn't do that to my wife and kids. Besides, I'm a devout Catholic and I know it's a sin to kill yourself.

Case Conceptualization/Crisis Resolution

There are several things that have transpired within this brief session. First, Antonio explains that he sought counseling, not only at the advice of his pain management specialist but because of how depressed he was that the surgery did not bring about the anticipated relief. It is common that patients will develop expectations about what their treatment or surgery will do for them. When these expectations are not met, or when the treatment is unsuccessful, the let down is difficult to cope with. In Antonio's case, this let down is exacerbated by the fact that the surgical procedure and recovery were such an ordeal. Therefore, when the expected relief was not forthcoming, it was normal for him to feel angry and depressed. It is noteworthy that in exploring alternatives there are basically two options that emerge. First, Antonio knows that more healing time may help him. It is often helpful in educating patients regarding surgical procedures to have them talk with other people who have gone through the same ordeal. Although their experiences may differ, it gives the patient some idea of what to expect. The internet has been very useful in helping to put potential surgical patients in touch with others who have had the procedure. Secondly, Antonio had also recently become aware of a device that could help him manage the pain, without the side effects of pain medication. Although Antonio had tried several other pain management techniques before (such as Tens Units, which deliver electrical stimulation to the effected area in order to "short circuit" the pain), he was hopeful about the morphine pump because intuitively, it made sense to him. In ongoing crisis therapy counseling with Antonio, it would be helpful to gain more information about this new pain management device and to make certain that Antonio does not let his expectations get too high.

cases of cardiopulmonary obstructive diseases (COPD). Chronic conditions also have serious implications for any individual, as would be the case with diabetes, an injury which often results in permanent physical disability, an amputation, or a colostomy. Chronic conditions will often result in permanent changes in the way in which the individual defines him or herself. This naturally will often result in a crisis.

Bellak and Seigel (1983) have devised guidelines for crisis counselors, psychiatrists, psychologists, medical social workers, or medical personnel working with people who are experiencing a medical crisis. These are the most relevant:

1. Explore the patient's concept of the illness or impending surgery.
2. Explore the personal meaning and role of the illness (such as secondary gains).
3. Educate the patient.
4. Establish contact with the treating physician or surgeon.
5. Explore the meaning of anesthesia.
6. Explore specific notions and fears of death.
7. Explore specific types of illnesses and surgery.

Bellak and Seigel (1983) suggest that the counselor explores the specific meaning of the illness or surgery to the patient. For example, does the illness impact this individual's self-concept as a man or woman? Does the patient associate the illness with significant others who may have had similar illnesses? It is also important to explore the personal meaning and secondary gain aspects of the illness. Is the patient gaining additional attention from being ill, or are others doing things for them that they had not done before? If so, this might represent the secondary gain aspects of the illness. There is also an exploration of the patient's anxieties and apprehensions. In other words, how is the patient responding or reacting to being ill or needing surgery? It is important that nurses, counselors, and other human service workers help to educate the patient about the illness and the potential risks and benefits. The assumption is that the more informed, educated patient is usually the more cooperative patient. It is also important that the counselor establishes contact with the treating physician and/or surgeon. As Bellak and Seigel suggest, it is best not to work at cross purposes with other medical professionals, therefore, it is highly recommended that the attending physician be kept appraised of your work with the patient. Hopefully, the physician will then reciprocate and report any changes in the patient's medical condition or changes in treatment regimen. This helps to facilitate the notion of a treatment team approach, as opposed to having several specialists working independent of one another and being uninformed of each other's findings and treatment plans.

It is important to deal with those aspects of the illness or surgery in which the patient may have other specific fears. For example, with anesthesia, many patients fear the burning and choking sensation they experience in the throat, or struggling for air. Others fear not being in control to keep an eye on things. Again, the more educated the patient is about both preoperative and postoperative procedures, the better. The fear of death also arises often from the experience of not being in control—that a mistake will be made or the patient fears not waking up. Bellak and Seigel talk of the importance of discussing these fears of death and dying and the patient's associations regarding death (such as being alone in a cold grave).

In the two cases described earlier, the counselor highlights some of the methods typically employed to establish rapport in doing medical crisis counseling.

Though certainly not complete, the crisis intervention counselor typically relies upon several key features for establishing rapport, which is of key importance in providing crisis intervention services (DeWolfe, 2000). They are as follows:

Listening with genuine concern to those in crisis as they talk about and often re-experience the crisis is paramount to establishing a rapport with the client. Doing so establishes a client's confidence such that they feel their experiences are understood, respected, and not judged in a negative way. It encourages those in crisis to unburden themselves with minimal self-consciousness. A skilled listener often adheres to the following guidelines:

Allowing for silences. Very often those in crisis reach a point where there is a long silence. An experienced listener does not rush in to fill the silence with comment or further questioning right away. The crisis counselor knows that such silences often allow those in crisis to reflect on and sometimes re-experience the intense emotional reactions to what they have endured. It is not uncommon for silences to be followed by a cascading of intense emotional affects that may have been suppressed and are now relived by the client.

Nonverbal attentiveness. Counselors can express concern and their "being" with the client in nonverbal ways. Good listeners are empathetic to their clients. They maintain good eye contact, nod their head in a knowing fashion at important junctures, and convey their attunement to the clients' momentary state by donning caring facial expressions that are in accord with the content of what is said and the emotional state of the clients. These nonverbal communications often come about quite naturally when listeners are attuned not only to the clients' words, but also to the accompanying affect and their nonverbal body language.

Clarifying or identifying feelings. Nonverbal gestures by clients or a change in the tone of their voice serve as markers for counselors to reflect back to clients what they may be feeling. This is most helpful when clients are either flooded by emotion or unable to put into words what he or she is feeling. Comments like "You look terrified," or "You sound angry" help clients identify and frame vague feelings that he or she may be detached from. Identifying feelings for clients who are unable to do so on their own encapsulates, makes concrete, and places boundary markers to feelings that are free-floating and otherwise intolerable. Those in crisis usually have a sense of greater control when able to identify and label a feeling state that is otherwise vague and free-floating. It may be less frightening to identify a specific fear than to try and deal with more generalized, non-focused anxiety.

Paraphrasing. Counselors can convey that they are attuned to clients by reflecting back what they have heard their clients say. Comments such as "If I've understood you correctly you are saying that…" confirm for clients that they are understood. It serves to validate what is being expressed by the client, and provides an opportunity for counselors to check on the accuracy of the information they have processed by seeing if it is consistent with what the clients say they are saying.

Emotional Release. Crucial to the healing work of crisis intervention is the emotional venting or release of intense feelings by clients. Crisis counselors may feel uncomfortable with their clients' venting of very intense emotions such as anger, grief, sadness, and so on. Crisis counselors may inadvertently communicate their discomfort with their clients' abreaction by way of subtle facial expressions of disapproval, prematurely timed verbal reassurances, interjections that do not mirror what their clients are feeling, or less subtle cues such as active redirecting of their clients' focus. Such cues serve to derail clients from free expression of what they are feeling. It stifles the flow of clients' emotional upheaval and in doing so, may obstruct the real working through of such intense feelings that are prerequisite for the constructive problem-solving that eventually follows.

RECOMMENDATIONS FOR CHAPTER ENRICHMENT

SUGGESTED FILMS

Whose Life Is It Anyway? **(1981)** Richard Dreyfuss plays a sculptor, named Ken Harrison, who is involved in a car accident that leaves him paralyzed from the neck down. The film portrays the crisis brought on by his medical condition and his wish to be allowed to terminate his life.

The Doctor **(1991)** This film focuses on the medical crisis of cancer, when a physician, played by William Hurt, is diagnosed with cancer. This film is unique in its portrayal of a doctor who is now in the role of being the patient and the reactions he experiences as a result.

Philadelphia **(1993)** Tom Hanks plays a gay attorney who is dying from AIDS-related complications. In this Oscar-winning performance the issues of the psychological-emotional crises surroundings AIDS is well-portrayed, as well as the bias and discrimination issues that individuals with AIDS often face.

The Savages **(2007)** A brother and sister are faced with the crisis of needing to put their estranged, elderly father in a nursing home. This film accurately depicts the devastating impact of Dementia (Alzheimer's) on both the elderly parent and his adult children.

SUGGESTED ACTIVITIES

1. Find someone who has gone through a major illness or accident that will agree to talk with you. Ask how he or she reacted at the time of the illness or accident. How is coping with that illness or accident now? How did the

accident or injury change his or her life? What helped him or her to cope with the illness or accident? What did not help?

2. In July 2007, Michael Moore released his documentary *Sicko*, which deals with the state of healthcare in America. After watching the film, discuss your reactions. What stood out most about the film? What would you do to change our current healthcare system?

3. Interview people who deal with those who are experiencing healthcare crises, such as nurses, doctors, EMT workers, police, or first aid squad volunteers. What do they find to be the most difficult aspect of their job? What is the most gratifying part of their work?

10

Bereavement Crisis

DISCUSSION QUESTIONS

Usually when people think of bereavement, they tend to think of losing a loved one who has died. What other kinds of losses can people experience that may produce a similar type of grief reaction?

Many cultures, and racial and ethnic groups have their own special ways of grieving the loss of a loved one. We often see this in funeral rituals. Can you think of some ways in which your culture, race, or ethnicity influences grieving rituals? Give examples.

INTRODUCTION

Bereavement issues present special challenges for crisis counselors. Naturally, not everyone who experiences a loss will go into a state of crisis and even if they do, they may not necessarily seek crisis counseling. However, there are particular times when grief can be intense, such as in the case of an unexpected, tragic death of a loved one or when the death involves a young child, toddler, or infant. Parents, other family members, and friends may be inconsolable in the face of this type of grief. If one thinks of a *crisis* as an event or situation that upsets an individual's sense of organization or equilibrium, then it is easy to see why a loss such as a death of a loved one can throw a person's life into chaos and turmoil. It is also important for crisis and bereavement counselors to take into consideration that people tend to grieve differently. Although Kubler-Ross (1969) eloquently described the various stages that people often go through when they are coming to grips with a terminal illness and how family members often go through the same type of grieving stages, it is also noted that reactions differ and that people often experience these stages differently. Therefore, some individuals may be in a state of Denial and Isolation for several weeks, while others may experience Anger or Depression for many months or even years. In the vignettes described in this chapter, various types of bereavement cases will be explored, along with how crisis counselors help these individuals to manage these crises.

C A S E   P R E S E N T A T I O N : **George, a Husband Grieves the Loss of his Wife**

George is a 56-year-old sales manager and the father of two daughters, ages 24 and 22. Three months ago, his wife Joan died of pancreatic cancer. Approximately eight months ago, she had been complaining of nausea and upper stomach pain, and was losing weight even though she was not dieting. Her physician suspected cancer and had Joan see an oncologist who made the diagnosis. After going through two months of radiation and chemotherapy, Joan died approximately six months after the initial diagnosis was made. George has been devastated by the loss. He and Joan were very proud of their two daughters, but one is married and living in Paris where she and her husband work for a large investment firm. The youngest daughter is currently in her junior year of college. George feels a lot of loneliness, especially when he's not occupied with work. He was referred for bereavement counseling by the minister of his church as George has been inconsolable at all their meetings and during church services.

In this case, George has just experienced the loss of his wife and his daughters are grown and on their own. The goal of this initial session is to **Listen** to George's grief and to get a sense as to what feelings he is most grappling with at this point. Here it is helpful to determine if he is experiencing one of the stages of grief, such as the stages described by Elizabeth Kubler-Ross (1969), such as Denial and Isolation, Anger, Bargaining, Depression, or Acceptance.

Intervention

COUNSELOR: Hello George, my name is Susan Reilly, I'm from the counseling center here at Southern Regional Medical Center. I understand that your minister had suggested that you come in today. Do you mind if we talk for a while?

GEORGE: No, I don't mind. Reverend Paul is a great guy. He could see I was having a tough time.

COUNSELOR: What have you been struggling with?

GEORGE: Well, my wife Joan died a few months ago. As a matter of fact, she was receiving chemo treatments here at Southern. We spent a lot of time in this place. I guess we were hoping for a miracle cure, but everything I had read on pancreatic cancer was not good. It advances and spreads so quickly. Joan put up a brave fight though. (George starts to weep)

COUNSELOR: You must miss her a great deal?

GEORGE: Sometimes I can't believe she's really gone. There are times when I'll come home from work and I'll see her car in the driveway and I'll think to my-self, "Oh look, Joan's home from work," and then it'll hit me that she's gone. It's weird how you always think about how you'll grow old to-gether, you never expect that things will turn out like this.

(continued)

C A S E   P R E S E N T A T I O N : George, a Husband
Grieves the Loss
of his Wife (*continued*)

COUNSELOR: This must have come as quite a shock to you.

GEORGE: She was fine, and then one day she began complaining of some pains up around her stomach area and it seemed like the next thing we knew she was diagnosed with cancer and then the treatment started. That was the worst part.

COUNSELOR: How so?

GEORGE: The chemo really knocked her for a loop. She couldn't keep any food down. It seemed that she had already lost a lot of weight, but the chemo made her look emaciated, like a concentration camp victim. She hated wearing that wig too. She said it made her look like one of those Barbie dolls the girls used to play with when they were kids. It was really horrible.

COUNSELOR: Sounds like you have very painful memories of those months. How are your daughters taking the loss of their mother?

GEORGE: They're taking it hard. They were both very close to their mother. She was such a good mother. She was always there for them. My one daughter who lives in Paris with her husband was able to take a few weeks off, but she hated going back. My younger daughter Jamie is in college. She'll be home for winter break soon. She's having a tough time also.

COUNSELOR: George, how have you been managing your days since your wife passed away?

GEORGE: I'm okay when I'm at work, I keep pretty busy; but once I get home I get really depressed. Sometimes I feel like I'm numb or like I'm on automatic pilot or something. Just going through the motions. Weekends are really tough. (George starts to tear up)

COUNSELOR: In what way?

GEORGE: Well I just lay around the house. It takes me hours just to get going to do simple chores or errands like going to the bank or post office.

COUNSELOR: Did you and Joan do things on the weekends?

GEORGE: That's what makes weekends so tough. Joan and I used to do everything together. We had a lot of friends that we used to get together with, you know like go out to dinner or the movies. Now I feel like the third wheel. They ask me to go out with them, but it's not the same.

COUNSELOR: Have any weekends been less difficult for you?

GEORGE: Actually I did have one decent weekend. My sister and brother-in-law invited me to go to a movie and out to dinner. It really helped to take my mind off of things for awhile. They really understand what a loss she is to me, and I'm not embarrassed if I tear up over nothing.

COUNSELOR: It sounds like most days are a struggle, though, which is normal. It's good to hear that you had a pretty good weekend when you saw your sister and brother-in-law. It also sounds like a lot of what you're going through is part of the painful grief that people go through when they lose someone they loved very much. Do you know of anyone who has gone through something similar to what you're experiencing?

GEORGE: I do have one friend that I used to work with. His wife died of a brain tumor. It was really awful. I remember Joan and I saying to each other, how horrible it was and we didn't know how our friend Victor got through it.

COUNSELOR: Are you still close to Victor?

GEORGE: Yes, he did come to the funeral. It was so nice to see him. He told me to call him if I wanted to talk or go out for dinner some time. I guess I should take him up on it, huh?

COUNSELOR: Do you feel ready to?

GEORGE: It actually does feel good to talk with somebody—like talking with you today.

COUNSELOR: Then let's set up another time to meet. I also know of some small groups for people who are going through similar grief as yours that you could attend when you feel ready. And call Victor, if you're ready; he may be a good support.

Case Discussion/Crisis Resolution

George's case presents an interesting illustration of how grieving can often be compounded by other losses, (such as the empty nest of the daughters living away from home, and the loss of friends and social contacts). George describes the loss of his wife Joan and how she managed to just keep going through all of it, yet his life is now in crisis. It is important that the counselor not label George's reactions as being unusual. He is the one to use the word *depression*, for example, not the counselor. Since grief reactions vary from person to person, it is inadvisable to label grief as pathological unless the person's functioning is severely impaired for lengthy periods. The goal of the session, then, becomes to establish a plan for ongoing support for George, which will help him to re-establish some equilibrium in his life. It sounds like his job is helping him to keep busy but nonwork hours are most difficult for him. It is important to note that the counselor does not push George towards any one crisis plan, but rather presents him with some alternatives that he can choose from. A collaborative crisis plan is always preferable to a plan that is imposed by the counselor.

**CASE PRESENTATION: James and Barbara,
a Couple Grieves the
Loss of their Son**

---

*James and Barbara have sought counseling following the death of their son in a car
accident. The accident took place two months ago when their son, Dave, was driving
home from work late at night. According to the police report, Dave either had fallen
asleep at the wheel or was picking up a CD or cell phone from the floor of his car
when he veered off the road and hit a tree. Both James and Barbara are devastated
by losing their 19-year-old son. They have a 21-year-old daughter who is away at
college. Since the accident, both James and Barbara have been unable to function.
Just getting through the first two weeks with planning the funeral had been an ordeal. Now most of the family and friends that have supported them through this
difficult time have gone home and moved on with their lives, and James and Barbara
find themselves feeling lost, isolated, and angry.*

Accidents such as this are among the three leading causes of death in individual's ages 15–24 (suicides and homicides being the other two causes). James and
Barbara find that they are unable to function, and unable to communicate their grief
to one another. The following is the crisis session that takes place approximately two
months after their son's death. In grieving, there are unspoken *milestones*. It is said
that these milestones occur temporally, coming at "two weeks, two months, and two
years." In the first two weeks, one is coming to grips with the reality of the death;
however, there is usually a lot of support, family, and friends around who help to
buffer the grief. The next milestone—two months—occurs when the reality of the
loss sets in. At two years, the person has experienced a year of "firsts" without the
loved one, as in the first birthday, the first Christmas and New Years, the first summer holiday, and so on. In the Jewish religion, these milestones vary because the deceased is often interred before sunset. The family often sits Shiva for the first week
following the death and the surviving loved ones formally grieve (refrain from social
activity) for at least one month. The unveiling of the headstone occurs at the one-
year anniversary of the death. Therefore, the milestones under Jewish tradition
would more appropriately be "one week, one month, one year."

Intervention

COUNSELOR: Hello Barbara and James, my name is Bob Kane. I understand from your
phone call that you're here because of having recently lost your son. I'm
so sorry for your loss. When did this happen?

JAMES: This has been the worst thing we have ever been through. No parent ever
expects to bury their kid. (James starts to cry)

**CASE PRESENTATION: Ryan, a Child Grieves
the Loss of his Mother**

---

*Ryan is 8 years old and is in the third grade at Middlebrook Elementary School.
Last month, his mother died in a car accident. Ryan's parents divorced when he
was 4 years old, and his father moved out of state last year when his company
transferred him to a new office in another city. Ryan's maternal grandparents
have been taking care of Ryan since his mother's death, in order that he could*

BARBARA: It seems like the past two months have been a blur. Like we were both on automatic pilot, just going through the motions. At least that's how I felt.

COUNSELOR: What was the worst part of these past two months?

JAMES: I just keep going back to the night we got the phone call from the police. At first I thought it was one of David's friends playing a joke or something, and then it sank in that it was for real. We still don't really know what happened. How the accident happened. We just know that there was no other driver involved, no alcohol or drugs in his system, and they say it was unintentional.

COUNSELOR: But that doesn't tell you what did happen, only what didn't happen. Barbara what was the worst part for you?

BARBARA: Like James said, getting the call, but then going to the Medical Examiner's office to identify David. I'll never get that image out of my mind. James didn't want me to go in, but how could I not see my baby for the last time.

COUNSELOR: This is such a tragic loss. You both miss David so much.

Here the counselor is joining with Barbara and James by hearing the story of their son's death, what they remember, and what was the worst part. These are tough memories to relive but necessary to the grief process. The main goal of the counselor is to create an environment where Barbara and James will feel comfortable in expressing their feelings.

Case Discussion/Crisis Resolution

It is important that the counselor stay with James and Barbara, and that he conveys to them that their feelings are being heard. If they express guilt, it is important not to rush to lessen their guilt, but, again, to let James and Barbara know that their feelings are being heard. Often, the impact of grief is determined in part by how the death occurs. It is obvious that a horrible tragedy, like a car accident, is difficult to come to grips with. It is also important that James and Barbara are aware that it is normal for couples to grieve in different ways, and not to judge each other harshly because of these differences.

remain in the same school. Ryan's teacher noticed that since returning to school he has been getting into fights with other students and that his grades had gone down. The teacher also noticed that Ryan was avoiding playing with his friends and would not join in any activities, so the teacher referred him to the school counselor.

(continued)

**CASE PRESENTATION: Ryan, a Child Grieves
                              the Loss of his Mother**
(*continued*)

In Ryan's case, we address the differences in childhood bereavement. Children and adolescents often have distinct grieving patterns. Much of how a child copes with grief will be determined by how much preparation they may have had received prior to the death, and how mourning is addressed after the death (Furman, 1974). Generally, it is thought that the older the child, the better their chances of understanding the permanence of death and, therefore, the better their overall adjustment. This naturally depends on how independent and emotionally stable the child is prior to the parent's death. Coping will also be determined by how the child's questions and curiosities are handled. On the one hand, if a child's questions are met with harshness or anxiety, this will only increase the child's confusion. On the other hand, too much or too little information can also be detrimental to overall adjustment. For example, Furman (1974) points out that children will often express concerns about losing the surviving parent by asking, "Will you die too, Daddy?" Although concerns about misleading or deceiving the child by replying, "No, Daddy will not die," are valid, giving too much information about the unpredictability of life or our shared ultimate fate will only serve to increase the child's anxiety. Similarly, even with younger children, when the parent has a terminal illness, it is best to properly label the disease—"Daddy is dying because of cancer"—as opposed to saying, "Daddy is sick." By not giving proper information, one runs the risk that the next time anyone in the child's life gets sick (including the child), he or she will fear that they too will die, much like Daddy did. In a sudden, unexpected death of a parent, the surviving parent or guardian can broach this by saying, "I have something very sad to tell you." Sometimes, all the details are not known; however, children seem to feel better when the parent promises that details will be shared with them as soon as they become available (Furman, 1974). Naturally, children cannot deal with a flood of frightening details, but they can cope with the surviving parent's or guardian's upset and tears. The child also benefits from reassurance that they will be well taken care of and explaining the arrangements will be very important. There are often questions about whether a child should attend the wake or funeral service. With very young children, it is usually advised that they not attend the wake, however, older children may attend even an open-casket viewing providing that they are allowed to set a distance they are comfortable with and that an adult is with them to support and comfort them, as well as to respond to their questions and concerns. It is also important to recognize that the child's longing to be with their deceased parent is part of the normal grief process, as would be the accompanying feelings of sadness and/or anger. Part of successful grieving in children (and adults for that matter), is their ability to withstand these feelings of longing or yearning to be with the deceased. The following is an excerpt of the initial crisis session with Ryan.

Intervention

COUNSELOR: Hi Ryan, my name is Heather Marks. Your teacher asked that I talk with you for a little bit. Do you know why she asked me to talk with you?

RYAN: Yeah, she said she was worried about me because I beat up John at recess.

COUNSELOR: Is that all she is worried about?

RYAN: No, she also said she's worried about my grades and my not doing my homework.

COUNSELOR: What's been happening with your grades?

RYAN: I'm not doing too good lately. I really hate Mrs. Burke nagging me. I'm doing the best I can.

COUNSELOR: I understand that you had been doing really well in your classes, up until the time that your Mom died.

RYAN: I guess she told you that too. Yes, my Mom died in a car accident last October (about a month ago).

COUNSELOR: I was so sorry to hear about your Mom, Ryan. This last month must have been especially tough for you.

Here, the counselor is trying to get Ryan to talk about his mother's death, even though he seems to be reluctant to do so, given the circumstances surrounding the referral. The counselor tries to roll with the resistance and not focus too much on Ryan's grades or his fights with peers.

RYAN: The accident happened right before Halloween. It was really bad. My grandparents have come to my house to stay with me ever since.

COUNSELOR: What is it like living with your grandparents?

RYAN: I like my grandparents but they've been really sad since Mom died. I hate to see them so sad, Grammie cries a lot but tries to hide it from me by going in another room. They say I should talk about how I feel about losing my Mom, but I don't want to upset them. It's hard to talk about. I just want my Mom back.

COUNSELOR: You must miss her a lot?

RYAN: Yes. I still can't believe this happened. I wish she never went to the mall that day. She said she was going to pick up some things for the Halloween party we were going to have. I wish she never went.

COUNSELOR: I can see how much you miss her. Have you been able to see your father since the funeral?

RYAN: My father flew in from San Diego to spend some time with me, but he had to go back. He thinks he'll be able to get transferred back home to be with me.

COUNSELOR: How would that be for you?

RYAN: I think I'd like that, but I still want to live with my grandparents too.

COUNSELOR: I guess some of those details will need to be worked out. What's important is that you're able to tell your father and grandparents what you want, too.

RYAN: I just don't want to hurt their feelings I guess.

COUNSELOR: I think I understand what you mean. Right now everyone's very upset and sad.

RYAN: Yeah.

Fortunately, Ryan was willing to talk about some of what he's been feeling since his mother died in the car accident. The counselor is able to get Ryan to talk about what he is experiencing by not focusing on his grades or the fighting issues. There will be time to focus on that later, for the present, it is more important to allow Ryan to talk about his loss and not feel judged.

(continued)

CASE PRESENTATION: Ryan, a Child Grieves
the Loss of his Mother
(*continued*)

COUNSELOR: Ryan, I'm glad you came in to talk to me today. I can see you're going through a difficult time right now and you're being really brave. I'd like for us to speak again. Would you be willing to come in later this week so we can continue our talk?

RYAN: Sure, do I need to get a pass to come down to your office?

COUNSELOR: I'll let your teacher know, and she'll excuse you from class to come down to my office. Is that O.K. with you?

RYAN: Yeah. I just don't want the other kids to know I'm coming here. They'll think I'm in trouble or something.

COUNSELOR: Sure, you're not in any trouble and if you just want to come down here after recess on Friday, I'll tell your teacher so she knows not to look for you.

RYAN: O.K., I'll see you Friday.

CASE PRESENTATION: Tara and Bill, Parent's
Grieving the Loss of their
Newborn Daughter

Tara and Bill have been married for two years. Tara is 24 years old and Bill is 26. They were both looking forward to having a baby and becoming parents. After having two miscarriages, Tara finally gave birth to a baby girl. She and Bill were both ecstatic; however, the neonatologist told them that their baby had been born with "respiratory complications" and was having difficulty breathing. A pulmonary neonatologist was called in on a consultation and told Tara and Bill that the baby had major heart and lung abnormalities and "would not be expected to live." Their baby died approximately two weeks later, never leaving the hospital.

The death of a child is probably the singular most traumatic event that a parent can face. It is universally assumed that a child will outlive both parents. As Rando (1984) points out, when an adult loses a parent they lose their past, but when they lose a child, they lose their future.

The divorce rate for grieving parents is higher than that of parents who do not suffer the loss of a child. Some estimates suggest that the divorce rate for bereaved parents who do not receive professional help is as high as 92% (Kanel, 2003). This can be attributed to a number of factors. For example, after the loss of the child, couples no longer feel that they are the same. Also, each parent tends to grieve differently and because of this, they may feel that the other partner is being callous. For example, if the husband (or male partner) views the death as something the couple can get over, or says that they can try to have another child, the spouse may perceive this as cold and invalidating. Likewise, if the wife (or female partner) is experiencing tremendous grief, then the husband may feel that he is not doing enough for her, or, in contrast, he may want his wife to move on with their lives as a couple. Finally, since both partners are experiencing grief, they often are unable to support one another through this process. They begin to feel isolated and disconnected from each other. In the case example described above, it is Tara who seeks counseling approximately four days after their baby died. Having experienced two miscarriages prior to the birth of their daughter compounds her grief. A miscarriage can be as emotionally devastating as any other tragic

Case Discussion/Resolution

It is very common that children will grieve differently than adults. Ryan's fights with his classmates are a good example of how children's grief can be displaced behaviorally. It is easy to see how his anger at his mother's death is being displaced onto his classmates through his fighting. The role of the school counselor is to help validate Ryan's anger and frustration, and hopefully to get him to accept counseling. Although the school counselor can still be of assistance to Ryan, it will be more appropriate for a bereavement counselor to work with Ryan, his father, and grandparents to process their feelings as they move through the grief. The role of the school counselor is to help Ryan with his adjustment at school and to deal with the immediate crisis surrounding his mother's death.

loss, and may intensify her current feelings. Unfortunately, there have been only a few medical centers and crisis intervention providers who have been attuned to the need for some more formal way to grieve the termination of a pregnancy by miscarriage or abortion. Some medical centers now provide grief counseling for those who have experienced a pregnancy loss. Some even provide a grieving ritual (such as planting a tree), to memorialize these losses.

Intervention

The following is an excerpt from the initial crisis session with Tara.

COUNSELOR: Hi Mrs. Smith, my name is Robert Torres, I am a counselor here at the Medical Center. I think you said your doctor referred you here?

TARA: (Begins sobbing) My baby died here last Tuesday morning. I've not been able to sleep. We buried her yesterday. I feel I can't go on.

COUNSELOR: I am so sorry to hear about your baby. Tell me what happened.

TARA: The doctor said she couldn't breathe because her lungs were not fully developed. She also had problems with her heart. Her heart stopped beating. (more sobbing)

COUNSELOR: (Handing Tara some tissues) This must be so horrible for you. Did you have any help in making the funeral arrangements?

Here the counselor begins to find out who is in Tara's support network.

TARA: Yes, my husband, Bill, and my mother. I just couldn't do it. The worst part was seeing that little white casket. I couldn't stop crying. I still can't stop crying; I don't think I will ever be able to stop.

COUNSELOR: I can see how hard this has been for you. How is your husband coping with losing his daughter?

(continued)

CASE PRESENTATION: Tara and Bill, Parent's
Grieving the Loss of their
Newborn Daughter
(*continued*)

TARA: Bill has been all over the map. One minute, he's angry with the doctors, the next minute he's quiet and won't talk to anyone, he just stares into space, and the next minute, he's talking on the phone with his business partner. He went back to work today. I can't even remember what I'm doing. I walk into a room for something and I forget why. Is this normal? Am I cracking up or something?

COUNSELOR: Yes, that's quite normal given what you're going through.

Here the counselor offers more reassurance to Tara as a means of normalizing her grief. The counselor also has a sense, at this point, that Bill is coping much differently than his wife. This may have gender implications, which will be explored later in the session.

TARA: I just wish that Bill hadn't gone back to work right away, but he said he had to get back so they wouldn't fall behind.

COUNSELOR: It sounds like he takes his work very seriously.

The counselor is being careful not to criticize Bill, as it is not the counselor's role to be judgmental.

TARA: Yes, he is good at his job and he is a good husband. I just wish he could talk about his pain, at least with me. I feel like he is blaming me for her death.

COUNSELOR: What gives you this feeling?

TARA: It's nothing he's doing, I guess. It must be me. My father died of a heart attack when I was 13 years old, so he may blame me for the baby having a bad heart because this runs in our family. He was really upset when I had the miscarriages also. He thought I was trying to do too much. I was working and taking a college course at night to finish my Bachelor's degree. Bill thought I needed to slow down.

CASE PRESENTATION: John, the Grief of Divorce

John is a 46-year-old married father of two daughters ages 20 and 18. Both daughters are away at college. He and his wife, Mary, had been married for the past 21 years. They met at work and were engaged for about a year. John thought that they were both happy and content in their relationship, however, one day Mary confronted John to tell him that she no longer loved him and that she had fallen in love with someone she met in one of her yoga classes. John was devastated. He tried to get Mary to go for counseling with him, but she refused. She felt that throughout their marriage she was always low on John's priority list. She saw no reason to rehash these issues that had been sources of conflict throughout their marriage. John did get Mary to agree to go to one marriage counseling session, however, he soon

COUNSELOR: It sounds like you're carrying a lot of the guilt and pain of your baby's death. Tara, you are not responsible for your baby's death.

TARA: Yes, I guess you're right. I just feel like I'm weak because I can't pull myself together like Bill seems to be doing.

COUNSELOR: It's O.K. that you and Bill are grieving differently. That doesn't make one of you right and the other wrong. It's just different. But is there anything that you need from Bill right now?

TARA: I need to know that he loves me and that he doesn't blame me for our baby's death or for the miscarriages. I just need for him to hold me and be with me.

COUNSELOR: What is the best way for him to hear your needs?

TARA: Well, I asked him to come in with me today, and he said he would come but that we would have to schedule something in the evening when he's off from work. Is that possible?

COUNSELOR: Sure, let's set something up. I'm glad to hear that Bill is willing to come in with you, that sounds like a good step. But if something comes up and Bill is not able to make the session, why don't you come in and we can always include Bill for the following session.

Case Discussion/Crisis Resolution.
The counselor makes the comment that Bill's willingness to come in with her is positive, however, he doesn't want Tara to become disappointed or to lose hope if he reneges on his agreement to join her. Towards the close of the first session, the counselor also mentions to Tara that there are support groups specifically for parents who have lost newborns. It seems that of all the treatment available, support groups are one of the most beneficial modes of treatment because it allows for honest sharing with those who have experienced the same loss and can better understand the pain that Tara and Bill are going through.

realized that she no longer loved him and there was no hope of salvaging the marriage; the separation was final. John sought crisis counseling at the urging of his brother, after John told his brother that he saw no reason to go on with life, and that he was so depressed he had not even been to work in the past three weeks.

In the case of John, a different type of loss is presented—separation and divorce—however, there are many who feel that the emotional pain associated with a divorce is tantamount to losing someone through death. In addition, just as there are hidden losses that one experiences when a loved one has died, so too do divorced individuals experience many other losses, such as loss of time with children, loss of income, loss of a home, loss of friends, loss of contact with in-laws, and loss of

(continued)

**C A S E   P R E S E N T A T I O N :   John, the Grief of
Divorce** (*continued*)

---

companionship. Even in the most amicable divorces, the sense of loss is tremendous and overwhelming. However, in the case of a contentious divorce, there may also be accompanying feeling of anger, rage, guilt, envy, and jealousy. When children are involved, the pain of loss often becomes greater. Such is the case when the noncustodial parent is now faced with limited time with their son or daughter as was so vividly depicted in the movie, *Kramer vs. Kramer.*

Crises involving divorce are quite common, mostly because the United States has the highest rates of divorce (4.44 per 1000), compared to other countries (United Kingdom 2.97 per 1000; Sweden 2.40 per 1000; and Germany 2.07 per 1000) (United Nations Secretariat, 1996). It is estimated that approximately 50% of marriages in the United States will end in divorce. There are several factors that are hypothesized as accounting for these extreme divorce rates. First, there is a greater acceptance of divorce in the United States. Marriage is not viewed as having the same permanence that it once had. Second, women's roles have shifted. With more women in the workforce, they are no longer dependent on men, and, therefore, are less willing to stay in unfulfilling marriages. Third, the sanctity of marriage as a religiously bound union is not as strongly accepted as it was years ago. Fourth, there has been a greater emphasis on seeking satisfaction of personal goals and higher expectations for marital happiness (Weitzman, 1985). Finally, people are living longer; therefore, it is not unusual for people to divorce after their children have gone off to college or have married and moved away from home.

Overall, even in amicable separations, divorces tend to have a deleterious effect on one's mental health. Indeed, divorce is associated with higher rates of *depression* (Anthony & Petronis, 1991; Gallo, Royall, & Anthony, 1993; Weissman, Bruce, Leaf, Florio, & Holzer, 1991), *suicide* (Cantor & Slater, 1995; Trovato, 1986), and *substance abuse* (Beck, Wright, Newman, & Liese, 1993). Granvold (2000) recommends that a thorough risk assessment be done when divorced individuals present for crisis intervention services because of these risk factors.

As discussed earlier in this chapter, just as bereavement reactions are often determined by the factors surrounding the death—such as cause of death, the survivor's relationship with the deceased loved one, age, ethnicity, and so on—so too, in cases of divorce, the events and factors surrounding the divorce also play a role. For example, marital infidelity, physical violence, verbal and/or emotional abuse, alcoholism and substance abuse, physical and/or sexual abuse of the children, gambling, gross financial irresponsibility, and episodic violation of trust (such as lying, deceit) (Granvold, 2000).

Intervention

In this session, John has been brought to a counselor by his brother, Barry, who became aware of John's veiled suicidal threats and his absence from work.

COUNSELOR: Hi Barry, I know we've spoken over the phone. You must be John, (extending his hand) I'm glad you could both make it today. Did you have any trouble finding the office?

BARRY: No, your directions were fine.

COUNSELOR: John, I understand from talking with Barry on the phone that you have been going through a very difficult time. Could you tell me what's been happening?

JOHN: I just can't function any more.... I haven't been able to go to work. I'm not sleeping or eating. I guess Barry told you about the break up with Mary?

BARRY: I did John, but I didn't get into any detail. I only told him that you were going through a really bad break up.

JOHN: "Really bad"? That's an understatement. I found out that my wife was fooling around with a guy she met in her yoga class, and she leaves me. What a kick in the gut that was. We had our whole life planned out. Where we were going to retire, where we wanted to travel to. I feel like my guts were torn out, like my whole future was taken away from me.

COUNSELOR: When did you learn all of this?

JOHN: About three weeks ago. I guess that's when I stopped functioning too.

COUNSELOR: John, it's really important that you answer this question honestly. In many instances when people are going through the kind of thing you are, they begin to think suicidal thoughts. Have you been having any suicidal thoughts?

JOHN: You know I did right when I first found out about the affair, but then I thought to myself, "No, way am I going to give in." Besides that bitch would get the insurance money and she and her boyfriend would probably have a blast spending it, while I'm rotting in the ground. So, I remembered the saying, "don't get mad, get even."

COUNSELOR: So, let's make sure I heard you right, you did feel suicidal, but you don't at this point, right?

JOHN: You got it, Doc.

COUNSELOR: John, could we also have an agreement that should that change, for example, if you begin to think that suicide sounds like a way out, you agree to call me and/or come in immediately. Would you agree to that?

JOHN: Yes, no problem.

A "no-suicide contract" is something that many counselors use to help ensure the client's safety. While there are no guarantees that John would not act on impulse, the contract does specify a course of action that John agrees to take, should he feel suicidal again. In doing a suicide assessment, the counselor would first make certain that there has been no prior history of suicidal gestures or attempts and would also make certain that John did not have a specific plan or a means of committing suicide.

COUNSELOR: John, let's go back to what you meant by "don't get mad, get even."

JOHN: Don't get me wrong, I would not hurt Mary, after all she is the mother of my two daughters. What I meant is that I'm tired of taking the brunt of all this. I was a good husband and a good provider—I am putting the girls through college. It's not fair that I can be perceived as the flawed party. I think my daughters need to know why we're breaking up, don't you?

COUNSELOR: Are you sure that Mary hasn't told them about why she's seeking a divorce?

JOHN: I'm pretty sure she hasn't said anything. She wouldn't want to look bad in their eyes.

COUNSELOR: If you did tell them, what do you think would happen?

JOHN: I think they would hate her for doing this to me and to them. I want her to suffer like I have.

(continued)

**C A S E   P R E S E N T A T I O N :   John, the Grief of
Divorce** (*continued*)

COUNSELOR: You sound really angry John, and I can see why you're angry, but I'm
wondering if that would help in getting over your anger. Are there other
things that might help get you back to where you can function again?

*Here the counselor is trying to allow John to explore some alternatives. As was al-
luded to earlier, when someone is in the midst of intense grief reactions, it is usually
not the best time to make major decisions. The counselor is also trying to slow John
down by validating his anger.*

JOHN: Maybe you're right, I'll have to think this through a bit. I don't want this to
come back where the girls are angry with me because I'm the messenger
that delivers the "bad news." You know, I don't know what would help in
getting through this anger or rage that I feel. Do you have any ideas?

COUNSELOR: Let me throw some ideas out to you. I know that not everyone benefits
from all of these things, it's a very individual thing; what helps some folks
might not benefit others.

JOHN: I understand.

COUNSELOR: The first thing is that with all the feelings that you're experiencing right
now, it is a good idea to have some ongoing support. I know of a
psychologist in the area who specializes with people who are going

General Guidelines for Crisis Counseling in Situations of Loss and Bereavement

Although there are no "hard and fast" rules when it comes to doing crisis intervention in bereavement situations, there are some guidelines that might be useful
for counselors to keep in mind as they are working with people in the throes of
these types of crises.

1. Join bereaved individuals at whatever stage they present in. (For example, if
   the stage is anger, it is important to hear out their anger and let them vent.)

2. Do not try to force people to the next stage. Instead, gently guide them.
   (The stages of grief are meant as a guide, not as a directive. Counselors can
   sometimes "preview" what the next stage in what the grief may feel like or
   sound like, but, again, this is not meant to be a dictate.)

3. While it's important to be a good empathic listener, do not become overwhelmed in the grief to the point where you also become immobilized by
   their story of grief. In other words, don't become like the "deer caught in
   the headlights." It is most important that, as the counselor, you convey to
   your clients that you will help them through this grief process, no matter
   how overwhelming it may initially seem.

4. It is important to be cognizant of the tendency to idealize the deceased
   almost, as if elevating the loved ones to sainthood. This is easy when the

through really tough divorces like you are. I think he also runs a men's group in the evening. Some find individual counseling more helpful and some guys find the group more helpful. Would you be willing to try either one out, or at least call Dr. Stevens and see what he has to offer?

JOHN: I would, do you have his phone number?

COUNSELOR: Sure. There are also some self-help support groups for people going through divorce, these groups meet on a regular basis and the difference is that there is not a counselor leading the group, but they are free and meet on a regular basis. I can give you phone numbers and addresses for some of these groups as well.

Case Discussion/Crisis Resolution.
At this point, John appears willing to accept these referrals as alternatives to staying "stuck" with his depression and anger, which appear to be part of his grief reactions. It is fortunate that his brother, Barry, is attending the session with him, because Barry can help monitor whether or not John makes these contacts and a few follow-up sessions can be set up to make certain that John is safe and beginning to make progress. If necessary, a referral for psychotropic medication may also be needed to help move John out of the immobilizing aspects of the grief. In some instances, an antidepressant may be helpful on a short-term basis in order to get John functioning again.

person was indeed good and kind-hearted, however, this will also occur when the person was quite the opposite. Even a miserable, vitriolic, abusive spouse can be deified in death. This is a common reaction and it is helpful to be aware of this and not feel the need to confront these "misperceptions." Those types of issues may be addressed in long-term bereavement counseling.

5. Also, avoid giving directives and being critical of the bereaved (Dershimer, 1990). Here it is important to avoid making any statements that might result in exacerbating feelings of guilt, shame, or self-doubt. As Dershimer points out, bereaved individuals often have their "radar" set for anything that might suggest that their grief is abnormal, so statements that might be misconstrued as being judgmental or critical are to be avoided. For example, a well-meaning crisis counselor might suggest to a bereaved widower that eventually they will be able to move on and their grief will not be as intense. The grieving husband could misinterpret this type of statement as a criticism of their present feelings.

6. Do not become impatient if clients seem "stuck" in their grief (Dershimer, 1990). It is important to take into account that grief has no timetable. Grief counselors estimate that grief sometimes takes five to seven years to resolve. Also, people tend to grieve in their own way and at their own pace. Those in mourning may appear to be coping well at one moment, only to emotionally fall apart the next. This is common.

7. Be careful not to brush aside, offer platitudes in response to, or judge clients' deep-seated fears or doubts (Dershimer, 1990). Bereaved individuals most likely have received enough platitudes or well-meant advice from their friends or family members, so it best that they not feel dismissed by the counselor brushing aside their fears or doubts. They do not need to hear platitudes such as, "You'll meet someone new," "You'll be able to have another child," "You'll get over it," or "This was God's will."

8. No matter how many times you hear the same story about the deceased, treat it as if it is the first time you are hearing the story, instead of responding verbally or nonverbally with, "You already told me that." One of the differences between formal crisis counseling and grief counseling, is that counselors will listen when all the bereaved friends and family have gone away or may be saying, "It's time to move on," or "I don't want to hear the same stories about the deceased anymore" (which may be said overtly or covertly). As with posttrauma counseling, each time the individuals relive a story of the deceased, it usually helps to bring them closer to resolving their feelings of loss.

9. Listen for prior instances of resolved or unresolved grief. Unresolved grief issues will surely exacerbate the current bereavement crisis, while prior grief issues that have resulted in a positive resolution can help to illustrate prior coping styles that were effective.

10. Generally, it is best to refrain from physically touching clients, unless they reach out for you. Putting your hand on someone's shoulder or placing your hand over their clasped hands can be comforting, however, it is most important to honor clients' physical boundaries. Empathy and compassion can be easily conveyed and demonstrated verbally.

11. Assist individuals in determining whom within their social support system they can rely on. Here, it is important to begin to address the issues of who is in the clients' social support system. The old saying, "You really know who your friends are when the chips are down," is very applicable here. Some friends or family members may "head for the hills" and will avoid dealing with the person in mourning. Often, this may arise out of their discomfort in dealing with death and mortality or some unresolved grief issues. On the other hand, unexpected friends or family members may sometimes surface as empathic supports. Often, these are individuals who may have gone through some type of grieving process themselves and are willing to listen and help.

RECOMMENDATIONS FOR CHAPTER ENRICHMENT

SUGGESTED FILMS

Ordinary People (1980) This film provides an accurate and emotionally powerful portrayal of a family who is unable to grieve the loss of their oldest son, Buck. Donald Sutherland and Mary Tyler Moore play the role of the parents, while Timothy Hutton plays the role of Conrad—Buck's younger brother who survives the sailing accident in which Buck drowns. Conrad becomes the "symptom bearer" of the family, and at the beginning of the film has just come from a psychiatric hospitalization after a failed suicide attempt. The film sensitively portrays the family dynamic that takes place following the death of Buck, the family hero.

In the Bedroom **(2001)** This film portrays a very realistic depiction of the grief experienced by parents after the murder of their son. What is unique about this film is that unlike many films, which merely alludes to parental grief, this film delves into the parents' grief over the course of several weeks following their son's death, and well-illustrates how differently both parents grieve and how those differences lead to conflict and tension.

Monster's Ball **(2001)** This film is replete with death and grief issues. Halle Berry plays the role of a single mother whose son is killed in a hit-and-run incident that she witnesses, is powerless to help save her son's life. Billy Bob Thornton plays the role of corrections officer whose son commits suicide by shooting himself as he tells his father that he had always loved him. This film is a powerful portrayal of grief and exhibits how mourning becomes more complicated when the causes of death are so tragic.

Men Don't Leave **(1990)** This is the story of a young woman, mother of two, whose husband is killed suddenly in a construction accident. The film traces the life of this young widow as she tries to re-establish a life for herself and her children, as a single, working mother, while at the same time trying to cope with her own grief and that of her children.

Stepmom **(1998)** This film portrays the grieving of a divorced mother of two, whose ex-husband is dating a younger woman. The film provides a realistic portrayal of the transitions the family experiences as the mother is dying of cancer.

Kramer vs. Kramer **(1979)** This film portrays a couple's divorce and the impact of the divorce on their son. This film portrays the grieving process that the husband faces, and the feelings of hopelessness and rage that often accompany this grieving process, as he tries to cope with the grief of the lost marriage and then losing his son in the custody battle.

SUGGESTED ACTIVITIES

1. Watch the film *In the Bedroom*. How did the couple depicted in the film deal with the crisis of their son's murder? What differences did you see in how the mother and father grieved? What brings them to taking the drastic steps they did to avenge their son's death? How does this relate to their grief?

2. Watch the film *Ordinary People*. How did each member of the family grieve? How did they respond to the crisis created by Buck's death?

3. Find out how certain burial customs or rituals in our society came about. Discuss the purpose or function of these customs (such as wakes, sitting Shiva, funeral and burial customs, and so on).

4. It is said that when people grieve, they go through various stages. Elizabeth Kubler-Ross described some of the most widely known Stages of Grief: Denial and Isolation, Bargaining, Anger, Depression, and Acceptance. From your experiences with grieving various types of losses, do these stages ring true? Do they match with your experience of grieving a loss? Write about what you personally experienced regarding your own loss.

11

Crises Involving
Suicide & Homicide

DISCUSSION QUESTIONS

What would you do if a friend or family member was threatening to commit suicide? Would you know what to do or who to contact?

In Spring 2006, Virginia Tech experienced a horrible tragedy when a student murdered several students and faculty. From what you read in the newspapers and other media, could this tragedy have been prevented? If so, how?

INTRODUCTION

Of all the types of crises that are presented in this case book, crises involving suicidal risk, violence, and homicidal risk are probably the most difficult and most frightening to manage. Unlike other crises, where intervention plans are collaboratively agreed upon with the person in crisis, suicide and threats of violence may result in a safety plan being enacted without his or her cooperation. The overriding goal of any crisis intervention is to preserve life, however, if a suicidal or homicidal person refuses evaluation or treatment services then crisis counselors are often forced to take immediate protective action. Therefore, if someone threatens to harm themselves or someone else, the crisis counselor cannot just send this person home with instructions to return the following day. Therefore, enacting a crisis plan with those individuals who are either suicidal or homicidal requires decisive, clearheaded action. This is not the time for passive therapeutic reflection, as you will see in the cases presented.

Before exploring case examples, however, it is important to be aware of several factors surrounding suicidal and homicidal intent. First, what brings someone to the point of feeling suicidal or to the brink of violence? Schneidman (1985) notes that one of the driving forces behind most suicides is unendurable psychological pain. Not surprisingly, the three most painful emotions often associated with suicide are self-hate, loneliness, and murderous hatred (Maltsberger, 1992). The statistics regarding suicide are rather alarming. Not only in the United States, but in many industrialized countries, suicide ranks among the leading causes of death (Malley, Kush, & Bogo, 1994). In the United States, for example, over the past ten years there are approximately 30,000 suicide deaths per year, roughly equivalent to more than 80 suicides per day or one suicide death every 20 minutes. Approximately 90% of people who commit suicide have a diagnosable mental illness (National Institute of Mental Health, 2009). In 2006, suicides outnumbered homicides 3:2, and were twice as common as deaths related to HIV and AIDS (National Institute of Mental Health, 2007). Young people between the ages of 15 and 24 are considered to be a high-risk group because suicide ranks among the top leading causes of death in this age group (along with homicide and car accidents). In fact, between 1950 and 1996, suicide rates within this age group tripled (National Center for Health Statistics, 2001). Suicide is the 4th leading cause of death for the 25 to 44 year old age group. Firearms caused the majority of the suicide deaths in the 15 to 24 year old age group; however, it should be noted that firearms constituted the leading cause of death for both adult men and women (National Center for Health Statistics, 1998). According to Maris (1992), therefore, the issues of suicide prevention and gun control are very much intertwined.

Adolescents and young adults are not the only group considered to be at higher risk for suicidal behavior. Males 45 years and older constitute another high-risk group. The research literature suggests that the risk of suicide in men increases with age. This risk is compounded if there is a chronic medical condition that also involves chronic pain. Risk can also be compounded by several other factors including particular psychiatric illnesses, alcohol and drug abuse, and social isolation. Lifetime data indicate that men outnumber women, 4.6:1 in their suicide completion rates (Shaffer, Gould, & Hicks, 1994; Centers for Disease Control, 1998; Kochanek, Murphy, Anderson, & Scott, 2004), however, adolescent and adult women outnumber men in nonfatal suicide attempt rates and in overall rates of depressive illness (Andrews & Lewinsohn, 1992; Frierson, Melikan & Wadman, 2002; Garrison, McKeown, & Valois, 1993).

Of the psychiatric disorders most often associated with suicide, Schizophrenia, Depression (both Major Depression and Bipolar Depression), and substance use disorders (alcohol and drug dependencies) are often positively correlated with suicide. Research indicates that approximately 10% of Schizophrenics commit suicide. Risk factors for suicidality in this population include being male, less than 30 years old, unemployed, having a high level of education, a chronic relapsing course, prior depression in the last episode of active schizo-phrenic symptoms, and a recent hospital discharge. Schizophrenics who com-mit suicide are often painfully aware of their condition and, as a result, often feel inadequate and hopeless. In the majority of instances, Schizophrenic indi-viduals rarely communicate their suicide intent to others. In addition, alcohol and drug abuse exacerbates suicidal risk in this population (Tsuang, Fleming, & Simpson, 1999). In general, alcohol and drug abuse tends to increase suicidal risk in any of the aforementioned "at-risk" populations. Intuitively, drinking or drug use will often intensify an already existing depression, which will add to feelings of hopelessness and helplessness. Alcohol and drug intoxication will often have a disinhibiting effect, thereby making the likelihood of suicidal action much greater. Mood-altering chemicals can also increase the chances of "indirect" sui-cidality, as when someone "accidentally" overdoses or "accidentally" is killed in a single car motor vehicle fatality (Weiss & Hufford, 1999). Suicide is also in-creased in instances where people have endured severe psychological trauma. According to Chu (1999) individuals who have been subject to severe childhood physical or sexual abuse often manifest two traits that place them at substantial risk for suicide: profound mistrust and self-hate.

Naturally, these are just a partial list of discrete risk factors. Often, several predictors must be taken into account when assessing someone who may be suspected of being suicidal. For example, suicidal risk is considered to be much greater when the individual is male; 45 years old or older; separated, wi-dowed, or divorced; lives alone; is unemployed or retired; is in poor physical health; has a mental disorder; drinks heavily; has had medical care within the past six months; has a suicidal plan involving the use of firearms, hanging, jumping, or drowning; has made a prior attempt in the spring or summer months; made the prior attempt at home and was discovered immediately; and does not report his suicidal intention to others. The other difficulty is that a person may manifest three or four of these risk factors and might actually be at lower risk for suicide, while another person may have one of these risk factors and be at high risk for suicide (for example, a depressed teenager with undefined suicidal ideas might be at lower suicidal risk than a teenager who has a prior history of suicide attempts, has voiced a suicide plan, and has begun giving away prized possessions). Assessment of risk is therefore best accom-plished on a case-by-case basis. The dilemma of what weight to give to risk factors is perhaps best summarized by Shneidman (1999), one of the leading authorities on suicide:

> My central belief is that in the distillation of each suicidal event,
> its essential element is a psychological one; that is, each suicidal drama
> occurs in the mind of a unique individual. Suicide is purposeful. Its
> purpose is to respond to or redress certain psychological needs. There
> are many pointless deaths, but there is never a needless suicide. Suicide is

a concatenated, multidimensional, conscious and unconscious "choice" of the best possible practical solution to a perceived problem, dilemma, impulse, crisis, or desperation. (p. 85)

When individuals are assessed for suicidal risk in a crisis situation, usually their entire history and family history is taken into account, as well as their current mental status. A mental status exam usually includes an assessment of present physical appearance, behavior, speech, emotional expression, thought processes, perception, attention and concentration abilities, memory, judgment, intellectual functioning and ability to form insight (Maxmen & Ward, 1995).

Assessing the potential for violence and homicidal threat must also be made on a case-by-case basis and should take into account factors such as a prior history of violent behavior, age, social stressors, substance abuse, personality traits, and psychopathology. It is well accepted that the best predictor of future violence is a past history of violence. In terms of personality traits and psychopathology, there are particular personality characteristics that are often associated with violent, acting-out individuals. These traits would include low-frustration tolerance, impulsivity, immaturity, poor problem-solving, and individuals who see violence as glamorous or a viable solution to life's problems. Three types of psychiatric disorders are often associated with violence and homicidal behavior. They include: Intermittent Explosive Disorder, Paranoid Schizophrenia, and Antisocial Personality Disorder. While not all individuals with Antisocial Personality Disorders are violent, many will resort to violence to achieve personal goals, as would be the case with psychopaths who use violent assault in a robbery or rape, or the spouse abuser who uses violence as a means of control and intimidation. Some of this violent behavior is impulsive and, therefore, spontaneous, while other psychopaths can be very calculated in their violent behavior (Hare, 1993).

Given that one of the best predictors of violent behavior is a past history of such behavior (Litwack, Kirschner, & Wack, 1993; McNiel & Binder, 1991; Meloy, 1987; Monahan, 1995; Mulvey & Lidz, 1995; Slovic & Monahan, 1995; Truscott, Evens, & Mansell, 1995), it is vital to thoroughly explore past history and to gather prior legal and treatment records as quickly as possible. Individuals with criminal histories that include assault and battery offenses, arson, sexual assault, weapons possession, aggravated felonies, domestic violence, drunk and disorderly conduct, property damage, reckless and/or drunk driving, a history of assaultive behavior while hospitalized, and/or naturally prior homicidal threat are considered to be at high risk for violent behavior (Blumenreich & Lewis, 1993; Klassen & O'Connor, 1988). This risk is further increased when the individual is male and has a history of prior victimization (Cavaiola & Schiff, 1988). Although women can also become violent and assaultive, it should be noted that the majority of women imprisoned for murder have committed these acts as "crimes of passion"—a term that refers to the murder of a spouse, boyfriend, or lover in the heat of a jealous rage or as a self-defense against a physically abusive partner.

Violent behavior can also occur situationally. Such would be the case with "road rage" where a person will act out violently or in instances where a person may be outraged by a boss or coworker. Violent behavior can also be exacerbated when individuals are under the influence of alcohol or drugs. Because alcohol intake can have a disinhibiting effect, it is not unexpected that there are correlations between criminally violent behavior and alcohol use (Bradford, Greenberg, & Motayne, 1992). Other mood-altering chemicals associated with a propensity towards violence include stimulant drugs such as amphetamines and cocaine. It is noted that violent behavior (such as accidents, suicide, and homicide) are the leading causes of death among stimulant users (Warner, 1993). Violent behavior has also been associated with certain types of hallucinogens, particularly phencyclidine (PCP), however, some research suggests that PCP does not induce violence in individuals unless they are already prone to violence (Brecher, Wang, Wong, & Morgan, 1988). Steroids have also been known to increase violent behavior, as in the well-known "roid rages" (Pope & Katz, 1990, 1994). Similarly, some types of inhalant abuse has also been linked to violent behavior and delinquency in adolescents (Reed & May, 1984) and in adults who inhale solvents (Dinwiddie, 1994).

The ability to effectively manage individuals who become aggressive or violent is an essential skill for any crisis counselor, police officer, teacher, nurse, or anyone involved in human service work, including customer service representatives, consumer complaint representatives, human resource personnel, and flight attendants. All of the aforementioned individuals may be faced with people who become aggressive or violent. At one time, it was thought that the ability to manage violent or aggressive behavior was needed only for corrections and police officers working with violent criminal types, or for psychiatric aides working with potentially violent psychiatric patients, but the ability to manage violent behavior is essential for anyone working in any human service field.

The goal of crisis intervention with violent or aggressive individuals is to provide safe, non-harmful behavior management (Crisis Prevention Institute, 1999). In order to do so, it is important to fit the intervention with the type of aggressive behavior. In other words, given that individuals may act out either verbally or physically, it is important to match the intervention to the type of aggressive behavior being displayed. For example, with someone who is acting out verbally, it would be an inappropriate overreaction to respond with a physical intervention. Similarly, verbal interventions may be ineffective with someone who is acting out physically by hitting, punching, or biting.

The following case examples provide illustrations of ways that crisis counselors intervene when individuals are in the throes of a suicidal or homicidal crises.

CASE PRESENTATION: The Case of Maria

Maria is a 19-year-old college student in her sophomore year. She told her roommate that she has been feeling depressed over problems that she has been having with her boyfriend. Recently, Maria found out that her boyfriend had been cheating on her with a mutual friend. When she confronted her boyfriend, he denied the accusations and told Maria she was "just being paranoid and crazy," but then seized the moment to break up with her. This made Maria feel more angry and depressed. Maria now feels taken and used. She cannot get out of bed and has been missing classes. She did well in her freshman year, but is receiving a scholarship and is afraid that if her grades drop she will lose the scholarship and have to return home to attend a local community college. Maria reports that she feels overwhelmed. She feels that nothing she does will make things any better. She tried calling the hotline of the local mental health clinic today because she felt so "upset" that she was considering taking her roommates prescription medication and washing it down with vodka. Maria explained to the hotline crisis worker that she had been in counseling while she was in high school after her parents separated. Maria described feeling "lifeless and hopeless," having no energy to do anything. She also reported that nothing is really enjoyable to her anymore and that, as a result, she has become more and more reclusive, preferring to be alone. Maria also stated that she has not been eating or sleeping very well. Although she initially told the crisis worker that she was not feeling suicidal, she stated that since the problems with her boyfriend began she feels she has nothing to live for.

Maria's history and presenting complaint reveals someone who is considered to be at risk for suicide. She feels isolated, angry, hopeless, and helpless. Maria is experiencing the loss of the relationship with her boyfriend and is in danger of losing her educational opportunity. In addition, she has thought about a plan of how she would kill herself. What makes this case difficult to assess is that the initial contact occurs by Maria calling a psychiatric hotline. There would be many advantages to conducting this assessment face-to-face if she were to have been seen in a clinic or emergency room, however, the crisis counselor is usually quite limited in how much information they will be able to obtain over the phone. The crisis counselor would first need to establish rapport and try to connect with Maria. Also, the crisis counselor will need to convey a willingness to listen to Maria's problems nonjudgmentally and convey that she is willing to help Maria work out some solutions to the problems she is encountering. The counselor needs to be very definite in convincing Maria that treatment works and that she can help her get through the present crisis. It is of utmost importance to provide hope (Bohen, 2002). This is sometimes difficult, as many suicidal individuals feel that there are no solutions, therefore, suicide is perceived as their only viable alternative and solution. However, Maria did call the crisis hotline, which can be viewed as a positive step and a cry for help.

Intervention

The crisis counselor needs to ally with that part of Maria that wants to live and that part of her personality that gave her the courage to call the hotline. Once Maria reveals that she had been experiencing suicidal feelings and has thought of a plan, the counselor would then need to assess Maria's current feelings regarding suicidal intent as follows:

COUNSELOR: Maria, I was wondering, given what you've told me so far, if you're feeling like harming yourself or wanting to end your life.

MARIA: Well, what if I do? Does that mean you're going to lock me up? Then I know I'd be thrown out of school.

COUNSELOR: No, Maria, I want to help you find some answers to the problems you've been having, which is why you called, isn't it? From what you've told me, you've really been going through a tough time.

MARIA: I have. It's really been horrible. I can't sleep, I can't eat. When I do sleep, I wake up at like 3:00 a.m. and begin thinking about Jimmy having sex with one of my best friends. I can't stand it.

COUNSELOR: How long have you been feeling like this?

MARIA: It's been a few weeks I guess. I can't keep track of time. I've also been missing all of my classes and now I know I'll fail everything.

Maria has avoided answering the counselor's original question about feeling suicidal, so the counselor redirects Maria to the question.

COUNSELOR: With all that you've been going through, have you had any suicidal thoughts?

MARIA: I have been thinking that I would just be better off dead. At least it would be a way of ending all this pain.

COUNSELOR: Maria, are you feeling suicidal right now? Is that why you called today?

MARIA: No, I think I just needed to talk to someone. I was feeling really alone, and I'd heard about this crisis hotline and thought it might be helpful to talk. Besides, I don't think I really want to die. I just want the hurt to stop.

COUNSELOR: I'm glad you decided to call. From what you've told me, I can hear how much pain you've been in. It must be really tough to be trying to deal with all this on your own. Let's talk about some things that might help you begin to feel better.

MARIA: I'd like that. I really don't want to flunk out and have to go back home.

COUNSELOR: I know that your college has a counseling center. If you were to go and speak with one of the counselors there, they can often help with talking to your professors to let them know that you're trying to get back to your studies.

MARIA: Will the counselor have to tell them the details of why I've missed classes?

COUNSELOR: No, they won't give details; just that you've had to miss class.

MARIA: That sounds like it would be helpful.

COUNSELOR: The counseling center can also arrange for ongoing counseling at no cost because you're a student there. Usually they will refer students over here at the medical center, if they think that medication may be helpful. Have you ever been in counseling before or taken any medication?

MARIA: I saw someone for counseling when I was in high school and my parents were separating. They had me on medication for about four months, then my parents got back together and I began to feel better.

COUNSELOR: Was the counseling helpful?

MARIA: It was helpful to talk about how I was feeling. My parents were fighting a lot and I began to develop irritable bowel syndrome. I guess because of the stress.

(continued)

C A S E   P R E S E N T A T I O N :   The Case of Maria (*continued*)

Case Conceptualization/Crisis Resolution

Maria went on to explain to the crisis counselor more about her parent's separation. The counselor was able to use this information to illustrate to Maria how she was able to make it through previous crises in her life, therefore, she would be able to make it through the present crisis. They also go on to talk about Maria's relationship with Jimmy and some of the problems they had been having. Maria had begun to feel that Jimmy was taking her for granted and was being verbally and emotionally abusive to her. Maria felt that she couldn't break free of the relationship but she was not really happy either. At this point, the counselor had obtained a commitment from Maria to see someone in the college counseling center and Maria allowed the counselor to call so that she would be seen that day. Maria also agreed that she would come to the medical center and speak with someone if she felt suicidal again. If the counselor had determined that Maria was in danger of harming herself at that particular moment, it would have been necessary for the counselor to trace the call through the telephone operator and have the police or a mobile mental health outreach team sent to Maria's apartment. If that were the case, Maria would then be brought to the local emergency room or mental health clinic for assessment and likely be admitted to a hospital for observation. Whereas, if it was determined that she was not actively suicidal, then she might be treated on an outpatient basis with a combination of counseling and antidepressant medication.

The crisis hotline intervention with Maria raises three issues that are central to working with suicidal patients. First, suicidal individuals often view their deaths as a solution to their problems or as a means to end the psychological, emotional, or physical pain they are experiencing. Second, suicidal individuals often feel that their lives are out of control or often feel overwhelmed by their problems and think that the only way to take control is through taking their own lives. Third, some suicides are motivated by revenge. There is an old saying that "behind every suicide, there is a homicide." This notion is derived primarily from Psychoanalytic theory, which indicates that suicide occurs in instances where anger is "turned inward" or against the self. This is true with many adolescents and young adults who view suicide as a means of getting back at a boyfriend or girlfriend who has rejected them or getting revenge against an overbearing parent.

In providing crisis intervention to a person in the throes of a suicidal crisis, the LAPC model can be utilized as a format to help manage the crisis. In the **Listening** phase, the crisis counselor first establishes rapport with Maria by talking about non-threatening topics. The counselor then begins to gather information about the crisis by asking about the particulars regarding Maria's reasons for seeking help and the difficulties she has been experiencing. It is also important to determine when Maria first began to feel suicidal and if she has had any previous history of suicidal ideation, intent, or attempts. If so, what happened as a result of these feelings or actions? Suicidal risk factors can also be determined at this point.

In the **Assess** phase, the counselor notes Maria's predominant emotional reactions. Maria expresses feelings of hopelessness and also states that she feels overwhelmed and unable to function. It is also noted that although Maria has every right to feel angry and betrayed by Jimmy, she instead feels defeated and helpless. Given that the presence of past depression and current suicidal ideation, the counselor would gather information for a lethality assessment. A lethality assessment would involve a thorough exploration of the suicide risk factors that Maria is manifesting. A lethality assessment also includes questions pertaining to whether Maria has a suicidal plan and a means to carry out that plan. Usually, plans that are more concrete, specific, and feasible are considered more dangerous than the lack of a plan or a plan that is vague and unlikely. One of the ultimate questions of the lethality assessment pertains to whether or not Maria falls into high risk factor status. It is noted that Maria manifests several risk factors—she has a previous history depression when her parents separated, she currently manifests many symptoms of depression, she is isolated and is feeling the loss of her relationship with her boyfriend, and she is experiencing the psychological turmoil over Jimmy's affair with her best friend. Maria's thinking appears to be impacted by depression and suicidal thoughts, otherwise she is able to reason logically and express herself coherently. Her attention span is adequate and there are no indications of any current medical problems.

In the **Planning** phase, the counselor attempts to determine if there is anyone whom Maria can reach out to for help. Maria's safety is the main priority, and here the counselor is making certain that Maria has support, in this instance through the college counseling center. The **Plan** agreed upon is that Maria will see a counselor at the counseling center who will also help Maria get back into her classes without being penalized. With regards to **Commitment**, it appears that Maria does have the resources to carry through with the plan to begin counseling and appears to be motivated, at this time, to follow through with the plan that has been agreed upon.

The major concern in providing crisis counseling to a person who is suicidal is that they are SAFE. But what if the person refuses help? Most states provide some procedure for an involuntary hospitalization or commitment of persons who present as a danger to themselves or others. According to Frierson, Melikian, and Wadman (2002), there are essentially three categories of potentially suicidal individuals: 1) patients with suicidal ideation, plan, and intent; 2) patients with ideation and plan but without intent; and 3) patients with ideation but no plan or intent. Patients that fall within the first group (especially when they have accompanying psychosocial stressors and access to a lethal means of suicide), should be psychiatrically hospitalized (either voluntarily or involuntarily, if necessary). Patients that fall within the second group, (suicidal ideation and plan but without intent) may be treated on an outpatient basis provided they have a good social support network and no access to lethal means of suicide. Some patients within this group, however, may require hospitalization if the environment cannot be assured as being safe or if they are not adequately supervised. For patients in the third group, outpatient treatment is recommended, however, again only if the environment is safe (for example, all weapons are removed from the dwelling), and there is adequate social support and supervision. For patients in the second and third groups, their willingness and motivation to seek treatment and naturally follow through with therapy will play a role in determining their suitability for outpatient treatment.

What would happen, though, if the son or daughter is not a child or adolescent, but a young adult (such as a college student)? Confidentiality regulations and professional ethical guidelines clearly specify that patient-doctor privilege requires information discussed in counseling to remain strictly confidential, *except* in instances involving danger to self or others. Many counselors, psychologists, and treatment agencies use an Informed Consent to Treatment form (which is signed by patients at the onset of treatment), which specifies that confidentiality can be broken in instances of suicidal or homicidal threat or suspected child abuse. In a lawsuit filed against the Massachusetts Institute of Technology, it is alleged that MIT administrators had not acted responsibly in preventing the death of an MIT student who purposely set herself on fire in her dorm room (Sontag, 2002). The suit alleges that the MIT staff did not inform the parents of their daughter's suicidal threats.

CASE PRESENTATION: Richard

Richard is a 43-year-old separated father of two. He had sought counseling at the recommendation of a coworker who was concerned about Richard making "threatening remarks" and depressive statements. This coworker was also worried because of Richard's increased use of alcohol and explosive temper outbursts at work. Richard explains that he recently separated from his wife after 20 years of marriage and that he does not know if he can go on without her. He is restless and angry as he describes how his wife "kicked him out of his home" because she wanted to "find herself." Richard suspects she is seeing a guy she works with at her part-time job. Richard states that the thought of them together "drives me crazy" and apparently, this is where his threats are focused. Richard had made some vague threats about killing his wife and lover, if he ever caught them together, and has also threatened to wait for him after work and beat him up. Richard denies any domestic abuse history in his relationship with his wife. Richard is currently living alone in a rented room and has few friends, other than his coworker, whom he seems to trust and confide in. Richard also confided in his coworker that he has both a handgun and a rifle in his possession.

Intervention

The crisis counselor working with Richard must make an assessment of both the potential for violence/homicide as well as suicide, and come up with a strategy that will ensure the safety of all involved. In the following session excerpt, the crisis counselor has already established a rapport with Richard and is now trying to assess the potential for acting out. What if Richard had walked out? What would the crisis counselor do? In an instance of either homicidal or suicidal threat, the counselor would need to consider reporting these threats to the police. In keeping with the Tarasoff (1976) ruling, the counselor would also need to consider whether or not to report the threats to both Carol and her boyfriend. Even if Richard agrees to go into the hospital as planned, there would still need to be a consideration of whether or not to notify Carol and her boyfriend of the threats. It is likely, given the homicidal and suicidal threats, that if Richard were to try to sign himself out of the hospital that he would be involuntarily committed, however, under the Tarasoff ruling potential victims may still need to be notified of the threats.

COUNSELOR: So, Richard you've given me a lot of background about yourself and your marriage to Carol, I can see how devastated you are by the separation.

RICHARD: You have no idea what this has been like for me. I can't sleep; I can't eat; I know the alcohol is not helping. I'm a mess.

COUNSELOR: From what you were telling me before, it sounded like you were seriously thinking about harming Carol and the guy you suspect she is seeing?

RICHARD: If I tell you, you promise you won't lock me up or anything?

COUNSELOR: Richard, my main concern right now is making sure you and Carol are safe. I want to help you come up with a plan that will make that possible.

RICHARD: Well, I was planning on going to where she works and if I saw her with that wife-stealer, I was going to shoot both of them and then myself.

COUNSELOR: Had you planned when you were going to do this?

RICHARD: Not really, maybe within the next few days. I waited outside of her work the last few nights and I didn't see them leave together, but I know he goes over to the house. That drives my up a wall, that's my house.

COUNSELOR: Richard if you did shoot them and then yourself, what would happen to your two daughters?

As suggested by Linehan (1999), the counselor is trying to get Richard to look at the possible consequences of his actions and that his plan is not a good solution to his problem.

RICHARD: I don't know, good question. Well I guess they would end up with my mother-in-law, both of my parents are dead, I have one sister and she has multiple sclerosis, so she's in no shape to take care of them.

COUNSELOR: What would it be like for your daughters knowing that their parents are dead, that their father killed their mother, and that they now are living with their grandmother?

RICHARD: Horrible, overwhelming; I couldn't do that to them. Besides, my mother-in-law is such a bitch, the girls would turn out just like her.

COUNSELOR: So let's talk about how to get you back to where you can function and think clearly again. It sounds like you could use a break from all this, after all you're not eating, not sleeping. What about going into the hospital for a break?

RICHARD: If you told me that a few minutes ago, I would have walked out of here, but now that you put the consequences out there, it does make sense.

Case Conceptualization/Crisis Resolution

Richard's situation represents a crisis that has the potential for violent acting out, with both homicidal and suicidal outcomes. This type of crisis would be one of the most frightening to work with because of its many inherent dangers; yet, one should also note that Richard does not appear to fit into any of the diagnostic groups that are most likely to act out aggressively. Instead, the catalyst to his crisis was the recent marital separation and Richard's suspicions and fears that his wife is now involved in another relationship. His sexual jealousy fuels his anger and fear, and his alcohol abuse makes the likelihood of his acting out even greater. The fact that Richard has a means of carrying out his plans for vengeance (because he owns firearms) also lends more urgency to this crisis. The research literature on murder-suicide also suggests this to be a high-risk situation. Marzuk, Tardiff, and Hirsch (1992) found the average age of murder-suicide perpetrators is 39.6 years old. Approximately, 93–97% are Caucasian (Copeland, 1985; Currens et al., 1991) and 85% of the victims are female (Hanzlick & Koponen, 1994). The principal method used in most cases is firearms, which are used in 80–94% of the cases (Copeland, 1985; Currens et al., 1991). The central theme found in most murder-suicides is that the perpetrator is overly attached to a relationship and when the relationship is threatened with dissolution, this leads to the destruction of the relationship and self (Nock & Murzuck, 1999). Murder-suicide between spouses and lovers accounts for 50–75% of all murder-suicides in the United States (Dorpat, 1966; Palmer & Humphrey, 1980; Allen, 1983; Currens et al., 1991). These relationships are often differentiated by emotional abusiveness and sexual jealousy.

**C A S E   P R E S E N T A T I O N : A Case Involving the
Threat of Violence**

---

*Jason has been court ordered to the local mental health clinic for an evaluation after
his landlord claimed that he threatened to kill him over a dispute involving payment
of back rent. Jason is a 28-year-old single male, who is currently on parole after serving five years in the state penitentiary for a variety of offenses including sexual assault, attempted rape, robbery, and aggravated assault. His parole officer provided
information to the mental health clinic regarding these convictions. In addition,
Jason identifies himself as a "skinhead" and a member of the Aryan nation. His
landlord is from Jamaica. The threats of violence are therefore racially motivated and
may constitute a bias crime. In talking with Jason, the counselor notes that he is very
guarded in revealing any information about his prior convictions. Jason only states
that he was "framed" and that the woman whom he was accused of assaulting had
invited him into her house. The other conviction involved his assaulting an elderly
man and stealing his wallet. Jason has absolutely no remorse or guilt over these incidents. Jason's history reveals that he has been in and out of institutions since he was
eight years old. There were several instances where he broke into neighbor's homes
and stole valuables. He also set fire to another neighbor's garage without any
cause or provocation. When asked about these prior incidents, Jason just shrugged
his shoulders and replied, "I thought it would be a fun thing to do, besides it
wasn't like I was hurting anyone or anything." When he was 16 years old, he was
sent to a state reformatory for boys for allegedly beating up an elderly man and
stealing his car. What was noteworthy, however, was that for each offense Jason
had an elaborate story as to why he was not responsible for the offense or how
he was "framed" by someone else. When asked about the threats to his landlord,
Jason merely replied that he has been "buggin" him for the rent for the past three
weeks and "when I get mine, he'll get his." He refuses to elaborate further on this
remark.*

In this case vignette, the crisis counselor is trying to work with Jason who has
come in, not so much in crisis, but more because of the Court's recommendation that
he submit to evaluation and possible counseling. The counselor is again faced with
the dilemma of trying to assess the risk of violence, given the alleged threats that
Jason has made against his landlord. Unlike Richard who had no prior psychiatric history or history of violent behavior, Jason has a record of both. However, because the
session is court-ordered, there are certainly limits to how much truthful information
the counselor will be able to obtain.

Intervention

COUNSELOR: Jason, tell me something about the accusations and possible parole
violation you are facing?

JASON: Is this being recorded? I'd rather not have what I say recorded, you know,
for legal purposes.

COUNSELOR: No, there is no audio or video recording of our meeting.

JASON: Man, I swear to you, I just told the guy to get off my back, that's the way
it happened.

COUNSELOR: Do you have any prior convictions?

JASON: Yeah, I got jammed up a couple of times before. Once on a rape charge, that was back in '98, and about four times on assault charges. I also did time when I was 16 in Jamesburg State Reformatory for Boys on an arson charge.

COUNSELOR: Tell me about the other assault charges.

JASON: What's there to tell? I was working as a construction supervisor for about six months or so and after work some of the crew and I would go down to the bar for some drinks. One thing would lead to another and the next thing you know, somebody was calling the damn cops. I wasn't doing anything that the others weren't doing.

COUNSELOR: And what about the situation with your landlord? Can you tell me something about that?

JASON: Well, there's not much to tell. I've been out of work for the past two months, so, naturally, I can't make my rent and this guy won't give me a moment of peace. He is constantly on my back, so I said some things that would kind of shut him up for a while. The cops are also tryin' to pin a bias crime charge on me because the guy's from Jamaica. I just know he's black and I don't get along with blacks from the time I was in Jamesburg. White kids don't do well in the system if you know what I mean.

COUNSELOR: What do you mean?

JASON: Well, let's put it this way, if you didn't stand up for yourself or join the Aryans, you might as well cut your own throat.

COUNSELOR: So what will you do to your landlord if he doesn't get off your back?

JASON: Nothing, Doc, honest, I just want to get him to lighten up.

COUNSELOR: Do you have any weapons—guns or knives?

JASON: No, I don't because I'm on parole.

Case Conceptualization/Crisis Resolution

In this case example, Jason typifies so many of the attitudes and behaviors of those individuals with Antisocial Personality Disorder. For example, his attitude toward the current allegation of threatening his landlord is very glib and nonchalant. He does not take responsibility for his actions. In a crisis assessment situation such as that described, it would not necessarily be the counselor's role to confront Jason on his behavior or to try to do the therapeutic work that would be done in long term therapy. Unfortunately, as indicated earlier, people with Antisocial Personality Disorders do not often present in crisis unless they have been caught in the act of, accused of, or planning criminal actions, at which point, they may be referred for assessment.

In preparation for this evaluation, the counselor and the clinic should make some preparations. They should alert the office staff to be vigilant and listen for a code phrase that indicates the counselor is feeling threatened. They should occupy an office in a busy area of the building and the counselor should sit closest to the door. In the event that Jason were to become more agitated to the point of threatening violence (either verbally or through physical actions such as slamming his fist on the

(continued)

C A S E P R E S E N T A T I O N : A Case Involving the
                                    Threat of Violence (*continued*)

---

table), then the crisis counselor would need to employ some *defusing* techniques. The following are some defusing strategies that might be used with a potentially violent individual:

1. *Understand the mindset of the hostile or potentially violent person.* These individuals often have a compelling need to communicate their grievances to someone—now! Even if these individuals are wrong, they are acting on perceptions that are real to them. In the overwhelming number of cases, they just want to be heard and treated fairly.
2. *Practice "Active Listening."* Stop what you are doing to give these individuals your full attention. Listen to what is really being said. Use silence and paraphrasing. Ask clarifying, open-ended questions.
3. *Build trust and provide help. Avoid confrontation.* Be calm, sit still, be courteous, respectful, and patient. It is important to be open and honest, but do not make promises you can't keep. Never belittle these individuals, embarrass them, or verbally confront potentially violent people.
4. *Allow a total airing of the grievance without comment or judgment.* While they are airing their grievances, make eye contact, but don't stare (that can be perceived as a challenge). Let individuals have their say, while ignoring challenges or insults. Don't take venting personally; redirect their attention to the real issues.
5. *Allow the aggrieved to suggest a solution.* they will more readily agree to a resolution that they have helped to formulate.
6. *Move towards a "win-win" solution.* Preserve these individuals' dignity. Switch the focus from what they cannot do, toward what they can do.

There may be times, however, when you will need to call in additional resources such as a supervisor, security, another counselor, or, if necessary, call the police if you feel you are in danger. If danger is imminent then it is not necessary to obtain consent from the client in order to call for assistance (Bohen, 2002, p. 27).

RECOMMENDATIONS FOR CHAPTER ENRICHMENT

SUGGESTED FILMS

Dead Poet's Society **(1989)** This film depicts the suicide death of a student who feels trapped by a demanding, perfectionist father who refuses to allow his son to pursue his interests in acting. Robin Williams plays a teacher at the exclusive boys boarding school who is blamed for encouraging the student to pursue his interests and is subsequently fired from his teaching position.

Girl Interrupted **(1999)** A young woman is psychiatrically hospitalized following a suicide attempt. The film also focuses on how she then attempts to put her life together after her hospitalization. The film graphically depicts the suicide death of one of the main characters.

1. Is there a past history of any of the following?
   - violent behavior   y/n
   - property destruction   y/n
   - attempted homicide   y/n
   - stalking   y/n
   - other criminal behavior   y/n
   - intimate partner violence   y/n
   - other family violence   y/n
   - bullying of others   y/n
   - child abuse (client)   y/n
   - incarceration   y/n
   - job loss due to threats   y/n
   - school expulsion   y/n
   - fascination with weapons   y/n
   - fascination with explosives   y/n
   - animal cruelty   y/n
   - past psychiatric treatment   y/n
   - alcohol or drug abuse   y/n
   - steroid abuse   y/n
   - abuse of other substances (specify) _____

   Are there:
2. present threats of violence?   y/n
3. violent or homicidal plan?   y/n
4. recent homicidal plan or behavior?   y/n
5. violent obsessions or ideation?   y/n
6. means or method to carry out plan?   y/n
7. recent disruption in interpersonal relationships (such as a separation)?   y/n

FIGURE 11.1 Lethality Assessment Form—Homicide/Violent Threat

Falling Down **(1993)** A middle-class businessman becomes progressively violent as the film unfolds. It is interesting to see how a chain of events and catalysts seem to push the main character towards further violent behavior. In watching this film, look for various risk factors for violent behavior such as those presented in Figure 11.1 Lethality Assessment—Homicide/Violent Threat.

Cape Fear **(1991)** Robert De Niro provides an excellent portrayal of someone with Antisocial Personality Disorder who uses violence and threats of violence throughout the film.

SUGGESTED ACTIVITIES

1. Watch either *Dead Poet's Society* or *Girl Interrupted* and determine those factors that were the prime motivators for the character taking his or her own life.

_____	Gender (Male)
_____	Age (15–24 yrs old or > 45)
_____	History of previous attempts or suicidal ideation expressed
_____	Medical illness (especially a chronic condition involving pain)
_____	Psychiatric illness (especially Major Depression, Bipolar Disorder, Substance Use Disorders, and Schizophrenia)
_____	Decline in socioeconomic status (e.g. job loss, major financial loss)
_____	Relationship loss (e.g. separation, divorce, widowed)
_____	Lack of Social Support
_____	Suicide Plan with means to carrying out plan (e.g. presence of firearm)
_____	Hopelessness/Helplessness (feelings expressed that their situation is hopeless and/or they feel powerless to change their situation)
_____	Radical shifts in mood or behavior (e.g. person gives away prized possessions or begins to say "goodbye" to loved ones, family, takes care of unfinished business)
_____	History of severe trauma (e.g. history or sexual assault or other trauma)

FIGURE 11.2 Lethality Assessment Form—Risk Factors for Suicide

Does the character who commits suicide fit the profile of those considered at risk for suicide? In order to determine this, you should fill out Figure 11.2 Lethality Assessment—Risk Factors for Suicide form above. What steps could have been taken to prevent the suicide of this character?

2. Read each of the case vignettes listed below. Rank in order which individual you feel is at highest risk to lowest risk for suicide. Discuss why you ranked them as you did. In other words, justify your rank ordering.

   a. Case Vignette #1: Rebecca is a 22-year-old college student, who has been dating Justin for the past two years. Approximately three days ago, Rebecca overheard two other students in one of her classes talking about seeing Justin hook up with someone they know at a party. At first Rebecca thought her classmates were talking about someone else, but when she asked them to describe Justin, the description they gave, along with other information, confirmed for Rebecca that it was her boyfriend. Rebecca confronted Justin later that evening and, although he did not deny that he was at the party, he denied that he was with another woman and became angry that Rebecca would believe these total strangers over him. Rebecca was distraught and could not stop crying. That evening, when she got back to her dorm room, she took 50 aspirin and made some cuts on her wrist. Her roommate called the Resident Assistant who then called the Campus Counseling Center. Rebecca was brought to the local emergency room by Campus Police. The crisis screener interviewed Rebecca and found that she had been treated for depression while in high school and was given Prozac. She had not had any history of suicidal behavior but the family history reveals that her uncle committed suicide in the aftermath of being arrested for embezzling from the corporation he worked for. Rebecca indicates that she doesn't really want to kill herself, she just wanted to get back at Justin.

b. Case Vignette #2: Sal is 62 years old and recently retired from his job as a police captain in a small suburban town. He took an early retirement because his wife had recently died of liver cancer and also because of an injury he sustained about five years ago. Sal had been a shift supervisor when he received a call for backup from one of his patrolmen. The patrolman had been called to the scene of a domestic violence dispute where the husband was intoxicated and threatening. As Sal was about to put the husband in handcuffs, the man bolted out of the door and began to run to the back of the house. Sal fell as he ran through the yards to catch him and suffered a major knee injury, which required surgery. Sal experiences a lot of pain from his injured knee even though the injury occurred five years ago. He has been given Percocet for the pain, which he will often take in order to get to sleep. Sal was very proud of being a policeman and feels he has been "useless" since the injury. He did feel good about taking care of his wife during her battle with cancer, but felt lonely and empty when she died. Sal visits her grave everyday and says he cannot wait until he "joins" his wife. Sal still sees some of his coworkers from the police department and every so often they will go to the pistol range for the afternoon.

c. Case Vignette #3: Hans is 24 years old and had recently moved to the United States after having lived in Denmark all of his life. He spent a couple of years at the University of Copenhagen but ran out of money and could not continue his studies. He planned to become an architect, but decided to put his plans on hold until he could find a job in the U.S. and begin to save some money. The only job Hans was able to find, however, was working as a janitor in a department store. He does not speak English very well, and finds himself feeling lonely and depressed. He says that he feels like a failure and that he should just "give up."

This exercise was based on a classroom activity described by Madson, L. & Vas, C. (2003). Learning risk factors for suicide: A scenario-based activity. *Teaching of Psychology, 30,* 123–126.

3. You are looking for a parking space in the parking lot of the local mall when you see someone pulling out ahead of you. You put on your blinker as you approach the space, but see another car rounding the corner with their blinker also on. Because the car leaving the space is pulling out in direction of the other car, it allows you to pull into the space. You turn your car off and are about to get out, when all of a sudden you are confronted by the the other car's driver who is yelling and shouting obscenities at you and threatens to drag you out of your car and "beat you to a pulp." Using the defusing

techniques discussed in this chapter, how would you deal with this situation?

4. You are having a quiet lunch in the student center when you are confronted by another student who accuses you of "hitting on" their boyfriend/girl-friend. The student starts yelling and screaming and his or her anger is escalating. How would you manage this situation?

12

School Crisis: Prevention and Intervention

DISCUSSION QUESTIONS

In your own experiences in school, what would you consider the most disruptive crisis-type event you remember? How did the school staff and administration cope with it? What was your own reaction to it?

Think back to those individuals with whom you attended school. Were there any whom you "profiled" in your own mind who might be the type who would instigate some level of violence within the school? What contributed to your impression of that individual?

Who were those groups in your school who were the likely ones to engage in bullying of others? Who were the likely ones to be the victims of bullies?

INTRODUCTION

School crises come in many forms. They can be from internal or external sources, from the hands of individuals or from nature itself. Internal crisis types are varied: the student who brings firearms to school for the purposes of evening a score with a teacher, administrator, or other student; the random, unplanned shooting of rival gang members in the school corridors; the suicide of a popular student or staff member; the untimely death of any member of the school community. External crisis types are equally as varied: motor vehicle accidents that claim the lives of students and staff; armed school intruders; industrial accidents; natural weather disasters that devastate communities.

Nothing resonates more with the American public, however, than yet another evening news story of violence within its schools. School shootings, as rare as they are horrific, lead the list of such events that have forever shaken the image of schools as safe and secure environments in which students learn and flourish. Televised images of traumatized children being comforted by rescue workers and parents in the aftermath of such tragedies are encoded in the consciousness of the television-viewing public.

No images have cast a greater pall on the American public than those of the events of April 20, 1999, in Littleton, Colorado, when Eric Harris and Dylan Klebold, students at Columbine High School, entered the school with an arsenal of weapons and killed 12 students and one teacher before turning the guns on themselves. They also wounded another 23 of their fellow students in the rampage, making this event the nation's deadliest school shooting. Since that day, another 25 school shootings have taken place in this country.

Even though these high-profile shootings are the least representative of homicides at school (Cornell, 2006), it can be argued that the extensive media coverage of such incidents of school violence has significantly exacerbated fears about it, suggesting the probability of harm that is out of proportion to the reality of harm for the typical student (Reddy, Borum, Berglund, Vossekuil, Fein, & Modzeleski, 2001). Despite the coverage of such high-profile events as school shootings, however, schools remain the safest places that children go (Poland & Gorin, 2002). Only a few of the approximately 60 million school children in this country who attend the nation's 119,000 schools will ever fall prey to a serious instance of violence in the schools they attend.

The Indicators of School Crime and Safety (2006), the ninth annual report produced jointly by the National Center for Education Statistics and the Bureau of Justice Statistics, demonstrated that school violence had decreased in most areas among secondary students between the years 1993 and 2005. The numbers of homicides, suicides, thefts, and violent crimes declined during this time period. From July 1, 2004, to June 30, 2005, there was the equivalent of one homicide or suicide of a school-age child (ages 5–18) at school for every two million students enrolled. Youth were over 50 times more likely to be murdered and almost 150 times more likely to commit suicide when they were away from school than at school. Even immediately after the Columbine shooting, it was argued that the odds that a child would die in school from homicide or suicide were close to one in two million (Brooks, Schiraldi, & Ziedenberg, 2000). Students are simply safer at school than they are away from school (DeVoe, Peter, Noonan, Snyder, & Baum, 2005).

Nevertheless, the death or violent victimization of even one student is a tragedy, whether showcased on the evening news or not. Individuals, families, and entire school communities are sent reeling in the aftershock of most crisis events. The manner in which schools cope with such events, both during and immediately after them, often determines how quickly the schools return to some level of pre-crisis equilibrium. Nowhere is the need for coordination and teamwork in crisis response more apparent than in the schools where multiple levels of the system must be prepared to spring into action and to undertake a variety of tasks designed to mitigate the effects of the crisis. From the adoption of policies and procedures regarding crisis preparedness and response by local boards of education all the way through to the implementation of such procedures by all levels of school staff, the task of effective crisis response is a daunting one. Coordination of such efforts with local community agencies for law enforcement, medical, and mental health assistance also adds yet another level of need to the crisis response protocol.

This chapter will focus on the entire school community's response to crisis events, both internal and external, which have an impact on schools and school children. The primary crisis events discussed will be school shootings, the unanticipated deaths of students by accident and suicide, and a school's response to the events of September 11, 2001.

PREVENTION FIRST

No discussion of school crisis intervention should be held without first addressing those school-related and other factors that contribute to the prevention of such events. To wait until a crisis presents itself is to overlook more positive prevention practices that can actually reduce the likelihood of, albeit not eliminate, some of these events and that can mitigate the emotional upheaval of the post-crisis aftermath. The importance of prevention was underscored by the National Association of School Psychologists, which adopted *Prevention is an Intervention* as its theme for the 2005–06 school year. This section will briefly address those school factors that are preventative in nature and that can help to reduce instances of school violence.

SCHOOL VIOLENCE

In 2002, the United States Secret Service, in collaboration with the United States Department of Education, completed the Safe School Initiative (SSI), a study of school shootings and other school-based attacks that took place between 1974 and 2000. The study focused on what the agencies defined as "targeted school violence," those incidents of violence where an attacker selected a particular target (such as a fellow student(s), teacher, administrator, and so on) prior to the violent attack; in fact, in over half the incidents, the shooter had targeted at least one school administrator, faculty member, or staff member. Those other random, unplanned, and impulsive shooting episodes in the schools were not included in the SSI. Although there have been over 20 school shootings since the period included in the SSI, the report examined a total of 37 incidents of targeted violence involving 41 student attackers. The purpose of the study was to identify those aspects of school shooters and shootings that might be identifiable before other shootings occur, thereby preventing additional ones.

In addition to an exhaustive review of records from multiple sources, the SSI investigators also interviewed 10 of these school shooters. The study arrived at 10 key findings:

- *Incidents at school are rarely sudden, impulsive acts.* More than half of the shooters developed the idea to harm the victim(s) at least two weeks prior to the attack, and, more than half planned the actual attacks at least two days before they struck. Most shooters had revenge as a motive, and many communicated their grievances to others prior to the attack.

- *Prior to most incidents, other people knew about the shooter's intent and/or actual plan.* In almost all of the cases studied in the SSI, the shooters told a peer (friend, schoolmate, or sibling) about the plan; they told more than one person in over half the incidents.

    One attacker told two friends about what he had planned and had arranged for several others to be in a safe place at the time of the shooting. When the fateful morning arrives, the word had spread to a total of 24 students, all of whom had assembled on the mezzanine overlooking the school lobby (the site announced beforehand by the shooter). One of the students who knew of the attack in advance even brought a camera to take pictures of the event.

- *Most attackers did not threaten their targets directly before the attacks.* Instead, worrisome behaviors or communications from the shooter were not heeded by others and did not prompt a response from the schools before the attacks.

- *There is no accurate "profile" of students who engage in targeted school violence.* Ages ranged from 11 to 21. They came from a variety of racial and ethnic backgrounds, from a variety of family situations, and from a wide range of academic performance (from excellent to failing). Some shooters were socially popular, some were social isolates; some had no documented behavioral problems, whereas some had a history of such. In short, the SSI uncovered no school-shooter "type." The only common thread throughout all shooters was simple: they were all male.

- *Most shooters engaged in some behavior prior to the incidents that caused others concern, usually adults.* These behaviors included expressed wishes to obtain a gun and themes of homicide or suicide in conversations or in classroom writing assignments.

- *Most attackers had problems coping with personal loss or failure.* Many (nearly three-quarters) also had threatened or attempted suicide.

- *Many attackers felt bullied, persecuted, or injured by others.* A number of them experienced bullying and harassment that was chronic and severe.

- *Most attackers had access to and had used handguns.* In almost two-thirds of the cases, the shooter got the gun used in the attack from his own home or that of a relative. The gun also had been a gift from the shooter's parents in some cases.

- *Other students were involved in the attack in some capacity.* Although most shooters acted alone, in almost half the cases others encouraged them to complete the act. One shooter was convinced by his friends that the only way for him to get other students to stop harassing him was to actually shoot kids at school in order to appear tough.

- *Despite the response of law enforcement to the attacks, most attacks were brief and were stopped by people other than law enforcement.* In over half the attacks, faculty or fellow students stopped the attack, or the attacker killed himself. Although the Columbine High School attack lasted over three hours, half of these incidents were over in 20 minutes or less, long before law enforcement arrived.

IMPLICATIONS FOR PREVENTION

The findings from the SSI strongly suggested that some school attacks might be preventable; many people, particularly students themselves, often the first ones to detect such threats, play a critical role in prevention efforts. Some of the preventive efforts that school districts can implement include:

Convincing students of their roles in the prevention of school violence   The silent "bystander" who directly or indirectly learns of threats, but alerts no one in a position to investigate or stop such events before they happen is complicit in these attacks. Schools must be proactive in convincing students that their roles are important in violence prevention and that they should bring any suspicions or other information gathered by their observations to staff members who can intervene. Perhaps redefining what is meant by "friendship" is also a goal, freeing students from the unwritten code of not "ratting out" a classmate to school authorities regarding suspicions of future violent behavior. Some of these attacks may indeed be preventable, provided that students take an active role in reporting their suspicions to the proper school authorities.

Eliminating barriers to effective student–staff communication   Students are inclined to seek out a school staff member to report suspicious behavior on the part of a fellow schoolmate if the school puts a number of factors in place, including:

a.   Disseminating information to school children regarding policies and procedures for reporting such suspicions; this information should include:

- an emphasis on the importance of student vigilance in violence prevention
- the types of unsettling behavioral and communication messages observed that should serve as "warning signs" worthy of reporting to a school official
- the manner in which this information should be reported, emphasizing ease of access to the proper authority
- the school resources available to all students outside the classroom, including school counselors, school psychologists, social workers, substance awareness counselors, and general school-based administration

b.   Instilling a sense of belonging to school in order for all students to feel connected to a system that values their welfare; this sense of belonging benefits both bystanders and potential perpetrators of violence alike. Students who feel bonded to their school will be inclined to report their suspicions since they would anticipate a positive outcome for their efforts and would expect school personnel to be willing and able to assist a fellow student in pain. The troubled students in question also would view themselves as being part of a larger system that is concerned for their welfare.

Reaching out in a proactive way to students in distress or in some need for assistance   Since most of the shooters in the SSI study exhibited some troubling behaviors prior to the attacks, it is incumbent upon school districts to reach out to such individuals beforehand and provide help in the form of counseling or referrals to local mental health or social service agencies outside the school district. A student observed coping with a major loss or any other perceived failure warrants attention. Caution should be exercised, however, in not alienating or stigmatizing the student in question.

Disaffected, disconnected students with no sense of bond with the school not only are more inclined to drop out but also are more likely to engage in antisocial behavior. If these students were asked the question, "If you were absent from school, who besides your friends would notice that you were gone and miss you?" their answers would reveal how connected to the school they felt. It is this type of student who requires some kind of outreach by school personnel.

Discussing with the school community, particularly with parent groups, the importance of gun safety and storage   Since most attackers obtained the firearms used in the attacks from their own homes or those of relatives, it is imperative that all community members understand the importance of making their weapons accessible only to those individuals who have the right to use them.

Establishing strong antibullying policies and programs in the schools   Although bullying was not a factor in every case examined by the SSI, in a number of cases the shooters described being bullied to the extent that it approached torment. Therefore, it is incumbent upon schools to adopt a formal antibullying policy and accompanying procedures to ensure that no student is bullied in the schools and to empower other students, the bystanders to such events, to notify other staff members of any instances of bullying.

Creating a warm, nurturing school climate   A school district is truly proactive in its attempt to prevent school violence if it promotes and communicates positive behavior clearly to all school community members, practices positive disciplinary approaches, and provides mental health services for students in distress. Also critical to student success and to building a student's feeling of connectedness to the school is a strong bond between the school and home; working together, a good home-school connection can address the needs of the whole child. Finally, training staff in crisis procedures and in the identification of potential sources of violent acts are critical for true violence prevention.

Echoing these conclusions were the findings of the American Psychological Association's (APA) Zero Tolerance Task Force (2008) which investigated the effectiveness of zero tolerance policies in the schools as an approach to discipline enforcement. These policies, originally developed as a means of drug enforcement, are those that require a predetermined consequence applied to a behavior, regardless of its severity, mitigating circumstances, or situational context. The kindergarten boy who pointed a "finger gun" at a fellow kindergartner during recess and said, "Bang, bang, I shot you," for example, was suspended from school pending a psychiatric evaluation attesting to the fact that he was not a danger to anyone. Eight days later he was able to return to school.

In concluding that these policies were ineffective and, in fact, did more harm than good, the APA Task Force echoed the importance of many of the prevention issues discussed above. It suggested that schools improve school climate, reconnect alienated youth to the school community, and evaluate threats of violence in the context of situational, developmental, and other factors.

SCHOOL CRISIS INTERVENTION

The schools' response to different types of crises typically does not occur in a vacuum. That is, for many crisis types, they must collaborate with heads of local government and with other community agencies including law enforcement, mental health, medical, and disaster-related groups such as the Red Cross. In fact, the United States Department of Education's Office of Safe and Drug-Free Schools requires such collaboration in order for local school districts to be eligible for Readiness and Emergency Management for Schools (REMS) grant monies designed to strengthen their crisis management capabilities. However, this chapter will focus on the typical school district's internal response to crisis, notwithstanding its appreciation of the roles and responsibilities of the outside agencies.

The National Association of School Psychologists (NASP) has developed a school crisis prevention and intervention protocol known as PREPaRE (Prevent and Prepare, Reaffirm, Evaluate, Provide and Respond, Examine) (Brock, Nickerson, Reeves, Jimerson, Lieberman, & Feinberg, 2009). It incorporates the crisis response model promoted by the Department of Homeland Security's National Incident Management System (NIMS), which provides an organizational structure and a common set of concepts and principles pertaining to crisis. Designed for school-based mental health professionals, PREPaRE also follows the Department of Education's four phases of Emergency Response and Crisis Management (ERCM): prevention/mitigation, preparedness, response (crisis intervention), and recovery.

Within the NIMS structure is the Incident Command System (ICS) designed to insure coordination of all participants who respond to a crisis. The ICS serves five functions of crisis response: incident command, planning and intelligence, operations, logistics, and finance/administration. Those mental health professionals who work in the schools comprise the "operations" function, and it is their responsibility to provide care for students, staff, and families during and after a crisis. The cases discussed below in this chapter are examples of the work of these operations professionals.

The other components of the PREPaRE program include:

Prevent and prepare for psychological trauma.

- Ensure building security and physical safety in schools.
- Foster internal and external resiliency factors in children.
- Create a warm, inviting school climate.
- Provide additional academic and psychological supports for at-risk children.
- Create a school crisis plan—Required for all schools by No Child Left Behind, it should be developed collaboratively with input from all members of the school community: students, parents, teachers, school administrators, and community members from various agencies. The plan should describe the activation of the ICS during a crisis, the roles and responsibilities of the crisis team members, and the protocol to be followed during and after a crisis (see Cavaiola & Colford, 2006, for a detailed description of crisis plans and teams).

Reaffirm physical health and ensure perceptions of security and safety.

- Reassure children after a crisis that they are safe and secure.
- Take care of their physical needs.

Evaluate psychological trauma.

- Conduct "psychological triage," the process of determining which children are most in need of services after a crisis event.
- Assess the presence of pre-existing internal and external vulnerability factors.

C A S E   P R E S E N T A T I O N : A Case Involving a School Shooting

---

Students at the local junior high overheard fourteen-year-old Victor complain bitterly about the perceived maltreatment he received at the hands of the school vice-principal, an out-of-school suspension for an assortment of transgressions which was to begin at the end of the school day. "Wait 'til they see what I can do!" he claimed as he left the vice principal's office; a number of students heard him, according to later reports. Later that same day, Victor was overheard by a teacher decrying his science teacher and swearing to "get even" for writing him up for a discipline in-fraction that ultimately lead to his suspension.

Three days later, one day before his suspension was up, Victor arrived at school in the middle of the day, anticipating that the vice principal and his science teacher would be in the school cafeteria providing supervision for approximately 100 students. He walked through the school corridors, much to the surprise of teachers and students alike that he was back in school prior to the end of his suspension. The heavy jacket he was wearing, considering the unseasonably warm day, also

- Internal: avoidant coping style, history of other trauma, poor regulation of emotion
- External: lack of family/social resources, family dysfunction, poverty/financial strain, not living with the nuclear family

- Assess children's physical and emotional proximity to the crisis and to the crisis victim. (Were they near the crisis when it occurred? Were that emotionally close to the victim?)

Provide interventions **a**nd **R**espond to psychological needs.

- Reestablish children's social support systems and return them to familiar routines and environments after a crisis.
- Disseminate facts of the crisis and dispel rumors.
- Identify and normalize crisis reactions.
- Teach stress management and coping strategies.

Examine the effectiveness of crisis prevention and intervention.

- Make sure that the crisis response was an effective one vis-à-vis a return to pre-crisis levels of school attendance, behavior problems, and academic functioning.

The following cases illustrate how crisis teams work. Teams consist of individuals to whom certain carefully circumscribed tasks will be delegated in an attempt to organize as much as possible the multitude of tasks that must be done during and after a crisis. Although school shootings are exceptionally rare events that will impact only a small percentage of students, their horrific nature and high profile make them an appropriate crisis type worthy of discussion first. Most crisis teams are more inclined to encounter the cases that follow: the suicide of a student at school and the deaths of students in a motor vehicle accident.

---

contributed to the suspiciousness of his appearance. Victor stormed into the cafeteria, pulled a handgun from his jacket pocket, and opened fire about 50 feet from the vice principal, sending students and other staff members screaming and scrambling for cover. When he finished firing, the vice principal lay dead and three students were wounded. When the gun emptied, staff members disarmed him and restrained him until the police arrived.

A post-mortem analysis of the event yielded this information: the day before the shooting he told a small group of students that he knew where he could get "a real gun with bullets." Some of his friends reinforced his disdain for the vice principal.

Case Discussion/Crisis Resolution
The above case is a composite of several actual school shooting incidents. Many of the components of school attacks are contained in this incident: a chronic history of

---

(continued)

C A S E   P R E S E N T A T I O N : A Case Involving a School Shooting
(*continued*)

---

school problems, a triggering event, verbalized threats overheard by several peers, and access to a firearm. When such an event takes place, safety of all members of the school community is paramount; collaboration with local law enforcement is critical in accomplishing this goal. Discussion of the case will include suggestions about what to do during the event as well as what the role of the school crisis team is, both immediately after and in the longer-term postvention period.

Once the shooting was over, approximately five minutes after it began, numerous tasks had to be accomplished. The crisis coordinator, the school principal, was involved with coordinating law enforcement efforts at the crime scene, so another administrative designee was assigned as the crisis team coordinator. She called a formal meeting of the crisis response team, which made a quick assessment regarding the collective emotional state of both students and staff. The functions of the team members were reviewed and assigned.

The team made a list of all the wounded students' classes and assigned members of the team to make special visits to each class to address the tragedy with them and to ascertain those students in need of more individual attention. Additionally, the team summoned other crisis teams from its own district schools and alerted another team from a neighboring school district to stand by to assist with these special needs. These team members maintained high visibility throughout the school building, providing many opportunities for students and staff to express their own thoughts, feelings, and fears about what happened.

Other important tasks that must be addressed after a crisis such as this (Cavaiola & Colford, 2006) and that were part of the plan include:

Completion of a Crisis Fact Sheet: A factual account of the day's events was summarized in an announcement that was distributed to all classes, most of which were not aware of the cafeteria shooting.

Planning for the afternoon faculty meeting: In order to provide an update of the event and to allow the staff to process it, the meeting was held to better prepare the staff to offer comfort for the students upon their return to school.

Planning the schedule for the first day back after the shooting: Since the return to routine is helpful after a crisis, the team decided to follow a regular class schedule when students returned.

Guidelines for Responding to a School Shooting

Poland and McCormick (1999) suggest the following protocol when an armed intruder is inside a school building:

1. Call the police immediately.

2. Make an announcement over the intercom, using a pre-established, coded warning signal; if one does not exist, use a straightforward announcement ("We have an intruder inside the building. Go into lockdown mode.").

3. Have the custodians lock the appropriate inside doors so that the armed individual is isolated from students and staff.

Planning for the evening parent meeting: An important component for any crisis response is the parent/community meeting. Among other things, parents were given information about children's reactions to traumatic events and suggestions for dealing with them at home.

Planning follow-up for the next day: The crisis team decided that the counseling liaison would devote much of the day after the shooting to providing outreach to those thought to be most needy.

Scheduling of regular crisis team meetings: In order to allow the team to continue to function as efficiently as possible, regular meetings were deemed essential to allow the team to continue to keep pace with the changing demands in the days and weeks following the crisis.

Other responsibilities for crisis team members included the medical liaison, the school nurse, who kept in contact with medical personnel and with families for ongoing updates on the health of the wounded. The media liaison proved to have one of the more difficult of the crisis team tasks; her primary responsibility was to make sure that members of the media, upon arrival at the school, remained in an assigned location, preferably some distance from the school building itself, where they would receive updates on the event from the designated school staff member. Wandering media personnel looking for distraught middle school students to speak with on camera can be an overwhelming and intrusive act at times like this, thus the need for separation of media and schools after a crisis. The media liaison was advised to utilize local law enforcement personnel to enforce the "no media allowed in school" policy, if needed.

The parent/family liaison greeted parents who arrived at school to address their concerns and advised them on how to talk with their children about the shooting. The security liaison for the team maintained regular contact with the local police and with other law enforcement agencies; he also began the process of evaluating the district's own safety and security systems.

After several days had passed, a sense of equilibrium returned to the school. Many students attended the funeral along with their parents. The wounded students returned to school and teachers returned to academics as their primary function after days of crisis debriefing. Nevertheless, the crisis team remained available on an as-needed basis.

4. Alert school security (if applicable).

5. Instruct teachers to close and lock their classroom doors and turn off all lights. Teachers also should keep students away from doors and windows and take roll call to account for all students.

6. Administrators should carefully walk through the halls to round up isolated students and direct them to safety.

7. Direct everyone to lie down on the floor or get under a desk until the intruder is apprehended.

8. Make an "all clear" announcement when given the signal from the police.

Even after the shooting incident has ended, some of the major questions that must be answered are simple: Should the school be closed? If yes, how many days is an appropriate length of time to keep it closed? Should school be kept open for the rest of the day?

Guidelines (Poland & McCormick, 1999) suggest that school be reopened as soon as possible after the shooting. The sooner crisis intervention is provided to the students and staff, the better off they will be regarding their emotional reactions to the event. Being around trained school personnel immediately after the event and returning as soon as possible to the familiarity of a daily routine and to a class full of familiar faces are far preferable to children than having them remain at home alone. For these same reasons, there are arguments that favor keeping a school open after a crisis. The exception to this guideline, however, is the very young child (such as the kindergartner) who should be reunited with a parent soon after the crisis to minimize the effects of the trauma. The argument for

---

C A S E   P R E S E N T A T I O N :   Suicide and the School's Response

Note: See Chapter 3 for an introduction of the rates and causes of adolescent suicide.

As students and staff arrived at their high school for another day of class, they were turned away by police who were standing guard by the front gate while stretching yellow tape across the entrance to the school. Early in the morning, Frankie, senior-classman of this 700-student high school had leaped to his death from the roof of the building. His family had reported him missing when he did not show up at home the night before, and the first teacher to arrive at the school discovered the body. Rumors began to spread among the students and staff members arriving shortly after regarding the presence of the police and of the diversion to different entrances to the school building.

Left behind by the victim were writings consistent with suicide. He also had sent numerous e-mails and text messages to his friends telling them that he loved them and saying, in essence, "good-bye." Until these messages were discovered, none of his friends or classmates noted any disturbing signs in his comments or in his behaviors that alerted them that something was amiss. In fact, he was active in several clubs in the high school, was a straight-A student, and was known as personable, hard-working, and very bright. His acceptance into an Ivy League college, which he planned to attend, and a new relationship with a girl at school seemed to indicate, if anything, that all was well with him.

Case Discussion/Crisis Resolution

Time was of the essence in responding to this crisis. So many things had to spring into action before the remainder of the student body and staff arrived at school that morning. Diverting the incoming individuals from their typical front gate entrance to any one of several side entrances was important in order to keep potential onlookers from seeing the deceased. This unusual diversion, however,

closing school early the day of a crisis, however, is that it gives the school's crisis team an opportunity to meet to discuss its crisis response immediately after the event and in the days and weeks that follow.

Poland and McCormick (1999) consider the following to determine whether to cancel school for the remainder of the day or to keep it open:

- If the majority of staff are "together" enough to assist students, then school should be kept open. If they are too affected by the crisis, then it is best to close school for the rest of the day so that the staff has time to deal with their own emotional reactions. This decision should not be made by one person, but rather it should be in the hands of the school crisis team.

- If the school is severely damaged or if large areas of the building are designated a crime scene, then school should be closed.

---

raised many suspicions as to what had occurred, especially with the presence of the police yellow tape stretched across the better part of the entranceway. Rumors were rampant as the students and staff entered the building. The school crisis team members, notified of the suicide only an hour before the school day was to begin, gathered together to decide the distribution of responsibilities for crisis intervention that day.

Many things had to happen very quickly. Routine had to be established in the school, beginning with the typical morning homeroom; a factual account of what had happened also had to be communicated to the students and staff. Counseling had to be provided and access to this service also communicated to both these groups. Specific outreach services also were to be offered to those closest, both physically and emotionally, to the deceased. These individuals included the teacher who discovered the body, the teachers and friends of the deceased, especially those who received his farewell text messages beforehand and had not responded to his pleas, his girlfriend, and all other classmates who had known him for many years. Others who were at risk for many other reasons (see page 221) also were included in this outreach effort.

Counselors from the school decided to follow Frankie's schedule, sharing the class time with his teachers and allowing discussion of his death. However, the discussion included the notion that suicide was an unfortunate decision, one designed as a permanent solution to a temporary problem. The emphasis during these discussions was on utilizing better problem-solving and coping strategies than suicide as a solution. Other interventions would include providing after school and evening counseling and feedback sessions for students, parents, and other members of the school community regarding the meaning of the death and ways of coping with it.

Guidelines for Dealing with a School-Related Suicide

According to the National Institute of Mental Health (2004) statistics, suicide ranked as the third leading cause of death among children ages 10–14 (1.3 per 100,000) and among adolescents ages 15–19 (8.2 per 100,000). Young people were more likely than adults to use firearms, suffocation, and poisoning as the preferred methods of death, with firearms the most common choice among adolescents and suffocation among children. There may be as many as 25 suicide attempts for every completed suicide.

The challenge for any school crisis team is to act very quickly after being notified of a student suicide, whether it occurred on school grounds or somewhere in the community after school hours. The fear of suicide contagion (Brock, 2002) (imitative suicidal behavior), particularly among other adolescents, places others at risk of a "copy cat" suicidal attempt as well, thus the need for swift action. The following steps are to be taken.

Engaging the school crisis team   The first thing that should be done, typically by the crisis coordinator, is to summon together the school crisis team. If the school is a particularly large facility with a large student body, then additional mental health resources may be requested from other local crisis teams. The coordinator also should verify the facts of the case, making sure that a suicide has been pronounced by medical authorities; speculation should never replace fact-finding. If suicide has not been confirmed by these authorities, then the cause of death should be considered "unknown" at this time. Only verifiable facts should be shared with the crisis team and with others.

Contacting the victim's family   The team's parent-family liaison should reach out to the family to provide comfort and support and to determine its wishes with regard to student expressions of grief and outreach efforts to other students.

Calling together the school staff   Whenever possible, the school staff should assemble prior to the return of students to the school building in order for them to receive the information about the suicide and to be apprised of the school crisis team's plan for the students' re-entry. This meeting would also be an opportunity for the crisis team to assess those faculty members who might have difficulty addressing this issue with their students.

Informing students of the news   Students should be informed in small, intimate settings (such as individual classrooms) rather than in large, open venues (such as auditorium assemblies or via large-scale intercom announcements through the school). One of the reasons for the preference for small settings is to allow the teacher to be able to conduct a discussion of the facts of the case and to monitor students' reactions to the news. Should they find that some students had an inordinate amount of difficulty handling the news, they would then be able to summon additional counseling resources for these students.

All information must be truthful. A death by suicide must be described in those exact terms in any notification to the general student body. It also should include some mention of suicide being a poor decision by the victim in his or her attempt to solve a problem. The crisis coordinator, in collaboration with the crisis team, should compose an announcement to be distributed to the staff and read by teachers to their classes. The announcement should be relatively brief; a sample follows:

John Doe, a senior in our high school, committed suicide early yesterday morning. As a faculty and school community we extend our sympathies to John's family and friends. We encourage all students to consider the tragic nature of this death and to realize that death is final. John's death is a reminder to us all that the act of taking one's life is not an appropriate solution to any of life's problems, nor is it an act of courage. There will be counselors available in school today and for the next few days in (specify locations in the building where counselors will be found) for any student wishing to talk to someone about John's death.

Funeral services will be held in _____; expressions of sympathy may be sent to _____.

Brock, Sandoval, and Lewis (2001) provided a sample of an announcement designed for students' parents:

It is with a heavy heart that I write this letter to you today. I have some very bad news to share. I have just learned that the death of a member of our school family has been ruled a suicide by the coroner's office. John Doe, a senior in our school, killed himself yesterday. Our school staff has made the choice not to speculate on what it was that may have lead to the suicide. Rather, our focus will be on what we can do to prevent other such losses.

Part of what makes this death especially tragic is that it did not have to happen. Clearly, this was a permanent solution to problems that could have been dealt with in other ways. Perhaps some good can come from this loss if it generates a greater awareness of the signs of possible suicidal thinking and of school and community resources that are available to help people cope with their problems. To this end, I would like to share with you some of the signals or warning signs suggesting the need for counseling support. These warning signs include the following:

The letter would then close with information regarding warning signs as well as available counseling services during the day for any student wishing to seek them out, including information about where in the school building the counselors would be located. The letter would also include a list of local mental health agencies and their phone numbers and information regarding the funeral arrangements. In the event of a suicide, student attendance at the funeral during the school day should be allowed on an individual basis with parental permission only; the school district should not provide en masse bus trips to the funeral, nor should it cancel classes during the time of the funeral.

Identifying at-risk students   A variety of emotional reactions are noted in individuals affected by the death by suicide of a close friend or family member. However, there are some individuals who might be more inclined than others to imitate the suicidal act. Imitative suicidal behaviors account for approximately 1–3% of all adolescent suicides (Moscicki, 1995). Factors to consider when assessing the risk for imitative suicidal behavior, according to Brock (2006), include those who:

- facilitated the suicide
- failed to recognize the suicidal intent
- believed they may have caused the suicide
- had a relationship with the victim
- identified with the victim
- have a history of suicidal behavior
- have a history of psychopathology
- have suffered significant losses
- lack social support resources

Crisis team members themselves may not be aware of all such at-risk students, but they should be able to reach out to staff members including teachers, the school nurse, drug and alcohol counselors, and school staff responsible for discipline; each one of these individuals would undoubtedly know of students who fit into one of these risk categories. Once known, the counseling liaison should facilitate an outreach program for these students, calling them from class to ascertain their levels of distress and to make the appropriate referrals, if needed, to other mental health resources.

Reinforcing prevention and coping among all survivors   Providing ongoing information to students regarding a host of proactive practices:

- knowing where to turn for help for self or others (provide contact information for school and community mental health services)
- recognizing warning signs among friends and knowing when to make referrals for assistance
- understanding that problems can be solved without resorting to suicide

Arranging for appropriate memorials for the deceased   Postvention services and activities, those provided for people affected by a completed suicide, have the potential to do more harm than good by increasing the risk of contagion (Brock, 2003). It is essential that the victim's death not be sensationalized and that the victim not be glorified or vilified in any way, thus giving them more notoriety in death than they ever had in life. Too much attention to the victim and too many details of the death just encourage identification with the victim, thereby increasing the risk of contagion.

Postvention activities that are contraindicated and potentially harmful include permanent memorials like planting trees, installing plaques, dedicating yearbooks, flying the flag at half-mast, or having assemblies to honor the deceased. Rather, appropriate activities should be proactive and preventive in nature: contributing money to a local hot line, developing student assistance programs, or contributing in some way to suicide prevention programs in the school or community.

C A S E   P R E S E N T A T I O N : Accidental Death of Student

---

Two of the five high school students in the car were just five days away from their graduation in this large, sprawling urban school district in which the size of the high school alone approached 5,000 students. Three others, all juniors in the same high school, had cut class to join their older friends after graduation practice for a cele-bratory trip to a local fast food restaurant just a couple of miles from the school. Only one wore his seat belt.

After picking up their fast food fare, the students decided to visit a large shopping mall about 10 miles away. Their 80 mile-per-hour trip down a heavily traveled highway proved fatal to the driver, who was a senior, and to one passen-ger. A car entering the highway from a small strip mall caused the students' car to spin, hit a tree, and flip over several times. The two students were pronounced dead a short time later at the local hospital. The three other passengers suffered non-lethal injuries; one of them still planned to attend his graduation ceremonies later that week.

RESPONDING TO ACCIDENTAL DEATH:
THE SCHOOL'S RESPONSE

Sudden and unexpected deaths such as these are especially difficult, since the survivors have no time to prepare for the loss of the lives of friends and acquaintances (Jimerson & Huff, 2002). Complicating the school's response to this tragedy were several factors. The major ones included:

- **The immediacy of the event:** There was practically no time to prepare; news spread of the accident while school was still in session.

- **The size of the high school:** Student enrollment in this exceptionally large school exceeded 5,000 students.

- **Cultural differences among the deceased and the survivor family members:** One of the students who died was born in Poland. His parents spoke little English, and additional family members were en route from their homeland to attend the funeral services. The other victim was Latino. Sensitivity to cultural norms and practices at times like these was critical in order to provide culturally-sensitive support services to the surviving family members of the accident victims.

- **Loss of contact between the schools and the student body:** It would only be five days before all students would be gone for the summer break, making outreach by the counseling staff an immediate need, particularly for those vulnerable students (see page 221) who would soon be removed from the reassuring and predictable routine of the school day and from those counseling services offered by the school district.

The immediacy of the event   This tragic accident took place during the school day, and the cell phone and text message capabilities of today's youth allow news, both good and bad, to circulate quickly. Before the school day was over, a large number of students within the school building had heard of the crash and of the fatalities. The crisis coordinator had to act quickly in obtaining the facts of the event and communicating them to staff and students alike. This step in the district's crisis response was accomplished by distributing an announcement to each individual classroom to be read by the teachers to the class. The announcement (see page 220 regarding the notification of students in the aftermath of a suicide) included a brief description of the accident, the names of the deceased, and the counseling services available to any student wishing to use them. Although a hand-delivered announcement is the most frequent recommendation for distributing this type of tragic news (National Association of School Psychologists, 1998), the public address system also may be used in the event of a death while school is in session. However, the administrators or their designees must plan this announcement carefully and rehearse what they will say. The manner in which the message is delivered, including choice of words used and the tone of voice, can indeed set the tone for the school's management of the tragedy. An emotionally-charged announcement can exacerbate students' own emotional reactions to the news; a calm, dispassionate delivery can be reassuring to the student body. A school-wide announcement, however, is contraindicated if the death is due to a suicide.

Teachers were summoned to an after-school faculty meeting to address the tragedy as well as the district's crisis intervention plans. The decision also was made to have counselors available after the school day had ended and into the evening.

The size of the high school   Another daunting factor was the size of the student body; school size alone can present a significant obstacle to effective crisis intervention, however, the development of an effective crisis plan should have taken this factor into consideration. In the case of this high school, the student body was separated into five separate but connected sections, thereby reducing in size the number of students who may have been personally connected to the victims. Each section also had its own crisis team, all of whom assembled when notified of the tragedy; among the things discussed in this meeting was the likely section of the school that the deceased attended and which would be most affected by the tragedy. Counseling "drop in" centers were prepared for those sections, and notification of these services was communicated via individual classroom announcements (see above section). A list of vulnerable students, particularly close friends of the deceased, was assembled, and outreach was planned for them by the team's counseling liaison and other mental health personnel. A list of any siblings of the deceased who attended any of the other district schools also was prepared, and the crisis teams in those schools were alerted to the need to respond to them as well.

Cultural differences among the deceased and the survivor family members   Another consideration that had to be made in this tragedy involved the cultural and linguistic differences among the deceased, one Polish young man and one Latino. Any crisis plan developed by a school district also should include participation by community groups, particularly representatives of the different cultural and ethnic groups that make up the district's surrounding community. Among those issues addressed in the crisis plan would be the languages spoken in the community, its prevailing religious beliefs, and their cultural practices, especially as they pertain to the meaning of tragedy to the families involved and to the manner in which these families grieve and bury their dead (Athey & Moody-Williams, 2003; Sandoval & Lewis, 2002).

Prior to reaching out to the victims' families, the district first communicated with community groups for assistance; this assistance included securing the services of an interpreter for families that required one and consulting with them regarding the appropriate form of communication for the school district to use in its family outreach efforts.

Loss of contact between the schools and the student body   Plans also were made to provide counseling in the high school for several days after the graduation ceremonies, even though the school year had officially ended. Concerns over students' reactions after the graduation ceremony and after the funeral services themselves prompted the extension of this counseling service. The school district summoned the assistance of personnel from the local mental health community to assist in this endeavor.

MEMORIALS

It is a common sight for motorists to find along the highways throughout the country makeshift memorials marking the actual locations of a motor vehicle-related death consisting of flowers, posters and letters with emotional testimony, and an assortment of other memorabilia designed to honor the dead. Although it is unclear what value these commemorative practices serve in recovery from tragedy, society in general has established certain rituals and ceremonies for tragic events (Pagliocca, Nickerson, & Williams, 2002).

Young (2002) suggested that, in cases such as these, school crisis plans approach memorialization in two parts: memorial services immediately after an event, typically within a week; and permanent memorials. What must be emphasized, however, is that memorials of any kind should not be provided in the case of a death by suicide. Another suggestion (Young, 2002) is that permanent memorials also not be encouraged if the death is due to the victims' own misconduct including, among other causes, reckless driving. Determining the conditions surrounding the deaths of any young people might be germane to a district's decision regarding a permanent memorial in their honor.

In the case of these accidental deaths, the district administrator composed a tribute to the victims on the district website. He also provided symbolic empty seats for the two seniors at the graduation ceremony that was held just a few days after the tragedy. Representatives from each family also ascended the stage and received diplomas for them.

The decision regarding a permanent memorial should include student participation but should be guided by school administrators and other staff.

However, allowing for the passage of time and some emotional distance from the actual event before planning the memorial is advisable to allow an opportunity for emotions to subside and for reason to replace emotion in establishing a commemoration that is appropriate to the event (Cavaiola & Colford, 2006). Otherwise, permanent memorials that are too obtrusive only serve as daily reminders of tragedy, long after the event took place. Rather, they should be in a location where students may choose to look at it and where it would not confront students every time they enter the school grounds (Paine, 1998). Some of

---

CASE PRESENTATION: Middle School and 9/11

When the twin towers were attacked that day, resulting in the deaths of almost 3,000 people, schools in many parts of the country had just opened their doors for the beginning of another school day. A suburban middle school within just an hour-or-so commuting distance from New York City was in the early part of the first academic period. Only a handful of teachers were aware of the jet airliner collisions with the towers, since they were without an assigned teaching period at that time and were watching the news unfold on a television set in the teacher's room. Gradually, however, other teachers gained access to the television and spread the grim news to their colleagues and students. The crisis team's concern was that rumor would replace fact and that students and staff alike would experience considerable anxiety.

Case Discussion/Crisis Resolution

After some time had passed, the specific impact the event had on this middle school became clear: a student had a father who worked in the towers, and a secretary had a son in the same location. Two popular teachers in the school also had spouses employed there. Superimposed on the grand scale of nationwide horror were these personal stories of anxiety and fear over the unknown fate of these family members. The tasks facing the school's crisis team were significant.

Among the difficulties encountered by the middle school staff were:

- hoards of parents arriving at the school to pick up their children and take them home, despite the school psychologist's explanation to them that school was the best place for them to be at the time. Remaining in school among friends and in a familiar routine was a better alternative to going home and watching the televised horror over and over again. Parental prerogative superceded professional advice, however, and many children left school with their parents before the day was over.

- the school district's inability to summon additional district resources (counselors, psychologists, or social workers) to assist with the middle school staff, since all schools in the district were in the same crisis mode in their respective school buildings. Although each school should have its own contained crisis team, those schools with low enrollment and limited staff often enlist the services of crisis team members from neighboring school districts or from other schools within the district. However, the magnitude of the crisis on this day precluded any assistance from other sources.

- the sudden nature of the crisis which prevented the crisis coordinator, the school principal, from summoning the crisis team together to sort out roles and responsibilities. In most crisis cases there is a time interval between an event and the return of children to school (such as when a popular student dies in a motor vehicle accident over the weekend, allowing time for the crisis team to assemble before school resumes on Monday morning). In this case, however, the school was already midway through the first period when the attacks occurred.

the more common memorials are plaques, tree plantings, and annual events in honor of the deceased. Poland and McCormick (1999) suggest "consumable" gestures instead, such as the establishment of a scholarship in the names of the victims, whereas schools and communities, in the aftermath of a tragedy, look for activities and projects designed to make a difference and to prevent similar tragedies in the future. Activities and curriculum projects that address tolerance and bullying, for example, are appropriate "memorials" after a violent event in the schools.

Nevertheless, those crisis team members who were present in the middle school decided to get to work. First, the crisis coordinator composed a brief, informative note for the teachers to read in their classrooms; the note presented only the facts as known at the time, which had not yet included confirmation about a terrorism connection. Notes distributed during times of crisis must be dispassionate and objective in presenting facts about the crisis as well as reassuring for students that the familiar routine of the school day was going to continue. The principal had his secretarial staff distribute the notes to each of the classrooms with instructions that they be read aloud in each class.

Throughout the entire day, the crisis team's counseling liaison, the school psychologist, the school counselors, and the school social worker made themselves available by being very visible in the school building, monitoring students' and staff members' reactions and intervening with those individuals who exhibited particularly strong reactions to the news. Besides attending to the needs of all members of the school community, however, the crisis team also had to reach out to those groups of people who were particularly vulnerable to the current crisis. The groups included any student or staff member who had a parent, other relative, friend, or loved one working in the Twin Towers. Although deaths were not confirmed until later in the day, the team sought out these individuals, both students and staff alike.

One teacher whose husband worked in the towers, overcome and inconsolable at the news, asked to leave school to be with her family; she was escorted home once it was clear that there would be some other relatives waiting for her there. Yet another teacher with a spouse employed in the towers was asked to leave his class to meet with the school psychologist and principal in order for them to offer support and reassurance. He stated emphatically that he felt strongly that his wife was indeed safe, and he then asked to return to his class to continue teaching. The team continued to monitor him during the remainder of the school day. The team, after consulting with many staff members, determined that one student only had a parent working in the towers. His mother decided to pick him up from school and take him home. A school secretary also had a son working there; she, too, left school to be with her family. Both the student and the secretary had the deaths of their father and son confirmed the next day.

In the days following the attacks, the school crisis team continued to monitor the emotional health of students and staff. Teachers who requested assistance from one of the school mental health specialists were able to secure their assistance in the days that followed to help them address the attack-related issues in class discussions. Crisis team members also were able to determine who those students were who had some special personal connections to the deceased; follow-up consultations with them was accomplished by the team members. It would be days before everything would settle down for most members of the school community.

RECOMMENDATIONS FOR CHAPTER ENRICHMENT

SUGGESTED FILMS

The Killer at Thurston High **(2000)** This documentary film chronicles the life of Kip Kinkel, a teenager who entered his high school cafeteria in September 1998 with a semiautomatic rifle, and fired 50 shots into the crowd, killing two students and wounding 25 others. He also killed both his parents at home the night before. The film includes family videotape footage and interviews with those who knew him.

Untold Stories of Columbine **(2000)** The two teenage gunmen entered Columbine High School armed with numerous weapons and roamed throughout the building firing at students and staff members who tried to run away and hide. Before turning the guns on themselves, they left 13 dead and 23 wounded. This documentary focuses on the death and life of one of the murdered students, Rachel Joy Scott; it features interviews with her father and excerpts from her diary. The issue of her Christian faith provides a focus as well.

SUGGESTED ACTIVITIES: WHAT WOULD YOU DO?

School had just ended for the day for this suburban high school. It was the beginning of the fall season, and the freshman and sophomores headed for the school buses to take them home. Meanwhile, the upper class students, those juniors and seniors with permission to park on campus, hurriedly raced through the parking lot to get to their cars for a quick trip home. One of the school security officers took to the parking lot and directed student traffic out of the lot and into the local street in an orderly fashion.

Sandra, a popular senior and member of the student council, was one of those who exited the lot. She was only several blocks from the school when she reportedly failed to stop for a stop sign and went through an intersection; a car driven by another high school senior, an acquaintance of Sandra's, hit her broadside, killing her instantly, according to the coroner's report. An analysis of the accident by the local police revealed that Sandra had been changing a CD in her CD player and probably never noticed the stop sign. The school day had only ended 20 minutes prior to her death.

Answer the following questions as if you were a member of Sandra's school district's crisis team:

1. What should the crisis coordinator do right away?
2. What issues should be addressed with Sandra's friends? With the driver of the other car?
3. What should the counseling liaison's primary responsibilities be in the immediate aftermath of the crash?
4. From what other agencies might the crisis team request assistance?

5. With school not in session at the time other students hear of this tragedy, what are your biggest concerns about making sure that all students are provided counseling or other supports?

6. What kinds of memorials, both immediate and permanent, might be appropriate?

7. What school-based prevention practices might come out of this event?

13

Crises in the Workplace

DISCUSSION QUESTIONS

You may have heard of the term *going postal*. What types of jobs or workplaces do you think have the highest incidence of workplace violence? What jobs are the most dangerous?

In times of economic recession, massive layoffs are common. What types of crises might an employee experience if they have just received notice that they are being laid off from their jobs?

INTRODUCTION

This chapter will address different crisis situations that commonly occur in various types of work settings. For many individuals, the workplace has become an environment filled with tensions and stressors. Also, given that most Americans devote one-third of their waking hours to work, it is not unusual to find that the workplace has become a breeding ground for stressors that give way to various types of crises. Work stress is exacerbated during times of economic recession; however, even during times of a booming economy, the United States continued to experience the stresses and strains of downsizing, corporate takeovers, increased work demands, long commutes, and longer work hours. Many families find that in order to meet ever-increasing daily expenses both parents must work outside the home. Unfortunately, "cradle-to-grave" jobs have become a thing of the past. Most employees feel that holding a job for a few years is all that can be expected in today's job climate. Just as employees feel that their employers hold no sense of loyalty towards them, in many cases, employees feel the same lack of loyalty towards their employers. The downfall of corporations (such as Enron and WorldCom) or brokerage institutions (such as Lehman Brothers) due to fiscal mismanagement or corporate greed have only served to strengthen these attitudes.

In response to the various crises and stressors common to the workplace, many companies have employee assistance counselors or employee assistance professionals (EAPs) on staff or available to their employees to help them deal with some of the crises discussed in this chapter. Some companies provide excellent in-house employee assistance programs, while others—often smaller companies—will outsource employee assistance counseling to managed care companies who provide brief, over-the-phone assessments and referrals to employees in crisis.

The cases presented in this chapter will address three common types of workplace crises, including crises pertaining to violence, downsizing or job termination, and supervisor-employee and coworker conflicts.

C A S E   P R E S E N T A T I O N : When Violence Threatens

Ted has been employed by a large telecommunications company for the past five years. During that time, he has been assigned to a work unit where Sandra Jones is his direct supervisor. Ted has been increasingly agitated by Sandra's treatment of him over the past few months. He feels that she has been unreasonable when assigning him extra work assignments with impossible deadlines. Ted was also promised a faster computer in order to do his work more efficiently, however after several months, he still has not received the computer. As Ted has become increasingly upset, he reports that he has been unable to sleep. He has been drinking more frequently and neglecting his personal hygiene. One day after being reprimanded by Ms. Jones for missing a deadline, Ted stated in front of several coworkers "If Ms. Jones dumps one more job on me, I'm going on a rampage that will make Columbine look like a day in the park." Background information reveals that Ted had been fired from a previous job for having a physical altercation with his former supervisor. Ted claims that he did not make a direct threat to Ms. Jones and that his comments about wanting to hurt her were "misunderstood." Because Ted's company does not have an on-site employee assistance counselor, he was referred to a counselor in the Human Resources Department who usually handles conflicts between employees and supervisors. The following is a brief sample of that meeting.

Intervention

HR COUNSELOR: Hi Ted, I understand that you've been having some difficulties with Ms. Jones. I thought we might talk about what's been happening and see if we could come up with some solutions.

TED: Well the first thing you could do is tell Ms. Jones to stop dumping work on me. I get all the jobs that no one else wants.

HR COUNSELOR: Do you feel that she's treating you differently from your coworkers?

TED: I do, no one else gets all the work I do ... but that's not the only problem I've had with her. About three months ago, I was promised a new computer to get my work done faster. I've yet to see the damn thing, but everyone else in the department has a new computer.

HR COUNSELOR: So your coworkers have the new computers, but they have fewer work assignments than you. Is that what you're saying?

TED: Yeah, can you see why I feel like I'm being treated like dirt?

HR COUNSELOR: So mainly, Ted, there are two things that you're most angry about: you're given more work than your coworkers and also you were promised a new computer but never received one.

(continued)

CASE PRESENTATION: When Violence Threatens (continued)

TED: Yes, those are the two main things that I'm really pissed off about and then there's the deadlines. Jones must think I'm superhuman or something. She gives me a project to work on and wants it done yesterday. I guess I just blew up. I don't want to hurt anyone. I just want to be treated fairly.

HR COUNSELOR: Ted, I hear what your saying and how frustrated or angry you must be. You said you don't want to hurt anyone right? What exactly did you say after Ms. Jones confronted you?

TED: I just got all steamed up, I guess. I said if she dumped one more job on me I'd come back and make Columbine look like a day in the park or something like that. I don't remember exactly ... I was just really pissed off.

HR COUNSELOR: Do you own any guns or weapons?

TED: I used to but I got rid of them. I really wouldn't do anything to hurt anyone. I just want to be treated fairly.

HR COUNSELOR: Ted, here's what I'm willing to do. I'll talk with Ms. Jones and I think I can get her to take some of the pressure off of you by distributing the workload more fairly and with more reasonable deadlines. I'll also find out what's holding up your new computer. But here's what I need from you. In situations like this when there's a threat made against another employee, it's company policy to have that person evaluated by a doctor just to make sure that there's no danger.

TED: Like I said, I wouldn't hurt Ms. Jones, I only spoke out of frustration.

HR COUNSELOR: I realize that Ted, and I hear you; this is done as a precaution. The evaluation is done by private psychiatrist and the company pays for it. Plus you're paid for those days that you'll be off between now and when the evaluation takes place.

TED: If it's something I have to do, I'll do it. You're sure you can get Ms. Jones to back off and you're pretty sure you can get my computer?

HR COUNSELOR: Yes, I'm pretty sure about both things, but only provided that you follow through with the evaluation.

TED: I'll do it.

HR COUNSELOR: O.K., I'll set the evaluation appointment up. I need to know that you'll be okay and that you have no intention of harming yourself or anyone else.

TED: No, I'll be fine. Really.

HR COUNSELOR: Here's my phone number in case you have any questions or concerns. I'm going to be in touch with you about the appointment and will give you directions to Dr. Randolph's office.

Case Conceptualization/Crisis Resolution

In this case illustration, Ted feels that he has been wronged by his supervisor, Ms. Jones, and treated unfairly. His frustrations and complaints have resulted in his making a threat to commit acts of violence. All threats of this nature must be taken seriously and not ignored or minimized in such a way to conclude that "Ted is just blowing off steam." In fact, Ted had voiced his frustrations to another supervisor and to his coworkers and he feels that he has gotten nowhere and that no one is listening to his complaints. In this crisis session, the Human Resource counselor is listening to Ted's complaints and conveying to Ted that he is willing to help and intervene on his behalf. The HR Counselor also knows that given Ted's threats, he cannot merely send him back to work. Therefore, he makes an agreement with Ted that he will intervene on his behalf provided that Ted goes for a psychiatric evaluation. The HR Counselor is careful not to use the term "psychiatric evaluation" immediately because he does not want Ted to become more agitated or respond with something like, "You think I'm crazy?" The HR Counselor alludes to the evaluation being "company policy," however, the counselor is also careful not to overemphasize this. The HR Counselor is trying to get a preliminary idea as to the level of danger by asking if Ted has a plan and whether or not he has access to weapons. Ted would be escorted to his desk and out to his car by security. The last thing the HR Counselor wants is for Ted to leave agitated and hostile, go out to his car to get a weapon, and return to the building. (This happened in a meatpacking plant in Grandview, Missouri in 2004 (Johnson, 2004))

There are two important questions to consider. What if Ted refuses the HR Counselor's mandate that he must have a psychiatric evaluation? In an instance like this, Ted would most likely be terminated from his position, the police would need to be called, and a restraining order would be requested from the courts. The restraining order would specify that Ted could not come near any company building, nor could he contact or come near Ms. Jones. The other question pertains to the psychiatric evaluation. What if the psychiatrist assesses Ted as having a high potential for committing violence? In this instance, inpatient psychiatric treatment may be court ordered until such time that Ted is no longer a threat to others. There is a possibility that inpatient treatment may be the safest option, given that Ted is not sleeping, he has increased his use of alcohol, and he has had a history of violence in the past.

According to recent statistics, more than 1,000 people are murdered annually on the job, while more than 2 million suffer physical attacks and an estimated 6 million people are threatened (Toufexis, 1994). Of course, when considering that more than 120 million people in the United States are employed, the total number of deaths per year may seem like a small percentage, yet the number of workplace assaults is more commonplace. It is also important to note that most workplace deaths occur during the course of robberies (such as convenience store clerks or cab drivers), while only 9–10% are attributed to business disputes, and only 4–6% were committed by employees or former employees. According to the Bureau of Justice Statistics (2009), it appears that workplace violence resulting from disputes with coworkers may make up the minority of instances of workplace violence. For example the rate of violence for various occupations was highest for law enforcement officers, followed by corrections officers, taxi drivers, private security guards, bartenders, mental health professionals, gas station attendants, and convenience or liquor store clerks. Therefore, the potential for violence is much greater for those who deal with the general public than it is for those who only deal with coworkers or supervisors, as in the case described above.

Lewis and Zare (1999) have outlined several factors that may exacerbate workplace violence. One of these is referred to as a *toxic* work environment: jobs that lack upward mobility and job security, and have limited benefits, low wages, heavy workload, long hours with weekends required, unexpected shift changes without input, expected or mandatory overtime, no autonomy, no say in decisions, and managers who are inconsistent, inflexible, untrained, and who show favoritism. Any organization or company that manifests these toxic workplace characteristics may be placing themselves at greater risk for workplace violence according to Lewis and Zare.

Obviously, not all individuals in toxic work environments commit acts of workplace violence. Therefore, it is important to determine what distinguishes the potentially violent employee from those who will cope with toxic workplaces. Although there are no foolproof ways to predict who will become potentially violent workers,

(continued)

C A S E   P R E S E N T A T I O N : When Violence Threatens *(continued)*

---

there are some signs that need to be taken into account. In terms of work-related behavior, Lewis and Zare (1999) suggest that absenteeism, tardiness, ignoring work assignments, frequently missing from one's workstation, leaving work early, or being late for work are significant factors. Coworkers or managers may begin to notice faulty judgments, poor decision-making, inconsistencies in work quality and productivity, and failure to remember instructions. From an attitudinal and emotional perspective, frequent mood swings; negative attitudes; frequent complaints from customers, vendors, or coworkers; and overreaction to any criticism. The aforementioned mood swings may be characterized by irritability, high anxiety, depression with crying jags, and hostility. The potentially violent individual often feels that they have been wronged or betrayed by their boss or employer (as in Ted's case). As their behavior escalates, they may display temper outbursts, frequent arguments with coworkers or supervisors, violence by throwing or smashing things, or they may abuse alcohol or drugs flagrantly. Alcohol and certain drugs (such as cocaine, amphetamines, and steroids) tend to exacerbate the potential for violent acting out. As these behaviors escalate over time, the potentially violent individual may or may not verbalize threats. If and when this happens, responsible individuals in the work setting, whether it be human resources staff, employee assistance professionals, or supervisors or managers, must be prepared to take action.

In an attempt to predict (and prevent workplace violence) it is also helpful to view workplace violence as arising from a combination of Personality Factors AND Workplace Factors AND Instigating Situations, because instances of violence rarely occur as a result of one isolated incident that pushes a person over the edge (see Table 13.1).

T A B L E 13.1   Factors Predictive of Workplace Violence

Personality Factors

prior history of violent behavior
Antisocial Personality Disorder
explosive personality
Schizoid Personality Disorder
Paranoid Personality Disorder
Borderline Personality Disorder

Toxic Workplace Factors

autocratic management
lack of control over workload
no upward mobility
lack of job security
lack of input into job
mandatory overtime

Instigating Factors

divorce or separation
being fired or laid off
verbal altercation with boss or coworker
feeling "wronged" or cheated by company
major job change or stressor
corporate merger

Even with what is known about profiles of individuals who may be prone to workplace violence, there are still those exceptions to the rule; therefore, sometimes individual coworkers, bosses, or supervisors must learn to trust their instincts or reactions when faced with individuals they feel uneasy about.

In order to prevent workplace violence, steps should be taken when some of the aforementioned behaviors are first noted. Sometimes, a nonthreatening meeting with a managing supervisor early in the process can help "clear the air" and come up with strategies for making this person's work situation more tolerable. One difficulty is that once the potentially violent worker feels "wronged," there is sometimes very little that can be done to diffuse this person's anger at a supervisor, coworkers, or the organization. This would especially be true if the person has some other mental disorder. Individuals who manifest any type of psychotic thinking, especially paranoid thinking, or who seem estranged or loners may be prone to increasing violence or may perceive violence as a means of achieving their goals. It is always best to intervene with these individuals as early as possible, for example, when peculiarities in their behavior or attitudes first begin to become evident. When a potentially violent employee is referred for psychiatric evaluation, one of the first things to be done is a *lethality assessment* (see Table 13.2). In assessing someone for potential violence, one of the best predictors of future violence is *a past history of such behavior*. Although the violence-prone individual may not be forthcoming about such information, in some instances the person may sign a release so that the counselor may speak with a trusted family member or a mental health counselor who may have previously treated this individual. In examining past violent behavior (which includes both verbal and physical assaults), it is important to determine what might have provoked these incidents and whether the individuals have any insight into whether or not their behavior was inappropriate.

T A B L E 13.2   Factors Associated with Increased Risk of Violence

Think of the acronym "ARM PAIN"

Altered state of consciousness such as delirium
Repeated assaults or history of violence
Male Gender (males are more prone to violent acts than females)
Paranoia (as in schizophrenia, mania, or delusional disorder)
Age (younger individuals are more likely to become violent)
Incapacity (brain injury or psychosis)
Neurological disease

Or think of the acronym: MADS and BADS

Mania (high energy level and poor judgment)
Alcohol (intoxication or withdrawal)
Dementia
Schizophrenia (especially paranoid subtype)
Borderline Personality Disorder (intense anger)
Antisocial Personality Disorder (disregard for safety of self or others)
Delirium (with hallucinations or delusions)
Substance abuse (especially PCP, cocaine, methamphetamines)

Reprinted with permission from S. Bohen, (2002) *Psychiatric Emergencies* (p. 24–24), PESI Healthcare: Eau Claire, WI.

Guidelines for Crisis Intervention with a Potentially
Violent Employee

The following are some defusing strategies that might be used with a potentially violent individual:

1. *Understand the mindset of the hostile or potentially violent person.* These individuals often have a compelling need to communicate their grievance to someone—now! Even when wrong they are acting on perceptions that are real to them. In the overwhelming number of cases, the indivuduals just want to be heard and treated with fairness.

2. *Practice "Active Listening."* Stop what you are doing and give your full attention. Listen to what is really being said. Use silence and paraphrasing. Ask clarifying, open-ended questions.

3. *Build trust and provide help. Avoid confrontation.* Be calm, courteous, respectful, and patient. It is important to be open and honest, but don't make promises you can't keep. Never belittle, embarrass, or verbally attack potentially violent people.

4. *Allow a total airing of the grievance without comment or judgment.* While the individuals are airing their grievances, make eye contact but do not stare (that can be perceived as a challenge). Let them have their say, while ignoring challenges or insults. Do not take venting personally; redirect their attention to the real issues.

5. *Allow the aggrieved party to suggest a solution.* People will more readily agree to a resolution that they have helped formulate.

6. *Move towards a "win-win" solution.* Preserve the individuals' dignity. Switch focus from what you cannot do toward what you can do. With permission, call in additional resources such as a supervisor, security, another counselor, or police. (Bohen, 2002, p. 27)

Lewis and Zare (1999) also recommend the use of "Crisis Response Teams" that can be activated in extreme instances of violent behavior in the workplace, such as a shooting. A Crisis Response Team may be composed of employee assistance counselors, representatives from management and labor, occupational health, legal and safety/security personnel, and outside liaisons to community resources such as mental health professionals. Each member of the team is designated a specific role. For example, one member of the team might be designated as the media liaison, another would provide information to employees, and another would set up debriefing sessions. The U.S. Department of Labor Occupational Safety and Health Administration, also provides valuable information on workplace violence that can be accessed on their website (www.osha.gov). Certainly, the old adage, "an ounce of prevention is worth a pound of cure" applies to workplace violence. In a majority of cases early intervention can prevent potentially volatile workers from acting out and harming others.

CRISES PERTAINING TO DOWNSIZING AND JOB TERMINATION

Downsizing has become one of the most pervasive yet understudied phenomenon in the American workplace. In October 2009 the unemployment rate hit a high of 10.2%, the highest level since 1983. Job loss and downsizing are common during times of economic recession (Andrews, 2008) and it is common that corporations differ in the ways they reduce their workforce. Hickok (2000) refers to the notion of "corporate culture" as a reflection of the ways in which companies will downsize. According to Hickok, "culture is to an organization what personality is to an individual." Therefore, it is not unusual to find many ways that corporations handle how they downsize their workforce. Some companies conscientiously plan a layoff and allow employees time and assistance (such as executive coaching) to make the transition smoother. These companies often initiate voluntary reductions as a first-step measure (such as job buyouts, job sharing, early retirement). Some companies will provide explicit criteria for who is laid off versus those who will stay on (Hickok, 2000). This type of downsizing is far different from the company that reacts impulsively to declining profits by arbitrarily laying off employees, giving them a cardboard box to clean out their desks, and having a security guard escort them to the parking lot. "Survivors" of corporate downsizing often experience high stress (Leana & Feldman, 1992); lower morale (Armstrong-Stassen, 1993); and a "syndrome" characterized by anger, envy, and guilt (Noer, 1993). Work relationships also suffer during periods of downsizing that can take the form of backstabbing, blaming, and failure to cooperate (Mohrman & Mohrman, 1983).

The stages that employees experience when they lose their jobs are somewhat similar to those experienced with other types of loss, in that employees go through a grieving process. The outcome of this process is that the person either becomes apathetic, depressed, and angry or they accept the loss and begin to move on with their lives. What is important for crisis counselors working with individuals who have experienced job loss it to determine what will help them move on. Leana and Feldman (1992) mention in their research with workers who had experienced job loss that "many had used metaphors of death and dying in their descriptions of the experience" (pg. 50). One worker stated, "Besides the death of a loved one, losing my job was one of the greatest hurts I have had in my life" (pg. 51). Eisenberg and Lazarsfeld (1938) were among the first to recognize that workers go through various stages in response to job loss. They were studying individuals who lost their jobs during the Depression of the 1930s. The stages that workers went through began with shock, which was then followed by an active job-hunt, at which point the person is usually optimistic and hopeful. When these efforts fail, however, the person experiences pessimism, anxiety, and active distress. This stage is followed by a fatalistic period where job attainment is viewed as hopeless or unattainable. Kaufman (1982) describes a four-stage model of response to unemployment. *Shock, relief, and relaxation* characterize this first stage. In the second stage, the person begins to *search for a new job*, however, if these attempts prove futile, the person then moves into a third stage of *self-doubt, anger, and vacillation*. In the fourth stage, the unemployed person experiences *resignation and withdrawal*. Kaufman suggests that this process may occur over a five to seven month period. Leana and Feldman (1992) researched what factors account for whether or not people succumbed to a state of apathy following their job loss or whether they viewed the job loss and re-employment as a challenge. Generally, they found that individuals with higher self-esteem (prior to the job layoff) and Type A Personality were predictive of those individuals who would take a more problem-focused coping approach. Problem-focused coping behaviors include making an active job search, retraining for another type of work or to increase employability skills, or relocating to another town or city where jobs are more plentiful. Type A personality is characterized by traits such as competitiveness, ambitiousness, and aggressiveness. These

---

CASE PRESENTATION: "I've been downsized"

Roberta worked for a financial investment firm for 20 years when she was promoted to senior vice president. Unfortunately, about three months after her promotion, the investment firm experienced major financial setbacks. As a result, Roberta and three other senior vice presidents were laid off. Roberta was emotionally devastated by the layoffs. What makes matters worse was that she was within five years of retirement and she has two children attending expensive private universities. Since Roberta was given notice of the lay-off approximately two weeks ago, she just sits and stares out of the window all day. She feels immobilized, angry, and betrayed.

Roberta can probably best be described as being in the stage of shock or depression. She is immobilized both by the news of her layoff as evidenced by her sitting and staring out of the window all day. Roberta is also experiencing regret for taking the promotion however the saying, "hindsight is always 20/20" applies here. She knows she also would have regretted not taking a promotion that resulted in higher pay, more prestige, and better benefits. The most important question is how to begin to mobilize Roberta's internal resources and her external network resources to begin the road to healing from this loss. Roberta has sought counseling through her health insurance plan, which she was allowed to keep as part of her severance package. The following is an excerpt of how such a session might go.

COUNSELOR: Roberta, I understand that you were laid off from your job as a result of the financial problems your company is experiencing.

ROBERTA: I still can't believe this is happening to me. I had just been promoted to senior vice president. I was finally at a point where all the hard work and overtime I put in had finally paid off and bang, they give me my pink slip.

COUNSELOR: When did all this happen?

ROBERTA: Three weeks ago. I have an O.K. severance package. I'll be on board for another few months, which allows me to train my replacement. Do you believe that? And then I'll get a year's severance pay with full benefits. I'm thinking of moving to Tahiti for a year—just kidding, of course. I have two kids in college, so I'm not going anywhere, least of all Tahiti!

COUNSELOR: Have you given any thought to what you'll do during this upcoming year?

ROBERTA: Well, that's why I agreed to see you. I admit I was resentful at first when my ex-husband suggested I come and speak with you, but then I thought to myself, why not take advantage of my health insurance while I still have it?

individuals are often driven, exhibit a great deal of goal-directed behavior, and often have a high energy level. In contrast, the Type B Personality is more laid back and less likely to become stressed. They tend to be more cooperative than competitive. With regards to the job search process, it is recommended that an active job seeker, will treat the search process as they would a full-time job.

It is difficult sometimes for crisis counselors to work with individuals who have recently been laid off, especially if the person is floundering in a mass of emotions that keep them immobilized such as blame, self-doubt, or pessimism. As with individuals who are going through a bereavement crisis, the role of the crisis counselor is to help facilitate the grieving process or to help the person experience the myriad of emotions that people naturally feel after going through such a loss while continuing to take active steps in their job search.

COUNSELOR: You mention you have two kids in college? How are they coping with the news of your layoff?

ROBERTA: They were pretty upset but like most college kids they're more focused on their own lives and how this will impact them. My son was pretty supportive. He works all summer to save money in order to pay for his expenses during the school year. My daughter is less motivated to work. She still thinks we have a money tree growing in the backyard. She's not as realistic when it comes to the harsh realities of life.

COUNSELOR: And your ex-husband, does he help with college expenses?

ROBERTA: He helps a little, but he was laid off from his job as a computer programmer about a year ago. His company downsized and outsourced their computer work to a company in India. He was never great when it came to helping out with the kids.

COUNSELOR: Had you ever been through a layoff or anything like this before?

ROBERTA: Well, not exactly like this. What it feels like is when I went through my divorce about ten years ago. That was pretty bad also. We had to sell our condo, I had no money, no place to live, I felt like a lost soul I guess.

COUNSELOR: Roberta, what helped you to get through that crisis? They say that going through a divorce is like grieving a death. How did you get through it?

Here, the counselor is not as interested in the details of the divorce as in talking about how Roberta was able to get through the emotional pain of the divorce. This might provide some clues for how Roberta coped with the loss and what might help her through the present crisis. It is not unusual for those who react the most intensely to a job loss crisis to have gone through some other major loss.

ROBERTA: Well, after I sulked and moped around for a couple of months, I finally found myself feeling angry at my ex. You know it was similar; here I was thinking I was a good wife, I worked hard and then one day, he says "I don't think I love you anymore, I need time to figure this out." About a month later he moved in with a woman he worked with. I guess he "figured things out."

(continued)

CASE PRESENTATION: "I've been downsized" *(continued)*

COUNSELOR: What helped you to get through all this?

ROBERTA: Well, I was able to talk with friends a lot. I spent time with my kids. I got into a support group at my church. I just got out of the pity pot and began doing things, like dating again.

COUNSELOR: Do you think you'll get to that point with this crisis?

ROBERTA: I see where you're going with this. You mean. I got through that crisis, I can get through this one, right? I don't know though, this one is pretty bad. Besides, who is going to hire me at 56 years old? I don't see things turning around, at least not in the near future anyway.

COUNSELOR: Are you ready to throw in the towel and move to Tahiti?

ROBERTA: I don't see many options here. The economy sucks. I don't even know how to tackle a job search. Where do I start?

COUNSELOR: There are a number of things we can work on. For example, I know of a headhunter who specializes in your industry, providing that you see yourself working in this industry.

ROBERTA: Yes, I don't want to make a total career change, I know investments inside and out, and I like the work.

COUNSELOR: O.K., I will give you her phone number so you can set up a meeting with her. What about networking? What I mean is that over the years you have met many people in this industry. What about putting out feelers, making some calls?

ROBERTA: Funny you mention that, I've kept every business card of everyone I've met in this business since I started out. I just feel lousy about calling them. Like I'm some sort of failure or charity case or something.

Guidelines for Crisis Counseling with a Downsized Employee

1. *Listen to the person's story and understand his or her reactions.* It is important to hear the events leading up to the downsizing and listen for various emotional reactions such as feelings of betrayal, sadness and loss, and anger. This is key to understanding how and why the person is reacting to the job loss.

2. *Assess whether there is depression, anxiety, or anger, which has become immobilizing.* There are many instances in which individuals can become totally immobilized by a job loss. If so, the crisis counselor will need to plan strategies according to the primary reaction. For example, would this person benefit from an antidepressant medication to help with mobilization?

3. *Facilitate the feelings of loss.* As with bereavement counseling, the role of the counselor is not to "push" the person, but rather to help facilitate expressions of grief.

4. *Refer for additional resources as appropriate.* In Roberta's case, the counselor saw that she had fought her way through other crises (her divorce) and was open to using support systems. Therefore, Roberta may have been open to job-finding self-help groups or, in this instance, a referral to a headhunter.

COUNSELOR: That's the first thing we'll need to work on. You know that the work-place has changed. Very few people have lifelong jobs anymore, so what makes you different? What's wrong with you asking if these contacts know of any job openings? What if one of the people whose cards you have called you looking to see what you knew about possible openings?

ROBERTA: I would try to help the person, unless they were a total loser or something.

COUNSELOR: So, you're not a "total loser." Don't you think some of your friends or colleagues would be willing to help you?

Case Conceptualization/Crisis Resolution
In the case illustration above, there are both emotional and practical goals. As with any grief counseling, the counselor tries to facilitate the grief process. By facilitation, we mean that the counselor tries to get the person to express the feelings associated with the particular stage of the experiencing. If the individual is angry, then the counselor tries to facilitate the expression of this anger. If depressed, the counselor tries to facilitate the expression of these depressive feelings. In the latter part of the session, the counselor uses a cognitive behavioral strategy. Roberta indirectly expresses one of Ellis's Irrational Beliefs (Ellis, 1952), "I must be thoroughly adequate, competent, and achieving in everything I do," therefore Roberta feels that losing her job is a sign that she is incompetent and flawed. The counselor is trying to get Roberta to refute this irrational perception.

5.   *Watch for signs of apathy.* As indicated earlier, there are many instances where job hunters become apathetic and will stop searching or become isolated. It is important to keep watch to make sure the person actively searches for a job.

6.   *Assist the person to become open to other options.* In some instances the job outlook for certain careers may not be as promising as others. If that is the case, it may be more helpful to encourage the person to be open to other possibilities.

CRISES PERTAINING TO SUPERVISOR—
COWORKER CONFLICT

Another aspect of workplace crises are those brought about by interactions between managers and employees, and interactions among coworkers. Because this area involves power, we have found that the abuse of power can often lead to crises in the workplace. There are many different types of power that each individual in the workplace may have. It is obvious that certain administrative or managerial positions give one the authority to make decisions involving others. Naturally, there are some bosses or managers who will flagrantly abuse this power. Sexual harassment is probably at the top of the list of such abuses. It is also not uncommon for supervisors or administrators to demand more work for less pay. When the worker tries to rectify such a situation he or she may be confronted with a statement such as, "You should consider yourself lucky you have a job." When someone's job responsibilities are not clearly defined, delineated and agreed upon, this can be abusive. When workers are subjected to demeaning comments, excluded from decisions that directly affect their ability to do their jobs, or their expertise is diminished in some way, then this too becomes abusive. When an administrator makes decisions arbitrarily, promotes arbitrarily, or raises or bonuses are doled out arbitrarily, then this too may feel abusive to those who are passed over. In some instances promotions can merely be an insignificant title which translates to more work, more responsibility, and the same pay. We have also witnessed several instances where companies have merged and many managers were given increased responsibilities for other departments within the newly merged company, with no increase in pay, no recognition, and no promotion.

Keep in mind, however, the abuse of power can run both ways. For example, the employee who refuses to complete a needed work assignment on time may use passive-aggressiveness to wield power. An employee who is continually negative about every idea for change even when positive, uses negativity to wield power. People's attitudes towards others can be very abusive. The employee who goes after an administrator by criticizing him or her at every opportunity or who sneaks around to other administrators is abusively wielding power. On the surface it may appear that the supervisor or manager has all the power, but this is not always true. Workplace bullying is a topic that has received a lot of attention lately (Rayner, 2000).

Sexual harassment and sexual abuse often involve yet another form of an abuse of power. All too often, people in positions of power use that power to take sexual advantage of a subordinate. Two forms of sexual harassment have been described in the literature, "quid pro quo" and "hostile working environment" (Sexual Harassment: Fact v. Myth, 1994). In the quid-pro-quo type, the harassment message is straightforward, "Sleep with me or you're fired." In other words, employment (hiring, promotions, raises, retaining one's job) is contingent on the victim's providing sexual favors. In defining a hostile workplace environment, the job becomes permeated with discriminatory intimidation, ridicule, and insult that are sufficiently severe or pervasive to alter the conditions of the victim's employment and create abusive working conditions. In determining whether a work environment is hostile or abusive, the U.S. Supreme Court handed down some guidelines by which all circumstances could be taken into account, such as: a) the frequency of the discriminatory conduct, b) its severity, c) whether it is physically threatening or a mere offensive utterance, and d) whether it unreasonably interferes with an employee's work performance. In the interpretation of the law, (Sexual Harassment: Fact v. Myth, 1994), a "hostile work environment" can be defined by "speech and/or conduct, of a sexually discriminatory nature, which was neither welcomed nor encouraged, committed by or permitted by a supervisor, which would be so offensive to a reasonable person as to create an abusive working environment and/or impair his/her job performance." Unfortunately, when sexual harassment does occur in the workplace, many companies "will still deny that the event occurred, admit no wrongdoing and turn against the victim. The harasser will deny the allegations. Coworkers will then place blame on the victim, saying it was something they wanted or asked for. Some coworkers will even become angry with the victim for coming forward with the complaint and will quickly run to the defense of the harasser, instead of offering assistance and understanding to the victim. The victim is then left standing alone" (www.join-wash.org). Unfortunately, many cases of sexual harassment go unreported. As with other forms of sexual assault, such as rape or intimate partner violence, there is fear that reporting the incident will result in reprisal. Victims of workplace harassment fear that they will lose their job, that others will not believe them, and that they will be attacked for having come forward.

CASE PRESENTATION: A Case of Sexual Harassment

Sandra works for a major airline in the maintenance department. Her job is to help guide planes into their gates and she is also responsible for setting up refueling and baggage unloading. Her boss Jack Pritchard often makes remarks about how slow Sandra is in getting her work done, but does this by making sexual innuendoes. "What's the matter, didn't you get any last night?" or similar remarks are common, and Sandra finds herself being the brunt of other jokes made by male employees. When Sandra confronted Mr. Pritchard about his remarks, he became defensive and said she was being "too sensitive" and remarked that jet maintenance was no place for women anyway. Sandra is a single parent who cannot afford to lose her job or benefits. She feels frustrated and trapped.

In Sandra's case, she is faced with the dilemma of whether or not to report the abuse. She decides that she will speak to the employee assistance counselor because she heard that whatever is said in the session will be confidential. The role of the employee assistance counselor is to first validate Sandra's feeling. Sandra reports that she feels trapped and powerless, but more so, she feels humiliated whenever she is at work and also feels that her coworkers have either joined Jack Pritchard in his abusive remarks, or they have turned their backs on Sandra totally. It is important that the employee assistance counselor validate these feelings—in other words, to make certain that Sandra's feelings are heard and understood. The counselor's role is not to play judge and jury, or to determine whether or not the abuse has occurred or the remarks constitute a violation of the law; rather the counselor's role is to help Sandra to define the problem and provide her with support. It is also important that the counselor not force Sandra to make any decisions as to what course of action to take, but rather to provide her with information by which she could make a more informed decision. The following session illustrates ways that the counselor might help Sandra through this crisis.

(continued)

CASE PRESENTATION: A Case of Sexual Harassment
(*continued*)

Intervention

COUNSELOR: Sandra, when you called earlier today to meet with me, you sounded really upset. Were you able to finish out your shift today?

SANDRA: Yeah, it was really tough going though; I haven't been sleeping very well since all this has been happening.

COUNSELOR: What type of problems have you been having?

SANDRA: First of all, before I get into anything, this is confidential right? I mean you can't tell my boss about what we talk about, or make me go to Human Resources, right?

COUNSELOR: Yes, it is confidential, the only time I am mandated by law to break confidentiality is in instances of threats of homicide, suicide, or child abuse. Anything else remains between us, and the only time I'm allowed to reveal anything is with your signed release. O.K.?

SANDRA: O.K.. Well what's been happening is that my boss, Mr. Pritchard, started (begins crying) ... this is really tough.

COUNSELOR: Yes, I can see it is. Why don't you take a minute to catch your breath? Do you want some water?

SANDRA: No, I'll be all right. About six months ago, Mr. Pritchard, my immediate boss began making remarks, sexual type remarks. When I was unloading baggage from the trucks he would say some really horrible things and make comments about my breasts. At first, I wouldn't say anything and just go about my business, then about a month ago, he started groping me, grabbing my butt, as I walked by, you know things like that. Some of the other guys on the crew also began making remarks. I warned them that I would talk with Mr. James, the VP in charge of maintenance, but they'd laugh and keep doing it. I was going to see Mr. James, but then I thought I would end up losing my job.

COUNSELOR: What made you think that you would lose your job?

SANDRA: Well, a friend of mine had the same thing happen at her job. She doesn't work here, she works at another airline and her boss said that if she didn't do "favors" for him, he'd fire her the next time she came in late. She refused and he fired her. She tried to report him, but the company denied it happened, and so did her coworkers.

COUNSELOR: Sandra, it must have been very tough for you to come here and talk about this. It sounds from what you've said this has been happening for several months. Have you told anyone besides me?

SANDRA: No, I felt like I couldn't tell anyone. I was afraid that if I told my brother or anyone in my family, they would put out a contract on Pritchard's life. My ex-husband split, not that he would care. I can't lose my job, he doesn't pay any child support so I bring in the only paycheck. If I lose this job, I'll lose my kids. My ex-husband's parents have already threatened to have them taken from me.

COUNSELOR: Why have they threatened to do that?

SANDRA: Because they want more time with the kids. I'm pretty good about making sure the kids spend time with their grandparents, but the more I give, the more they seem to want.

COUNSELOR: I can see the bind you're in. What have you done so far?

SANDRA: I talked with Mr. Pritchard. I told him I was uncomfortable with the things he was saying and his grabbing me, but he laughed it off and said I was being too sensitive. He said since women have been working the flight line, everything has to be "nicey-nice." I feel bad that I didn't try talking with him when this first started or with his boss, but I'm afraid they would just fire me.

COUNSELOR: You did the right thing by trying to talk with him first. Sandra, you are a victim of sexual harassment. There are laws that prevent any employee from harassment in the workplace and that protect them from being fired in retaliation.

SANDRA: The laws didn't help my friend though.

COUNSELOR: I guess not, but perhaps she didn't file an EEOC complaint.

SANDRA: What is an EEOC?

COUNSELOR: The EEOC is the Equal Employment Opportunity Commission. They are responsible for making certain that companies are in compliance with EEOC regulations. This covers things like making sure that companies do not discriminate against people because of gender, race, ethnicity, disability, and so on, and also enforces laws pertaining to sexual harassment and hostile work environment. You could file a complaint through the EEOC office here at the Airline or through one of the regional offices.

SANDRA: And then I suppose I would get my pink slip in my next paycheck — no way!

COUNSELOR: No, Sandra. Once you file a complaint, your job is protected. Mr. Pritchard could not fire you unless there was some major infringement of company policy. Basically, you would be safe.

SANDRA: What happens once I file a complaint?

COUNSELOR: Usually, the EEOC staff will investigate to determine if the allegations are valid. If they are, then the Airline would need to take steps to rectify the situation. Sometimes this might involve sitting down with a mediator.

SANDRA: But once this is all over, could Pritchard turn around and fire me?

COUNSELOR: Not if you're doing your job.

SANDRA: I do my job; don't worry about that. I'm never late, I never take a day off, my performance reviews are all "Outstanding."

COUNSELOR: That's in your favor. Sandra, what do you suppose would be the reaction of your coworkers if you were to file a complaint?

SANDRA: Well, I know the guys I work with would be ticked off. I don't care. There is one other woman that works part-time, though, and she has put up with some of the same stuff. I don't think as much as I have. I don't know how she would react. Why? Do you think it matters?

COUNSELOR: What is unfortunate in instances like this, is that it is not uncommon for coworkers to turn against the person that files the complaint. They often feel alone after filing.

SANDRA: So, are you telling me not to file?

(continued)

C A S E   P R E S E N T A T I O N :   A Case of Sexual Harassment
(*continued*)

COUNSELOR: No. I just want to give you as much information as possible in the event that you do file. Let's take the other case scenario. What if you don't file?

SANDRA: Well, I guess Pritchard will keep pawing me and making nasty remarks. I don't know if I can put up with that?

COUNSELOR: Sandra, there is nothing to say that you have to file a complaint today. Why don't you think on it a bit? Find out if your friend had filed an EEOC complaint. You don't have to do anything right now. Also, you can continue to come for counseling here, or I can refer you to a counselor close to where you live. Sometimes, it's helpful to get another opinion on something like this anyway. Your insurance plan will cover your seeing an outside counselor.

SANDRA: Can I think this over a bit and can we meet in a few days maybe?

COUNSELOR: That would be fine. Sandra, how are you feeling right now? Are you going to be O.K.?

SANDRA: Believe it or not, I do feel a little better. I feel like, at least I have some options. I don't feel as trapped.

COUNSELOR: Good. Let's meet on Thursday.

Sexual Harassment Complaint Filed Against Best Buy
Washington, DC: December, 13, 2000/PR Newswire

The Council on American-Islamic Relations (CAIR) announced today that it has filed an EEOC compliant against Minnesota-based Best Buy Co., one of the nation's largest electronics retailers, after that company failed to resolve a case of sexual harassment involving a female Muslim employee in Maryland. (Best Buy operates more that 350 retail stores in 39 states.) The filing of an EEOC complaint is necessary prior to a lawsuit.

According to the Best Buy employee, who wears a religiously-mandated headscarf, a supervisor repeatedly made sexually explicit comments, which she tried to ignore. On September 8, 2000, the worker says the supervisor approached her from behind in a state of sexual arousal and whispered, "This is (for) you, This is (for) you," while rubbing against her.

The next day, the supervisor again approached the Muslim woman, grabbed her hand and attempted to pull her close to him. She resisted and told him to stop and indicated that she was a married woman. The supervisor allegedly said: "That is good, because I am married too, I won't have to worry about my wife finding out

---

Before concluding, it is important to point out that sexual harassment and hostile work environment, although primarily a male-to-female phenomenon, can also include instances where men are subjected to sexual harassment by female supervisors or by fellow male coworkers. Such was the case with a male

Case Conceptualization/Crisis Resolution

In the case illustration the Counselor was careful to validate Sandra's feelings that she was being mistreated by her supervisor. Often victims of sexual harassment will doubt their own perceptions and feelings, and might feel that something they are doing is causing the harassment. They may also question whether they should report the harassment. For example, in Sandra's trying to deal directly with Mr. Pritchard, he downplays the harassment and accuses Sandra of being "too sensitive." This is unfortunately very common.

The counselor is also careful to provide Sandra with information about options, while not forcing her to make a decision. According to EEOC guidelines, a complaint must be filed within 180 days of the alleged act; however, in some jurisdictions, a complaint may be filed within 300 days of the alleged act. Since Sandra's harassment has been ongoing, it is likely that her case falls within these guidelines. It is also important that Sandra is given all the facts to weigh the merits of whether or not to file a complaint. This is why the EAP Counselor suggested that she may want to speak with a neutral counselor outside of the company.

because we could both have a lot to lose." He did not stop the harassment until another worker intervened.

Following the incident, the woman asked for time off because she no longer felt comfortable in the store. She said other workers who heard about the incident were avoiding her. Company officials allowed her to take time off but said she would not be paid and that the negative coworker reactions were a result of the employee "running her mouth" about the incident.

In two letters to Best Buy, CAIR demanded that the company: 1) Reprimand the supervisor for his actions. (The supervisor was subsequently terminated.) 2) Institute sensitivity training for Best Buy supervisors. 3) Offer the Muslim employees a formal apology. 4) Offer compensation for any humiliation and emotional distress that she suffered as a result of the harassment.

A similar case resulted in a female employee at a Missouri Wal-Mart being awarded 50 million dollars by a jury that found she was subjected to a hostile work environment.

employee who, while working for a construction crew, was continually subjected to ridicule and harassment by other male employees who taunted this individual by calling him "a pansy," "a fairy," and "a homo." This person was subjected to this ridicule because he was not as brash or vulgar as his coworkers.

Because he was quiet and nonthreatening, he was an easy mark for bullying and sexually demeaning remarks. Eventually, this person quit the job, but only after filing an EEOC complaint having alleged that his foreman condoned the "hostile work environment" that was created by his coworkers. Male-to-male sexual harassment has become more commonplace and, according to recent legal rulings, does constitute a form of "hostile work environment" that is often cited in sexual harassment suits (Talbot, 2002).

There are many other instances of coworker- and supervisor-created conflict. For example, there are many other types of discrimination that take place other than sexual harassment, which can place an employee in turmoil. In prior research, it appears that much of the stress created in the workplace by administrators, coworkers, or subordinates may be produced by individuals with personality disorders (Cavaiola & Lavender, 1999). Because individuals with personality disorders often lack insight into their behavior, this naturally leads to problems in interpersonal relationships. Since most workplaces involve social interaction, individuals with personality disorders often generate a great deal of stress for those whom they work with. For example, the narcissistic administrator (Levinson, 1994) is a classic example of how an individual with narcissistic personality disorders or narcissistic traits can create stress in the workplace. As an illustration of this, a 28-year-old administrative assistant to an up-and-coming vice president at an investment banking firm had become pregnant but lost the baby after three months. When she called her boss to let him know that she needed to take a few days off to recover both physically and emotionally from the miscarriage, he screamed, "This is unacceptable, you know we have the month-end report due by next week. If you're not in here by tomorrow, don't bother coming in at all." Narcissistic managers or bosses are known for their lack of empathy and compassion. Instead, they will see things only from the vantage point of how it will impact them or their careers.

It is possible, also, to have a narcissist working for you as an employee or a subordinate. In trying to manage this person, however, this type of employee will feel that they are "special" and should be treated in a special way. They may also feel that the rules that apply to others do not apply to them. A more pathological or problematic narcissist will think nothing of going after the boss's job or going behind the boss's back to upper management (Cavaiola & Lavender, 2000). These are just a couple of examples of how individuals with personality disorders can create stress and crises in the workplace, by the very nature of their personalities, lack of social skills, or lack of ethics and fair play.

Guidelines for Crisis Counseling in Instances of Supervisor-Coworker Conflict

1. *Listen to employees and hear out their complaints without judging them.* Individuals who experience conflicts with supervisors or coworkers are often attuned to who is "on their side" versus those who are not. Therefore, it is important that you listen without judging those seeking help. At the same time, it is important to get information about the events leading up to the crisis.

2. *Assess their primary reactions.* People differ in how they may react to this type of conflict. Someone being sexually harassed may feel anger, hurt, betrayal, rage, sadness, frustration, or humiliation. It is important to encourage expression of these feelings and to help identify these reactions as normal responses to often abnormal situations.

3. *Determine if they are being treated unjustly or if there is evidence of discrimination or harassment.* Although some types of supervisor-coworker conflict do not constitute a violation of one's rights in the workplace, other instances might— such as in the case of gender, age or racial discrimination in job promotion or of sexual harassment. Counselors should be familiar with laws pertaining to worker's rights (such as the Americans With Disabilities Act).

4. *Know what resources are available and refer as appropriate.* Just as it is important to know the laws pertaining to one's rights in the workplace, it is also very important to know what resources are available to individuals who may be victimized. For example, in Sandra's case, she was unaware that she could file a complaint with the EEOC and of what was involved in filing a complaint.

RECOMMENDATIONS FOR CHAPTER ENRICHMENT

SUGGESTED WEBSITES

Job Loss Resources

Guidelines for Thriving During Job Loss and Job Search
> This site provides useful tips for job search and surviving a job loss.

http://www.thrivenet.com/articles/jloss.shtml

Surviving Job Loss
> Site offers strategies, techniques, and tools to help survive losing a job. Includes information on personal finance, COBRA benefits, job searching, and places to get help.

http://careerplanning.about.com/od/jobloss/a/job_loss.htm

Job-Loss Grief Stages
> Detailed information about the stages of job-loss grief, including: symptoms, how to help, and suggestions for managing your own job-loss grief.

http://members.tripod.com/~jobnet/joblossc.htm

Managing after Downsizing
> Provides helpful suggestions and recommendations for people who have lost their jobs through downsizing. Once this website is reached, go to "Profile of Articles," "Business and Money," and then to "Managing after Downsizing."

http://www.JohnShepler.com

Workplace Violence Resources

Protecting Yourself and Preventing Workplace Violence
This site explores some of the sources and origins of violence at the workplace, what can be done to prevent it, and what to do when it happens.

http://www.uslawbooks.com/books/violence.htm

Guidelines for Preventing Workplace Violence for Health Care and Social Service Workers
U.S. Department of Labor Occupational Safety and Health Administration (OSHA) material contained in this publication: violence prevention program elements, work-site analysis, hazard prevention and control, training, and education.

http://www.osha.gov/Publications/OSHA3148/osha3148.html

Industrial Hygiene
Searchable database allowing for quick location of Internet resources about workplace violence.

http://www.industrialhygiene.com/links/Occupational_Safety/
Workplace_Violence

Sexual Harassment

Sexual Harassment in the Workplace: A Primer
This website provides a lot of information of types of sexual harassment in the workplace and steps that can be taken to deal with sexual harassment and ways for corporations to avoid sexual harassment.

http://www3.uakron.edu/lawrev/robert1.html

Sexual Harassment Support
This website provides a great deal of information about sexual harassment and support for those going through sexual harassment in the workplace. Many valuable guidelines and links to other information pertaining to this crisis.

http://www.sexualharassmentsupport.org/SHworkplace.html

Suggested Films

Nine to Five (1980) This film depicts the story of three women working for a egotistical, narcissistic, harassing boss, played by Dabney Coleman. The movie is loosely based on a true story and, although it is basically a comedy (due to the revenge that these women exact from their tormentor), it does give a good depiction of workplace harassment and the inappropriate boundary violations that can and do occur.

Office Space (1999) This film depicts office workers who are tormented by a narcissistic, exploitative boss. This film provides an excellent illustration of a narcissistic administrator.

Close to Home **(2009)** This documentary chronicles the impact of the economic recession on several families and provides an excellent depiction of the various crises that come about in the aftermath of layoffs and corporate downsizing. First aired on PBS Frontline.

SUGGESTED ACTIVITIES

1. The following newspaper describes an actual workplace shooting which occurred on December 26, 2000. Read through the article and determine if there are any Factors Predictive of Workplace Violence (described in Figure 1) present.

2. Imagine you have a family member who is laid off or downsized from their job. Would any of the guidelines described in the websites pertaining to job loss be useful to them? If not what would you suggest they do?

3. There have been many cases of sexual harassment allegations which involve celebrities. See what you can find out regarding cases involving actor Rob Lowe, Fox News anchor Bill O'Reilly, former Oregon Senator Bob Packwood, TV host Maury Povich. From what you've found, do you feel the allegations were warranted? What were the outcomes of these cases?

"Seven Die in Massachusetts Office Shooting"— Wakefield, MA, Dec. 26, 2000

A heavily armed employee shot and killed seven coworkers today in the offices of a suburban Boston Internet company, "an incredible workplace tragedy" that may have stemmed from a tax dispute with the IRS, according to prosecutors and witnesses.

Amid Christmas wreaths and other holiday decorations, authorities said, Michael M. McDermott, 42, was armed with an assault rifle, a 12-gauge shotgun, and a semi-automatic pistol as he methodically gunned down colleagues in the first-floor offices of Edgewater Technology Inc., an Internet consulting firm about 10 miles north of downtown Boston.

Four women and three men were shot dead, but none of the other 80 workers inside the building were injured, officials said.

"It appears to have been aimed at individuals, as opposed to random spraying," Middlesex County District Attorney Martha Coakley said tonight, calling it "an incredible workplace tragedy."

Coakley said detectives are investigating whether the shooting was related to moves by Edgewater and the Internal Revenue Service to garnish McDermott's wages for back taxes, just one of the financial and personal problems that had recently beset him.

McDermott, who has worked as a software tester at Edgewater since at least March, recently skipped out of one apartment while owing rent and moved into a new apartment without his wife, according to acquaintances and officials.

(continued)

"Seven Die in Massachusetts Office Shooting"—
Wakefield, MA, Dec. 26, 2000 (*continued*)

Prosecutors said the rampage began at 11 a.m.—more than two hours after McDermott arrived for work—when he calmly walked into the main reception area and from 10 feet away, shot the receptionist. Coakley said McDermott proceeded to the nearby accounting section, where he began using the assault rifle and the shotgun. Five of the seven killed were in the accounting department, authorities said, and the two were in the reception area.

McDermott had an angry outburst in the accounting department last week over the prospect of losing some of his wages, the Associated Press quoted an unnamed employee as saying. He apparently felt the company was not doing enough to take his side against the IRS, the employee said.

In a statement last night, the company said that "his actions apparently stem from occurrences in his personal life. We deeply regret that Mr. McDermott's problems manifested in actions against the company and its employees. There was no way to anticipate his actions or any apparent reasons to restrict his access to the building."

Mike Stanley, a team project leader at Edgewater, told reporters that McDermott had been coming in late and that his performance wasn't as good as it could have been. He said McDermott was kidding around with coworkers not long before the shootings.

"He was joking with a bunch of people before he went on the rampage," Stanley said. "It seems like a random, ridiculous thing." But Stanley also described McDermott as "strange" and "quirky," adding: "Of all the people that I thought could have done this, it was him."

(Source: *Washington Post* article by Dan Eggen & Pamela Ferdinand, *Washington Post* Staff Writers)

Major Shootings in the Workplace Since 1995

The following major workplace shootings preceded yesterday's killing of seven people at Edgewater Technology, Inc. in Wakefield, MA:

- March 20, 2000: Fired employee Susan Harris, 28, fatally shot five people at a Dallas-area car wash. Harris was convicted and sentenced to death.

- Dec. 30, 1999: Authorities said housekeeper Silvio Izquierdo-Leyva, 36, fatally shot five coworkers at Tampa's Radisson Bay Harbor Hotel. He pleaded not guilty.

- Nov. 2, 1999: Copier repairman Bryan Uyesugi, 40, fatally shot several people at a Xerox Corp. facility in Honolulu. He was convicted and sentenced to life in prison.

- Aug. 5, 1999: Truck driver Alan E. Miller, 35, fatally shot two coworkers at a Pelham, AL, office, then killed a former coworker. Miller was convicted and sentenced to death.

- July 29, 1999: Former day trader, Mark Barton, 44, killed nine people at two Atlanta brokerage offices and later committed suicide.

- March 6, 1998: Former Connecticut Lottery Corp. accountant, Matthew Beck, 35, fatally shot four lottery executives, then himself.

- Dec. 18, 1997: Fired employee Arturo R. Torres, 43, killed four former coworkers at a maintenance yard in Orange County, Calif., and was shot to death by police.

- Sept. 15, 1997: Fired assembly line worker Arthur H. Wise, 43, allegedly opened fire at an Aiken, SC, parts plant, killing four. His trial is pending.

- April 24, 1996: Former employee James Simpson, 28, fatally shot five people at a refinery inspection station in Corpus Christi, TX, then killed himself.

- July 19, 1995: City electrician Willie Woods fatally shot four supervisors at C. Erwin Piper Technical Center in Los Angeles. He was sentenced to life in prison.

(Source: *The Washington Post*, December 27, 2000)

"Murder Becoming a Real Job Hazard"
by Roland D. Maiuro (*Newsday*, Oct. 4, 1998)

Ever-increasing pressures in the workplace is creating a breeding ground for violence, says Roland D. Maiuro. Those of us who track the rise and fall of the tide of violence in our society know that the problem is not restricted to wayward youth in our schools, but is one that mirrors itself in adult institutions.

Contrary to recent headlines, there are numerous indicators that the most rapidly growing category of violence is in the workplace. In fact, murder has become the Number 1 cause of death for women on the job.... According to some researchers, the most common "profile" of a violence-prone employee is a white male, 35 or older, who has few interests and social supports outside of work, an affinity for guns, a history of family problems, and a tendency to harbor resentments and grudges, verbalize extremist opinions, and abuse drugs and alcohol during times of stress.

Some experts, however, argue that generic profiles are of questionable value as such acts may be committed by men and women of all races and ages, regardless of a history violence. More immediate or situational predictors such as acute paranoia and distrust, perceived attack by coworkers or supervisors, feelings of irreparable damage or loss, depression, actual suicidal or homicidal threats, and a history of unresolved conflicts associated with the filing of grievances and lawsuits may have greater value as red flags for workplace violence.

14

Community Response to Crisis

DISCUSSION QUESTIONS

Take a tour of your own community. What potential sources of crises are there? Consider all types of possible crises such as those posed by one's location to industrial areas, power plants, sources of natural weather-related events, potential terrorist targets, and so on.

What do you think should be the public's responsibility in responding to a crisis event that has a significant impact on the community?

Have you ever been involved in a volunteer effort to assist someone in need in the aftermath of a crisis? Has anyone assisted you after a personal crisis without your requesting the assistance?

INTRODUCTION

Who helps in times of crisis?

Many people do, according to *A Survey of Charitable Giving After September 11, 2001* (Independent Sector, 2001). This survey reported that seven in ten Americans donated money, blood, or time in response to the terrorist attacks of 9/11, whereas 30% of those surveyed claimed that they had participated in one or more community, spiritual, or local neighborhood events or activities commemorating the 9/11 event. Candlelight vigils, religious services, prayer vigils, and town meetings were only some of the activities they had attended in a spontaneous display of support.

Researchers have long distinguished between helping (spontaneous helping) and volunteerism (planned helping) (Clary, Snyder, Ridge, Copeland, Stukas, Haugen, & Miene, 1998). The helper is one who experiences an unexpected need to help someone and who makes an immediate decision to act; the volunteer, however, is someone who actively seeks out the opportunity to help others. The helper's act involves one relatively brief instance of helping, whereas the volunteer may commit to an ongoing relationship with a person, a cause, or an organization.

This sustained nature of volunteering is what distinguishes it from the more spontaneous act of helping, otherwise known as bystander intervention, the object of considerable earlier research efforts in investigating the reasons behind prosocial actions (Finkelstein, 2007). Later research (Clary et al., 1998) into volunteering, however, identified six potential motives of the volunteer:

- Values—expressing altruistic and humanitarian values
- Understanding—acquiring learning experiences and/or exercising unused skills
- Social—strengthening social relationships
- Career—gaining career-related benefits
- Protective—reducing negative feelings about oneself or addressing personal problems
- Enhancement—growing psychologically

Nevertheless, regardless of the motives that drive the helper and the volunteer to provide assistance to those in need, it is clear that volunteers represent an integral part of this country's workforce (Finkelstein, 2007). According to the Bureau of Labor Statistics' *Volunteering in the United States, 2006* report, about 61.2 million people volunteered through or for an organization at least once in the previous year, approximately 26.7% of the population. Almost half of these volunteers (43%) became involved with their primary volunteer organization after being asked to do so by a member of the organization, and a slightly smaller proportion of volunteers (40%) initiated contact with the organization on their own initiative.

A greater proportion of women than men (30% versus 23%) volunteer. People between the ages of 35 and 54 are the most likely to volunteer (31% of the group), whereas the least likely age group to volunteer were people in their early 20s (17.8%). Although the organizations where volunteers worked the most hours were frequently religious, educational, youth-service related, social or community service organizations were also the recipients of a large share of volunteer hours.

This large number of helper and volunteer hours must surely be considered a minimal estimate of the total number of hours given in the volunteer effort. Individuals who are not necessarily connected to an organization when they contribute time, effort, or money constitute another whole cadre of volunteers, the numbers of whom elude even rough approximations. People who organize their own bake sales, garage sales, or other fund-raising activities to provide donations to victims of a natural or man-made disaster are not counted among this number, nor are individuals who provide comfort, shelter, or any form of support to rescue workers or crisis survivors. Donations of all kinds done in anonymity ensure that the true numbers of helpers and volunteers, and their donated hours, will never be known.

Large numbers of volunteers, however, are not always without their share of problems. In the aftermath of 9/11, for example, the city of New York had to turn down offers of blood donations after it reached its capacity to test it and store it properly. It even had to refuse all but the most skilled and essential volunteers who offered their services, considering the vast numbers of individuals who appeared on the scene (Cavaiola & Colford, 2006). The National Voluntary Organizations Active in Disaster (NVOAD), a group created in 1970 to coordinate the efforts of volunteer groups responding to disasters, reported on the serious challenges presented by the large numbers of volunteers after a disaster, particularly those events of a significant magnitude like 9/11. In fact, just several months after 9/11, NVOAD sponsored the first National Leadership Forum on Disaster Volunteerism to discuss ways to provide guidance to the public on the management of volunteers in disasters.

The federal government's role in crisis response comes primarily through the efforts of the Federal Emergency Management Agency (FEMA), a former independent agency that became part of the Department of Homeland Security in 2003. FEMA is charged with responding to, planning for, recovering from, and mitigating against disasters. It often works in partnership with other organizations that are part of the country's emergency management system, including state and local emergency management agencies, other federal agencies, and the American Red Cross.

Once state governors assess the extent and level of a disaster to be beyond the capability of the states' resources to respond to it effectively, they can request that the president make a disaster declaration in order to insure FEMA's intervention. Since 2000, there have been 421 disaster declarations made.

The focus of this chapter is on one particular community's response to the events of 9/11. It will document the coordinated efforts of the municipal government and of two volunteer groups that sprang spontaneously from the needs of a community devastated by the attacks on that day. Although there have been more recent crises that have had profound consequences on different communities, such as the natural disasters of hurricanes Katrina, Rita, and Ike, the California wildfires, and the severe flooding in the Midwest, one of the current authors of this text is a resident of the community that is highlighted below. He thought it fitting that he tell this story.

MIDDLETOWN, NEW JERSEY:

A COMMUNITY IN CRISIS

Townships known as Middletown number approximately 35 and stretch across the United States, with 19 states claiming to have one or more of them listed among their rosters of municipalities. Urban and rural, large and small, the name connotes a settlement somewhere between two larger and more established ones, making the name appear as a mere footnote to more substantial, more important settlements. Middletown, New Jersey, a 42-square mile town and home to almost 70,000 residents, was once just another Middletown, named for its strategic geographic position midway between New York City and Philadelphia. Located approximately 43 miles south of the Manhattan site where the World Trade Center Twin Towers once stood, this Middletown was the perfect commuter town, sending many members of its 23,000 households into Manhattan each day by car, train, bus, or ferry. And so it was on September 11, 2001.

Thirty-seven of these same commuters were barely at their desks somewhere in the Towers that morning when the first attack came; 37 Middletown residents died that day, the largest concentration of victims from any town in America. Suddenly, this Middletown became the international representative for human tragedy; no longer would this Middletown be confused with any of its 34 namesakes.

Pictures of unclaimed cars in Middletown's bus and train station commuter parking lots, many of them belonging to those who would never again return to claim them, made the local newspapers the next day. One of the police department's first duties that week was to visit these lots and record license plate numbers in order to track their owners, all potential victims of the attack. Missing persons' reports filed by local residents as well as requests for prayers from the local clergy suggested early what later was confirmed: Many Middletown residents lost their lives that day.

Among the dead were youth baseball and basketball coaches, volunteer firefighters, the PTA president of a local parochial school, and 26 parishioners of the local Catholic parish. One of these coaches, Paul Nimbley, had been sworn in as the new Middletown Youth Athletic Association basketball commissioner just the night before; he was proud to be able to oversee a 500-player program, although his special interest was in enlarging the girls' league in town. He left behind a wife, two daughters, a six-month old son, and a household packed in boxes in anticipation of a move to a new neighborhood just days later.

News of the large number of Middletown dead soon spread around the globe. A front page story of the town's loss in the *Washington Post* insured international attention. Reporters and film crews descended on the town over the next few weeks looking for friends and family members of Nimbley, who had been featured prominently in the *Washington Post* story.

During a girls' basketball game at one of the town's middle schools in which Nimbley would have been coaching, a reporter from the *Baltimore Sun-Times* sat in the bleachers interviewing some of his acquaintances, while a film crew from the British Broadcasting Company set up shop in one corner of the gym and conducted a series of interviews with those who knew him. In yet another corner of the gym that night was a film crew from the Japanese Broadcasting System show described as the Japanese counterpart to America's own news magazine show, *60 Minutes*; Dai Koyama, the host, conducted on-camera interviews.

Reporters from other countries, including Belgium, Italy, France, and Australia also arrived in Middletown within days of the attacks. Best selling author, Gail Sheehy, spent much of the next two years in the township interviewing victims' family members as well as a host of others involved in the recovery effort for her book, *Middletown, America: One Town's Passage from Trauma to Hope*. This suburban setting would never be the same again.

MIDDLETOWN'S RESPONSE TO 9/11

The modest basement office was unassuming. Besides the requisite office furniture of a half-moon desk separating a swivel chair from three side chairs, there was little more to distinguish this simple office arrangement from any other in the bustling police department headquarters in Middletown, New Jersey.

There was little more, save for the constant reminders of that day, September 11, 2001, which were positioned prominently in this small, intimate room and kept it frozen in time. Were it not for the desk calendar, one might think that the day of this interview (November 28, 2007) was just shortly after the terrorist attacks on the Twin Towers of New York City over six years earlier.

All three of the framed pictures hanging on the office walls were of the Towers and of the 9/11 nightmare: a night photograph of the New York skyline with the twin beams of light commemorating the Towers not long after the attack, a *Remember the Heroes, September 11, 2001* framed poster picturing the Towers adorned with the colors of the American flag, and a framed artist's rendition of a police officer and a firefighter arm-in-arm inside a cloud of smoke above the Towers entitled *Always Honored, Never Forgotten, New Jersey State PBA.*

Propped up on the small window ledge was an article from the local newspaper, the *Asbury Park Press*, laminated onto a wood frame with the title, "Cop Calls on 9/11 Families and Helps." And resting atop the office desk was a glass and chrome clock given by FAVOR, a local volunteer group born in the aftermath of 9/11 (see page 259), with an inscription commemorating this same person for *Leadership and Initiative That Lead to Our Success.* Still somewhere else in this office was a Middletown *Employee of the Year* plaque honoring its occupant for his work in the year after 9/11.

The recipient of these honors and the keeper of all these memories is Joe Capriotti, currently Detective Lieutenant and Commander of the Detective Bureau. It was immediately after 9/11 that then Detective Sergeant Capriotti became the liaison between the police department and the Middletown families of all the victims of the attacks.

Detective Capriotti's job was to contact each of these families with offers of assistance.

A more gruesome series of tasks he assumed, however, included personal visits to notify families of victims whenever body parts had been identified. He performed 12 of these visits over a seemingly never-ending three year period; his last such visit was just days before the third anniversary of 9/11. Notifications then became the responsibility of the New York City Medical Examiner's office. Remains of only 16 of the 37 Middletown residents had been identified by that time.

The Attorney General's Office called for a specific protocol for death notifications; at least two police officers had to knock on the door of the deceased's family, one of whom had to be in uniform, to inform them of the death. Plainclothed Detective Capriotti typically took with him for these visits a uniformed officer, a neighbor, friend, or family member of those to be notified; and a member of the clergy. "Whenever I knocked, most people knew why I was there," Detective Capriotti claimed. Reactions varied among those who allowed him entry into their homes. "Some people could deal with it and didn't want me there, whereas others needed comfort and assistance, like calling a funeral director or the New York City medical examiner for additional assistance."

The reactions of others, however, were varied. Some respondents wanted to grieve privately, while others preferred hours of solace from Capriotti and his entourage before being able to let them go. One diminutive woman threw objects around her living room, including Capriotti and the parish priest when they attempted to calm her rage over the news of her loss.

At the time of the attacks, Detective Capriotti was a 44-year-old detective in his 19th year with the Middletown police force and in his 34th year as a township resident. A former little league coach and a frequent visitor to the local scholastic sporting events, he was quite familiar with the town's children and families. His identity around town, however, changed with the events of 9/11. Suddenly, he was no longer the coach or the team supporter, but instead the bearer of tragic news. "It's tough being remembered for the most traumatic event in your life," he claimed, sensing that those he knew before 9/11 looked at him differently now.

Capriotti undertook his responsibilities to the Middletown victims' families seriously, as documented by the accolades described above. Calling it "my proudest accomplishment in my 25 years as a police officer," he began this task in earnest. He became a partner with a grassroots group of "helpers" (see the next section) who banded together after the Towers fell to take care of the town's families.

MIDDLETOWN'S FAVOR ANSWERS THE CALL

It was the unforeseen response to the Boys Scouts' car wash, scheduled for the Saturday after the attacks, that got at least one Middletown resident thinking about what else she could do to help. Janet Dluhi, a scout leader in the local troop, thought that the car wash might be a fitting way for the Scouts to respond to the events of 9/11 by raising some money to donate to the American Red Cross. What she didn't anticipate, however, were the spontaneous donations that customers made to the Scouts that Saturday morning for the wash; contributions in the amounts of $10 and $20 rather than the more typical $5 were common. The Scouts also collected four donations of $100 that day.

Just under a mile from the car-wash site, Dluhi also commissioned other Scouts to man the entrance to the local donut shop to go "canning," the practice of soliciting donations, for the Red Cross effort. "People were just throwing money at us," Dluhi claimed; "Women would stop and kiss the kids and thank them for their work." The Scouts collected over $4,000 in just a few hours. It was as if the donators' generosity was the direct response to the attacks. Dluhi mused about the reason for such largesse, "Everybody felt so helpless, so they needed to do something. Giving was their way of doing something." With people in such a giving mood, she thought, it might be easy to raise money for the Middletown victims' families. And so it began.

Soon after the car wash, Dluhi ran into her friend Alysson Gilbert at the local health club. It didn't take long for the pair to come up with an idea to help the families of the 9/11 victims by capitalizing on this spirit of giving. Gilbert's business acumen from her years as a Certified Public Accountant and management consultant helped with the organizational aspect of what was to follow. Before long, Middletown's FAVOR was born, Friends Assisting Victims Of terroR. Friends Laura Wilton, Tracy Rogers, and Ellen Ruane soon joined the group, as did the chief of police, a state senator, and the superintendent of the Middletown schools. They decided that perhaps FAVOR could do more than just raise money for the families, the amount of which might not be substantial enough to make a difference. Rather, the group chose to provide goods, services, and money to those families according to need. "We wanted to restore those little things that make a difference, like pizza on Fridays; we wanted to keep normalcy as much as possible," Gilbert said. FAVOR's mission statement was clear. It stated, in part:

> Middletown's Friends Assisting Victims Of terroR is a not-for-profit organization created to help those residents of Middletown who have lost an immediate family member as a result of the horrific attack on the World Trade Center on September 11, 2001. It is our mission to provide our beneficiaries with services, goods, and monetary assistance donated by local businesses, Middletown residents, and other friends. We cannot bring back their loved ones. However, we hope to assist them so that they may continue in their normal lifestyle.

So off to local businesses and to other families and individuals the four FAVOR founders went asking for donations. Pizzerias donated gift certificates for pizzas, hardware stores provided tools and equipment for typical household repairs, clothing stores gave clothing, and local markets donated gift certificates and food supplies of all kinds. Families also received free counseling, financial and accounting services, memberships to a local health club, art classes, dry cleaning, and even an hour of massage therapy. The State Association of REALTORS even offered to pay three months rent or three months mortgage for the families.

Local community folk gave time and labor: They mowed the families' lawns, raked their fallen leaves, fixed their leaky roofs, shoveled snow from their porches and driveways, and ran all kinds of errands for them. Others gave according to their own specialty areas of interest: The captain of the nearby charter fishing boat took the surviving children of the victims to sea and taught them how to fish, a family with a house at the shore offered it to families for vacation time, the contractor refinished both bathrooms in the home of a 9/11 widow, and the local train enthusiast known for his elaborate model train display opened his home for a special showing and party for the families just before Christmas. The volunteers numbered 150 in all.

As word of FAVOR's existence spread, "FAVOR became the funnel of many donations from around the world and the country," Gilbert explained. "We couldn't envision what happened." Holidays brought yet more giving: turkeys and turkey dinners, more money, and toys galore. Gilbert recalled one family who drove four hours from their home in Pennsylvania to drop off teddy bears they had made for the families, only to turn around and return home without availing themselves of Gilbert's offer of hospitality after their ride. There also was the quilting club in Florida that made quilts for all the children in town who lost their parents.

The mayor, the police chief, and the chief financial officer from the town of Middletown, Virginia, arrived in town with a check for $10,100 for FAVOR; almost half the amount came from their community's yard sale, with the rest coming from a matching donor and assorted other contributors. In all, FAVOR collected between $200,000 and $300,000, according to Gilbert. Capriotti guessed that the value of the goods and services donated reached $500,000.

When asked why people were so generous, Gilbert echoed Dluhi's thoughts, "Giving makes people feel good. When you have no control, at least you can do something." FAVOR's efforts did not go unnoticed. The group was a recipient of one of New Jersey's Ramapo College's annual *Russ Berrie Award for Making a Difference*, a financial award "to recognize unsung heroes for New Jersey who made a significant difference to the well-being of their community." FAVOR used the $2500 award to fund a social gathering of the 150 volunteers and the surviving members of the 9/11 victims' families, the first time that both groups had ever been together as one.

MIDDLETOWN AND FAVOR WORKING TOGETHER

The process by which FAVOR offered these various donations to the town's families was an organized one. Gilbert, the Executive Director, and her other four FAVOR members each took primary responsibility for an equal number of the families to be served by the organization. "We each became advocates for our families," Gilbert said. "This way we got to know the families, and the families depended on us; there was a big connection." These core members each made from six to eight visits to their assigned families, sometimes to deliver a package of donated goods, sometimes just to respond to a phone call to visit and talk.

The group then created an introductory letter explaining FAVOR's mission and purpose along with an application form for any family wishing to be recipients of FAVOR's largesse. The application itself included questions pertaining to the names and ages of the surviving children as well as a checklist of the types of goods and services useful to each family. One woman from FAVOR, in the company of both Capriotti and the Chief of Police, visited the homes of the families and presented the paperwork to them.

All but one family completed the application to begin its participation in the program. Once received, the FAVOR members set about the task of matching those donated services, monies, and materials to the indicated areas of need on the application forms. Gilbert's basement, filled to the brim with boxes and packages of all kinds, became the base of operations for the distribution effort. She and her friends each created packages for the seven or eight families assigned to their care, lobbying each other for certain items that best fit their families' needs.

There was typically more than just one delivery per family; Thanksgiving and the Christmas seasons brought more donations to FAVOR for these families and yet more deliveries. Despite the clause in its mission statement that "FAVOR will exist for a very limited duration, up to six months," the group was unable to abide by this timeline. Well after this six-month period, donations continued to arrive, Gilbert claimed, some Easter-related gifts, beach-related paraphernalia for the upcoming summer season, and still more money. Each anniversary of the event also brought in donations. "You can't walk away from this now," someone said to the FAVOR members who made the last donations to the families a full five years later.

Some of the last checks given to the families remained uncashed. One recipient didn't take it but used it to send her son's friend to college instead. Capriotti's connection to FAVOR remained strong. As he prepared to make his own visits to families to notify them that their members' body parts had been identified, he always called FAVOR first. "Is there anything I should know about the family?" he asked.

Almost seven years later, the community's response to the attacks are literally written in stone; the memorial garden dedicated to the victims contains 37 granite stones, one per victim, emblazoned with their names and images along with a brief description provided by the surviving spouses or other family members. The experience, however, lingers. Gilbert and Dluhi recall the days of FAVOR tearfully, while Capriotti still sits in his office among various reminders of that day. From time to time he thinks that it's time to remove them and move on. "I looked at them the other day and said to myself, 'Maybe it's time to take them down,' but then I said, 'Nah!'"

A PARISH RISES UP TO HELP

Eileen Theall, a volunteer and a helper both, was at a loss to explain how she became involved in the recovery effort in Middletown. A registered nurse with a career of service to others, Theall served as the head of the Parish of St. Mary's Nursing Ministry for a few years before the attacks of 9/11. The parish was a busy one, the largest in the diocese, serving over 4,000 families. It was just such a position that placed her in the forefront of the parish response to the tragedy, a parish that lost 26 members that day.

The Parish of St. Mary had opened a 24-hours-a-day, seven-days-a-week Adoration Chapel just four years prior to 9/11; two parish volunteers were present in the chapel in one-hour increments all throughout the daytime and evening. The 100-seat chapel was open to anyone, parishioner or not, who wanted some time in silence to reflect or to pray. In the wee hours of a typical early morning, only a small handful of individuals tended to be present. And then came 9/11.

Attendance changed dramatically immediately after the news of the attacks; the number of people at the chapel increased to a "standing room only' crowd all day and night. Some sat or stood in silence and prayed, some sobbed uncontrollably, and others stoically tried to hold back tears. The overwhelming turnout was a surprise to Theall and to the parish clergy. Stunned by this unanticipated mass outpouring of grief, Theall and others thought that they should do more to assist with the emotional recovery of the community. Although she remains unclear to this day who first proposed the idea, she and others made the decision to open up a crisis center.

The chapel itself was adjacent to the former parish convent, a building that once housed as many as forty nuns. With declining numbers of the religious sisters over the years, however, the building had lain vacant and unused for some time. It consisted of a large, open community room with a kitchen area, and a long, narrow corridor that provided access to many small, dormitory-like rooms that were once homes for the nuns. This setting, Theall and others thought, would serve quite well as the site for the 24-hours-a-day, seven-days-a-week crisis center they envisioned.

"We all got together and said, 'We have to have some place for people to go, some place for people to talk,'" Theall recalled. And so this vacant space became the busiest crisis center in town for the next month. Theall put calls out to community members with professional training: psychologists, counselors, nurses, art therapists, and social workers. There was nary a moment for the next thirty days when there was not one or more of these helpers available to the center visitors whenever they stopped by, regardless of the hour. The community room served as the site of informal group counseling and support, while the smaller rooms accommodated those wishing for a more private setting for their expressions of grief. Approximately 50 people visited the center each day, Theall claimed, "and sometimes more." This number was Theall's best guess at the turnout, since "We kept no records; it was so unplanned, we just did it."

There were those friends and family members of the deceased who came, and there also were those who "just wanted to be around familiar people, they wanted reassurance," added Theall. In they came, sitting in groups with others or engaged in one-to-one encounters with one of the counselors. They offered support to others and gained support themselves. Many were repeat visitors; others were one-timers only. The center itself had a nonstop flow of visitors in the days immediately following the tragedy.

Just as the staff was discussing chipping in some money of their own to buy pizza for the visitors and staff members that first night, food arrived. Unsolicited and unexpected, individuals from the community dropped off trays of hot and cold food. These food donations went on throughout the life of the crisis center; one woman made a delivery of breakfast at 5:00 a.m. each day, and others made similar daily donations at lunch- and dinner-time. Most of the food was dropped off by anonymous donors. "At no point did we put out one penny," Theall recalled.

As word of the center spread, more people came. The volunteer staff also kept a watchful eye on the visitors to the Adoration Chapel, ushering those more visibly bereaved individuals into the crisis center. Soon community members began referring friends and neighbors to the center as well. As time passed and as the community returned to some sense of normalcy, the crisis center closed its doors. What continued for several years, however, was an ongoing support group for the spouses and other family members of those lost in the attacks, staffed by some of the volunteer counselors from the crisis center. The number eventually dwindled from the initial group of 14 members as some moved away and others "got their lives back," Theall said.

When asked to reflect on the experience, Theall had no explanation as to how it all started. "It's hard to explain," she said, "We were in awe. We never knew that this would happen. We all just did what had to be done at the time." She was equally unsure about why people help out in times of crisis; she posed, "It's just what people have to do; people are kind and care for other people. They want to help, it's as simple as that."

As simple as that.

RECOMMENDATIONS FOR CHAPTER ENRICHMENT

SUGGESTED FILMS

9/11 (2002) Hosted by actor Robert De Niro, this documentary film chronicles the attack on the Twin Towers in New York's World Trade Center. The reactions of the firefighters who were first responders are showcased as much in this film as were the actual minute-by-minute events of the day.

World Trade Center (2006) The film is the true story of two Port Authority policemen, John McLoughlin and William Jimeno, who were among the last saved from Ground Zero, and of their rescuers. The themes of courage, persistence, and personal resilience mark this film.

Triumph Over Disaster: The Hurricane Andrew Story (1993) In August of 1992, Hurricane Andrew, the most destructive U.S. hurricane on record, pummeled southern Florida with winds of 164 miles an hour. Twenty-nine people died, and property damage in three states reached almost $27 billion. This film examines the lives of several people affected by the storm and their attempts at recovery.

SUGGESTED ACTIVITIES

1. Log onto the Federal Emergency Management Agency website (www.fema. org) and find the listing of all emergencies to which FEMA has responded. What kind of crises prompted its involvement?

2. Hurricane Katrina devastated the better part of New Orleans. Even though there are parts of the city that are uninhabitable to this day, investigate those agencies that contributed goods and services to its recovery.

3. Make a list of local community groups, agencies, or organizations on a countywide level in your area that provide volunteer opportunities for its citizens. Categorize them according to the services they provide and the volunteer opportunities offered for people like you.

Case Book References

**Chapter 1 Crisis Intervention:
An Introduction**

Athey, J., & Moody-Williams, J. (2003). *Developing cultural competence in disaster mental health problems: Guiding principles and recommendations*. Washington, DC: U.S. Department of Health and Human Services.

Brammer, L. M. (1985). *The helping relationship: Process and skills* (3rd ed.). Upper Saddle River, NJ: Prentice Hall.

Brock, S. E. (2002). Crisis theory: A foundation for the comprehensive school crisis response team. In S. E. Brock, P. J. Lazarus, & S. R. Jimerson (Eds.) *Best practices in school crisis prevention and intervention*. Bethesda, MD: National Association of School Psychologists.

Brock, S. E., Nickerson, A. B., Reeves, M. A., Jimerson, S. R., Lieberman, R. A., & Feinberg, T. A. (2009). *School crisis prevention and intervention: The PREPaRE model*. Bethesda, MD: National Association of School Psychologists.

Caplan, G. (1964). *Principles of preventative psychiatry*. New York: Basic Books.

Carkhuff, R. (1969). *Helping and human relations: A primer for lay and professional helpers*. New York: Holt, Rinehart, & Winston.

Carlson, E. B. (1997). *Trauma assessments: A clinician's guide*. New York: Guilford Press.

Cavaiola, A., & Colford, J. (2006). *A practical guide to crisis intervention*. Boston: Houghton Mifflin Company.

Erikson, E. (1963). *Childhood and society* (2nd ed.). New York: Norton Press.

Fraser, J. S. (1998). A catalyst model: Guidelines for doing crisis intervention and brief therapy from a process view. *Crisis Intervention and Time-Limited Treatment, 4*, 159–177.

Rogers, C. (1951). *Client-centered therapy: Its current practice, implications, and theory*. Boston: Houghton Mifflin Company.

Saylor, C. F., Belter, R., & Stokes, S. J. (1997). Children and families coping with disaster. In S. A. Wolchik & I. N. Sandler (Eds.), *Handbook of children's coping: Linking theory and intervention*. New York: Plenum Press.

Young, M. (2001). *Victim assistance: Frontiers and fundamentals*. Washington, DC: National Organization for Victim Assistance.

Chapter 2 Child Maltreatment

Cavaiola, A., & Colford, J. (2006). *A practical guide to crisis intervention.* Boston: Houghton Mifflin Company.

Eigsti, I., & Cicchetti, D. (2004). The impact of child maltreatment on expressive syntax at 60 months. *Developmental Science, 7,* 88–102.

Fromm, S. (2001). *Total estimated cost of child abuse and neglect in the United States: Statistical evidence.* Chicago, IL: Prevent Child Abuse America.

Grych, J. H., Jouriles, E. N., Swank, P. R., McDonald, R., & Norwood, W. D. (2000). Patterns of adjustment among women of battered children, *Journal of Consulting and Clinical Psychology, 68,* 84–94.

Kolko, D. J. (2002). Child physical abuse. In J. B. Myers, L. Berliner, J. Briere, C. T. Hendrix, C. Jenny, & T. A. Reid (Eds.), *The APSAC handbook on child maltreatment.* Thousand Oaks, CA: Sage.

Mash, E. J., & Dosois, D. J. A. (2003). Child psychopathology: A developmental-systems perspective. In E. J. Mash & R. A. Barkley (Eds.), *Child psychopathology* (pp. 3–71).

McConaughy, S. (2005). *Clinical interviews for children and adolescents: Assessment to intervention.* New York: The Guilford Press.

National Center on Shaken Baby Syndrome. (2005). *All about shaken baby syndrome (SBS) and abusive head trauma (AHT).* Retrieved from: http://www.dontshake.org/sbs.php.

Prevent Child Abuse America (2006). *Annual report: Winds of change.* Chicago, IL: Author.

Runyan, D., Wattam, C., Ikeda, R., Hassan, F., & Ramiro, L. (2002). Child abuse and neglect by parents and other caregivers. In Krug, E., Dahlberg, L., Mercy, J. A., Zwi, A. B., & Lozano, R. (Eds.), *World report on violence and health.* Geneva, Switzerland: World Health Organization. Retrieved from: www.who.int/violence_injury_prevention/violence/global_campaign/en/chap3.pdf.

Sedlak, A. J., & Broadhurst, D. D. (1996). *Third national incidence study of child abuse and neglect: Final report.* Washington, D.C.: U.S. Department of Health and Human Services.

U.S. Department of Health and Human Services (DHHS), National Center on Child Abuse and Neglect. (2005). *Child maltreatment 2005.* Washington, D.C.: U.S. Government Printing Office.

U.S. Department of Health and Human Services, Administration for Children and Families. (1974). *The child abuse prevention and treatment act.* Washington, D.C.: U.S. Government Printing Office.

Weis, R. (2008). *Abnormal child and adolescent psychology.* Thousand Oaks, CA: Sage Publications.

Wekerle, C., & Wolfe, D. A. (2003). Child maltreatment. In E. J. Mash and R. A. Barkley (Eds.), *Child psychopathology.* New York: Guilford.

Chapter 3 Adolescent Crises

Anorexia and Related Eating Disorders Inc. (2004). *Statistics: How many people have eating disorders?* Retrieved May 15, 2007 from www.anred.com/stats.html

Berman, A., Jobes, D., & Silverman, R. (2006). *Adolescent suicide: Assessment and intervention* (2nd ed.). Washington, DC: American Psychological Association.

Bowman, S., & Randall, K. (2004). *See my pain! Creative strategies for helping young people who self-injure.* Chapin, SC: Youthlight, Inc.

Brock, S. E., Sandoval, J., & Hart, S. (2006). Suicidal ideation and behaviors. In G. G. Bear & K. M. Minke (Eds.), *Children's needs III: Development, prevention, and intervention.*

Bethesda, MD: National Association of School Psychologists.

Carnegie Foundation (1995). *Great transitions: Preparing adolescents for a new century*, p. 1. Carnegie Corporation of New York.

Center for Disease Control and Prevention (CDC). (2005). *Web-based injury statistics query and reporting system.* National Center for Injury Prevention and Control.

Elkind, D. (1967). Egocentrism in adolescence. *Child Development, 38*, 1025–1034.

Favazza, A. R. (1998). The coming of age of self-mutilation. *Journal of Nervous and Mental Disease, 186*, 259–268.

Froeschle, J., & Moyer, M. (2004). Just cut it out: Legal and ethical challenges in counseling students who self-mutilate. *Professional School Counseling, 7*, 231–236.

Havighurst, R. (1972). *Developmental tasks and education.* Essex, England: Longman Group United Kingdom.

Kaiser Family Foundation. (2003). *National survey of adolescents and young adults: Sexual health knowledge, attitudes, and experiences.* Menlo Park, CA: Henry J. Kaiser Family Foundation.

Kalafat, J., & Lazarus, P. (2002). Suicide prevention in schools. In S. Brock, P. Lazarus, & S. Jimerson (Eds.), *Best practices in school crisis prevention and intervention.* Bethesda, MD: National Association of School Psychologists.

Kress, V., Gibson, D., & Reynolds, C. (2004). Adolescents who self-injure: Implications and strategies for school counselors. *Professional School Counseling, 7*, 195–202.

Kroger, J. (2000). *Identity development: Adolescence through adulthood.* Thousand Oaks, CA: Sage.

Levenkron, S. (1998). *Understanding and overcoming self-mutilation.* New York: W.W. Norton & Co.

Lieberman, R. (2004). Understanding and responding to students who self-mutilate. *National Association of Secondary School Principals: Principal Leadership, 4*(7), 10–13.

Lieberman, R., Poland, S., & Cassel, R. (2008). Best practices in suicide intervention. In A. Thomas & J. Grimes (Eds.), *Best practices in school psychology V.* Bethesda, MD: The National Association of School Psychologists.

Marcia, J. (1994). The empirical study of ego identity. In H. Bosma, T. Graasfma, H. Grotebanc, & D. DeLivita (Eds.), *The identity and development.* Newbury Park, CA: Sage.

McVey-Noble, M. E., Khemlani-Patel, S., & Neziroglu, F. (2006). *When your child is cutting: A parent's guide to helping children overcome self-injury.* Oakland, CA: New Harbinger Publications.

Polivy, J. & Herman, C. P. (2002). Causes of eating disorders. *Annual Review of Psychology, 53*, 187–213.

Popenoe, D. & Whitehead, B. (2005). *The state of our unions: The social health of marriage in America.* New Brunsuick, NJ: National Marriage Project.

Rice, F. P. & Dolgin, K. G. (2008). *The adolescent: Development, relationships, and culture* (12th ed.). New York: Allyn & Bacon.

Ross, H. & Heath, N. (2002). A study of the frequency of self-mutilation in a community sample of adolescents. *Journal of Youth and Adolescence, 31*, 209–217.

Seligman, M. (1998). *Learned optimism.* New York: Pocket Books.

Smolak, L. (2005). Eating disorders in girls. In D. J. Bell, S. L. Foster, & E. J. Mash (Eds.), *Handbook of behavioral and emotional problems in girls* (pp. 463–487). New York: Kluwer Academic.

Steinberg, L. (2005). *Adolescence* (7th ed.). New York: McGraw Hill.

Suyemoto, K. & Kountz, X. (2002). Self-mutilation. *The Prevention Researcher,* 7, 4.

Tozzi, F., Thornton, L., Klump, K., Fichter, M., Halmi, K., & Kaplan, A. (2005). Symptom fluctuation in eating disorders: Correlates of diagnostic crossover. *American Journal of Psychiatry,* 162, 732–740.

U.S. Center for Disease Control and Prevention. (2005). *Youth risk behavior surveillance survey.* Washington, D.C.: Government Printing Office.

U.S. Department of Health and Human Services. (2006). *Monitoring the future; National results on adolescent drug use.* Investigators: Institute for Social Research: University of Michigan.

Winkler, K. (2003). *Cutting and self-mutilation: When teens injure themselves.* Berkeley Heights, NJ: Enslow Publishers.

Woolfolk, A. (2007). *Educational Psychology* (10th Ed.) Boston, MA: Pearson Education, Inc.

Zila, L., & Kiselica, M. (2001). Understanding and counseling self-mutilation in female adolescents and young adults. *Journal of Counseling and Development,* 29, 46–52.

Chapter 4 Crisis at Midlife

American Association of Retired Persons. (2004). *The divorce experience: A study of divorce at midlife and beyond.* Washington, D.C.: Author.

American Association of Retired Persons. (2004). *Boomers at midlife: The AARP life stage study.* Washington, D.C.: Author.

Brim, O. (1992). *Ambition: How we manage success and failure throughout our lives.* New York: Basic Books.

Ciernia, J. R. (1985). Myths about male midlife crises. *Psychological Reports, 56,* 1003–1007.

Jacques, E. (1965). Death and the mid-life crisis. *International Journal of Psychoanalysis, 46,* 502–514.

Jung, C. G. (1933). *Modern Man in Search of a Soul.* New York: Harcourt, Brace, & World.

Lachman, M. (2001). *Handbook of midlife development.* New York: Wiley.

Lachman, M. (2004). Development in midlife. *Annual Review of Psychology, 55,* 305–31.

Levinson, M. (1986). A conception of adult development. *American Psychologist, 41,* 3–13.

Levinson, D., Darrow, C., Klein, E., Levinson, M., McKee, B. (1978). *The seasons of a man's life.* New York: Knopf.

National Council on Aging. (2000). *Myths and realities: 2000 survey results.* Washington, D.C.: Author.

Neugarten, B. L. (1968). Adult personality: Toward a psychology of the life cycle. In B. L. Neugarten (Ed.), *Middle age and aging: Reader in social psychology* (pp. 137–147). Chicago: University of Chicago Press.

Sheehy, G. (1995). *New passages.* New York: Random House Publishing.

Shek, D. T. (1996). Mid-life crisis in Chinese men and women. *Journal of Psychology, 130,* 109–119.

U.S. Census Bureau. (2000).

Wethington, E., Kessler, R., & Pixley, J. (2004). Turning points in adulthood. In O. Brim, C. Ryff, & R. Kessler (Eds.), *How healthy we are: A national study of well-being in midlife.* Chicago: University of Chicago Press.

Chapter 5: Intimate Partner Violence & Domestic Violence

Bureau of Justice. (2009). Victim Characteristics. Washington, DC: U.S. Department of Justice, Office of

Justice Programs. Retrieved from: http://www.ojp.usdoj.gov/bjs/intimate/victims.htm

Edleson, J. L. & Tolman, R. M. (1992). *Intervention for men who batter.* Newbury Park, CA: Sage Publishers.

Evans, P. (1992). *The verbally abusive relationship.* Holbrook, MA: Adams Media Corporation.

Jacobson, N. & Gottman, J. (1998). *When Men Batter: New insights into ending abusive relationships.* New York: Simon and Schuster.

Roberts, A. R. (1998). Crisis intervention: A practical guide to immediate help for victims families. In A. Horton & J. Williamson (Eds.), *Abuse and religion.* (p. 606). Lexington, MA: D. C. Heath.

Schreder, C. (Producer), & Greenwald, R. (Director). (1995). *The burning bed.* (Motion Picture). United States: Anchor Bay Entertainment.

Sonkin, D. J., & Durphy, M. (1993). *Learning to live without violence* (3rd ed.). San Francisco, CA: Volcano Press.

Sontag, D. (2002, Nov. 17). Fierce entanglements. *New York Times.*

Tolman, R. M. (1989). The development of a measure of psychological maltreatment of women by their male partners. *Violence & Victims, 4,* 159–177.

Walker, L. (1980). *The battered woman.* New York: Harper & Row.

Walker, L. (1994). *Abused women and survivor therapy.* Washington, D.C.: American Psychological Association.

Walker, L. (1994b). *The abused woman: A survivor therapy approach.* Manual & Video, New York: Newbridge Communications Inc.

Walker, L. (2000). *The battered woman syndrome* (2nd ed.). New York: Springer Publishing Co.

Chapter 6 Sexual Assault

Bohner, G. (1998). *Rape myths.* Landau, Germany: Verlag Empirische Padagogik.

Cavaiola, A., & Colford, J. (2006). *A practical guide to crisis intervention.* Boston: Houghton Mifflin Company.

Kendall, P., & Hammen, C. (1998). *Abnormal psychology: Understanding human problems.* Boston: Houghton Mifflin Company.

Malamuth, N. M., & Check, J. (1983). Sexual arousal to rape depictions: Individual Differences. *Journal of Abnormal Psychology, 92,* 55–67.

Men Against Sexual Assault. (1998). *Test your knowledge.* University of Rochester: Author. Retrieved January 3, 2008, from http://sa.rochester.edu/masa/truefalse.php.

National Center for Victims of Crimes. *Sexual assault.* Washington, DC: Author. Retrieved December 12, 2007, from http://www.ncvc.org/ncvc/main.aspx.

Odem, M. E., & Clay-Warner, J. (1998). *Confronting rape and sexual assault.* Wilmington, DE: Scholarly Resources, Inc.

Rape, Abuse, and Incest National Network. *Statistics.* Washington, D.C.: Author. Retrieved December 12, 2007, from http://www.rainn.org/statistics/index/html

Scully, D. (1990). *Understanding sexual violence: A study of convicted rapists.* Boston: Unwin Hyman, Inc.

U.S. Department of Justice. (2001). *National violence against women survey.* Washington, D.C.: Author.

U.S. Department of Justice. (2004). *A national protocol for sexual assault medical forensic examinations.* Washington, D.C.: Author.

U.S. Department of Justice (2005). *National crime victimization survey.* Washington, D.C.: Author.

Chapter 7 Alcohol and Drug Crises

Anthony, J. C., Warner, L. A. & Kessler, R. C. (1997). Comparative epidemiology of dependence on tobacco, alcohol, controlled substances, and inhalants: Basic findings from the National Comorbidity Survey. In G. A. Marlatt & G. R. VandenBos (Eds.). *Addictive Behaviors: Readings on Etiology, Prevention and Treatment*, Washington, D.C.: American Psychological Association (pp. 3–39).

Conway, K. P., Compton, W., Stinson, F. S., & Grant, B. F. (2006). Lifetime co-morbidity of DSM-IV mood and anxiety disorders: Results from the National Epidemiologic Survey on alcohol and related conditions. *Journal Clinical Psychiatry, 67*, 247–257.

Drug Abuse Warning Network (DAWN) (2006). National estimates of drug-related emergency department visits. U.S. Department of Health & Human Services, Substance Abuse and Mental Health Services Administration, http://DAWNinfo.samhsa.gov

Gentilello, L. M., Ebel, B. F., Wickizer, T. M., Salkever, D. S., & Rivara, F. P. (2005). Alcohol interventions for trauma patients treated in emergency departments and hospitals: A cost benefit analysis. Annals of Surgery, 241, 541–550.

Hesselbrock, M. N., & Hesselbrock, V. (1992). Relationship of family history, antisocial personality disorder and personality traits in young men at risk for alcoholism. *Journal of Studies on Alcohol, 53*, 619–625.

Johnson, V. (1980). *I'll Quit Tomorrow: A practical guide to alcoholism treatment*. San Francisco, CA: HarperCollins.

Merikangas, K. R. (1990). The genetic epidemiology of alcoholism. *Psychological Medicine, 20*, 11–22.

Milzman, D. P. & Soderstrom, C. A. (1994). Substance use disorders in trauma patients. *Critical Care Clinics, 10*, 595–612.

Schuckit, M. A., & Smith, T. L. (1997). Assessing the risk for alcoholism among sons of alcoholics. *Journal of Studies on Alcohol, 58*, 141–145.

Steinglass, P., Bennett, L. A., Wolin, S. J., & Reiss, D. (1987). *The alcoholic family*. New York: Basic Books.

Substance Abuse & Mental Health Services Administration. (2002). Office of Applied Statistics. *2001 National Household Survey on Drug Abuse*. Retrieved from: www.samhsa.gov.

Trezza, G. R., & Scheft, H. (2009). Contemporary issues in the evaluation and management of alcohol and drug related crises. In Kleespies, P. M. Behavioral emergencies: An evidence-based resource for evaluating and managing risk of suicide, violence and victimization. Washington, DC: American Psychological Association.

Chapter 8 Psychiatric Crises

American Psychiatric Association. (2004). *Diagnostic and statistical manual of mental disorders* (4th ed., Text Revision). Washington, D.C.: American Psychiatric Assocation Press.

Asaad, G. (1995). *Understanding mental disorders due to medical conditions or substance use: What every therapist should know*. New York: Brunner/Mazel.

Bohen, S. (2002, June). *Psychiatric emergencies*. PESI Healthcare LLC., Eau Claire:

Carlson, J., Chemtob, C., Rusnak, K., Hedlund, L., & Muraoka, M. (1998). Eye movement desensitization and reprocessing (EMDR) treatment for combat-related posttraumatic stress disorder. *Journal of Traumatic Stress, 11*, 3–24.

Cornelius, J. R., Soloff, P. H., Perel, J. M., & Ulrich, R. F. (1993). Continuation pharmacotherapy of borderline personality disorder with haloperidol and phenelzine. *American Journal of Psychiatry, 150*, 1843–1848.

Freeman, A., & Fusco, G. (2000). Treating high-arousal patient: Differentiating between patients in-crisis and crisis-prone patients. In F. M. Dattilio & A. Freeman (Eds.). *Cognitive-behavioral strategies in crisis intervention*. New York: Guilford Press.

Horowitz, M. J. (1985). Disasters and psychological response to stress. *Psychiatric Annals, 15*, 161–167.

Kessler, R. C., Chiu, W. T., Demler, O., & Walters, E. E. (2005). Prevalence, severity, and co-morbidity of twelve-month DSM-IV disorders in the National Co-Morbidity Survey Replication (NCS-R). *Archives of General Psychiatry, 62*, 617–627.

Linehan, M. M. (1995). Treating borderline personality disorder: The dialectical approach (Program Manual) New York: Guilford Press.

Maxmen, J. S., & Ward, N. G. (1995). *Essential psychopathology and its treatment* (2nd ed.). New York: W. W. Norton & Co.

Murphy, M. D., & Moller, M. F. (1997). The three R's rehabilitation program: A prevention approach for the management of relapse symptoms associated with psychiatric diagnoses. *Psychiatric Rehabilitation Journal, 20*(3), 42–49.

Reiger, D. A., Narrow, W. E., Rae, D. S., Manderscheid, R. W., Locke, B. Z., & Goodwin, F. K. (1993) The de facto U.S. mental and addictive disorder delivery system. Epidemiologic Catchment Area prospective 1 year prevalence rates of disorders and services. *Archives of General Psychiatry, 50*, 85–94.

Robins, L. E. & Reiger, D. A. (Eds.). (1991). *Psychiatric Disorders in America: The Epidemiological Catchment Area Study*. (pp. 343–350). New York: Free Press.

United States Department of Health & Human Services. (2002). *Statistics on mental health*. Washington, D.C.: U.S. Government Printing Office.

Wolpe, J. (1982). *The practice of behavior therapy*. New York: Pergamon Press.

World Health Organization. (2004). The World Health Report 2004: Changing history. Annex Table 3. Burden of disease in DALYs by cause, sex and mortality stratum in WHO regions, estimates for 2002. Geneva: World Health Organization.

Chapter 9 Health Crises

Bachmann, L. P., Cooney, R., Schute, C. (Producers) & Badham, J. (Director). (1981). *Whose life is it anyway?* (Motion Picture). United States: Metro Goldwyn Mayer.

Beck, A. T. (1976). *Cognitive therapy and the emotional disorders*. New York: International Universities Press.

Bellak, L., & Siegel, H. (1983). *Handbook of intensive brief and emergency psychotherapy*. Larchmont, NY: CPS, Inc.

Bernal, G. (1982). Cuban families. In M. McGoldrick, J. K. Pearce, & J. Giordano (Eds.). *Ethnicity and family therapy*. New York: Guilford Press.

Centers for Disease Control & Prevention. (2009). Leading causes of death. http://www.cdc.gov/nchs/fastats/lcod.htm

DeWolfe, D. J. (2000). *Field manual for mental health and human service workers in major disasters*. Government Printing Office, DHHS Publication No. (ADM) 90–537.

DiTomasso, R. A., Martin, D. M. & Kovnat, K. D. (2000). Medical patients in crisis. In F. M. Dattilio & A. Freeman (Eds.). *Cognitive-Behavioral strategies in crisis intervention*. New York: Guilford Press.

Harwood, A. (1982). Mainland Puerto Ricans. In A. Harwood (ed.) *Ethnicity and medical care*. Cambridge, MA: Harvard University Press.

Landers, S. (2000, Aug. 28). The world's healthcare: How do we rank? Retrieved from: www.amednews.com.

McGoldrick, M. (1982). Irish families. In M. McGoldrick, J. K. Pearce, & J. Giordano (Eds.) *Ethnicity and family therapy*. New York: Guilford Press.

Ragucci, A. T. (1982). Italian Americans. In A. Harwood (Ed.) *Ethnicity and medical care*. Cambridge, MA: Harvard University Press.

Wegscheider, S. (1981). *Another chance: Hope and health for the alcoholic family*. Palo Alto, CA: Science & Behavior Books.

Chapter 10 Bereavement Crisis

Anthony, J. C., & Petronis, K. R. (1991). Suspected risk factors for depression among adults 18-44 years old. *Epidemiology, 2,* 123–132.

Beck, A. T., Wright, F. D., Newman, C. F., & Liese, B. S. (1993). *Cognitive therapy of substance abuse*. New York: Guilford Press.

Cantor, C. H., & Slater, P. J. (1995). Marital breakdown, parenthood, and suicide. *Journal of Family Studies, 1,* 91–104.

Dershimer, R. A. (1990). *Counseling the bereaved*. New York: Pergamon Press.

Furman, E. (1974). *A child's parent dies: Studies in childhood bereavement*. New Haven, CT: Yale University Press.

Gallo, J. J., Royall, D. R., & Anthony, J. C. (1993). Risk factors for the onset of depression in middle age and later life. *Social Psychiatry & Psychiatric Epidemiology, 28,* 101–108.

Granvold, D. K. (2000). The crisis of divorce: Cognitive-behavioral and constructivist assessment and treatment. In A. R. Roberts (Ed.) *Crisis intervention handbook: Assessment, treatment and research*. New York: Oxford University Press.

Kubler-Ross, E. (1969). *On death and dying*. New York: Macmillan.

Rando, T. A. (1984). Grief, dying and death: Clinical interventions for caregivers. Champaign, IL: Research Press.

Trovato, F. (1986). The relationship between marital dissolution and suicide: The Canadian case. *Journal of Marriage and the Family, 48,* 341–348.

United Nations Secretariat. (1996). *Demographics yearbook*. Department for Economic and Social Information and Policy Analysis, Statistical Division, United Nations. New York:

Weitzman, J. L. (1985). *The divorce revolution: The unexpected social and economic consequences for women and children in America*. New York: Free Press.

Weissman, M. M., Bruce, M., Leaf, P., Florio, L., & Holzer, C. (1991). Affective disorders. In L. Robins & E. Reiger (Eds.), *Psychiatric disorders in America* (pp. 53–80). New York: Free Press.

Suggested Readings

Boss, P. (1999). *Ambiguous loss: Learning to live with unresolved grief*. Cambridge, MA: Harvard University Press.

Bowlby, J. (1980). *Attachment and loss: Loss, sadness and depression,* (*Vol. III*), New York: Basic Books.

Donnelly, K. F. (2001). *Recovering from the loss of a child*. New York: Dodd, Mead & Co.

Edelman, H. (1994). *Motherless daughters*. New York, NY: Delta Press.

Gates, P. (1990). *Suddenly alone: A woman's guide to widowhood*. New York: Harper Perennial.

Huntley, T. (1991). *Helping children grieve*. Minneapolis, MN: Augsburg.

James, J. W., & Friedman, R. (2001). *When children grieve*. New York: HarperCollins.

Kubler-Ross, E. (1969). *On death and dying*. New York: Macmillan.

Kushner, H. S. (1981). *When bad things happen to good people.* New York: Avon Press.

Parks, C. M., & Weiss, R. S. (1983). *Recovery from bereavement.* New York: Basic Books.

Chapter 11 Crises Involving Suicide & Homicide

Andrews, J. A., & Lewinsohn, P. M. (1992). Suicidal attempts among older adolescents: Prevalence and co-occurrence with psychiatric disorders. *Journal of the American Academy of Child & Adolescent Psychiatry, 31,* 655–662.

Allen, N. H. (1983). Homicide followed by suicide: Los Angeles, 1970–1979. *Suicide & Life Threatening Behavior, 13,* 155–165.

Blumenreich, P. E. & Lewis, S. J. (1993). *Managing the violent patient: A clinician's guide.* Philadelphia, PA: Brunner/Mazel.

Bohen, S. (2002, June). *Psychiatric emergencies.* PESI Healthcare LLC. Eau Claire, WI:

Bradford, J. M. W., Greenberg, D. M., & Motayne, G. G. (1992). Substance abuse and criminal behavior. *Psychiatric Clinics of North America, 15,* 605–622.

Brecher, M., Wang, B. W., Wong, H., & Morgan, J. P. (1988). Phencyclidine and violence: Clinical and legal issues. *Journal of Clinical Psychopharmacology, 8,* 397–401.

Cavaiola, A. A., & Schiff, M. (1988). Behavioral sequalae of sexual and/or physical abuse in chemically dependent adolescents. *Child Abuse & Neglect, 12,* 181–188.

Centers for Disease Control. (1998). Suicide among black youths: United States, 1980–1995. *MMWR, 47*(10).

Chu, J. A. (1999). Trauma and suicide. In D. G. Jacobs (Ed.) *The Harvard Medical School guide to suicide assessment and intervention.* San Francisco: Jossey Bass.

Crisis Prevention Institute. (1999). Nonviolent crisis intervention: A practical approach for managing violent behavior. *Violence Prevention Resource Center.* Retrieved from: www.crisis-prevention.com.

Copeland, A. R. (1985). Dyadic death revisited. *Journal of the Forensic Science Society, 25,* 181–188.

Currens, S., Fritsch, T., Jones, D. et al. (1991). Homicide followed by suicide: Kentucky 1985–1990. *MMWR, 40,* 652–653, 659.

Dinwiddie, S. W. (1994). Abuse of inhalants: A review. *Addiction, 89,* 925–929.

Dorpat, T. L. (1966). Suicide in murderers. *Psychiatry Digest, 27,* 51–55.

Frierson, R. L., Melikian, M., & Wadman, P. C. (2002). Principles of suicide risk assessment. *Postgraduate Medicine, 112* (3), Retrieved from: www.postgradmed.com/issues/2002/09_02/frierson4.htm

Garrison, C. Z., McKeown, R. E., & Valois, R. F. (1993). Aggression, substance use and suicidal behaviors in high school students. *American Journal of Public Health, 83,* 179–184.

Hanzlick, R., & Koponen, M. (1994). Murder-suicide in Fulton County, Georgia, 1988–1991. *American Journal of Forensic Medical Pathology, 15,* 168–173.

Hare, R. D. (1993). *Without conscience: The disturbing work of psychopaths among us.* New York: Guilford Press.

Klassen, D. & O'Connor, W. A. (1988). A prospective study of predictors of violence in adult male mental health admissions. *Law & Human Behavior, 12,* 143–158.

Kochanek, K. D., Murphy, S. L., Anderson, R. N., & Scott, C. (2004). Deaths: Final data for 2002. *National Vital Statistics Reports.* 2004 Oct 12: *53*(5), 1–115.

Linehan, M. M. (1999). Standard protocol for assessing and treating suicidal behaviors. In D. G. Jacobs (Ed.) *The Harvard Medical School guide to suicide assessment and intervention.* San Francisco: Jossey Bass.

Litwack, T., Kirschner, S., & Wack, R. (1993). The assessment of dangerousness and prediction of violence: Recent research and future prospects. *Psychiatric Quarterly, 64,* 245–273.

Madson, L. & Vas, C. (2003). Learning risk factors for Suicide: A scenario-based activity. *Teaching of Psychology, 30,* 123–126.

Malley, P. B., Kush, F., Bogo, R. J. (1994) School-based adolescent suicide prevention and intervention programs: A survey. *The School Counselor, 42,* 130–136.

Maltsberger, J. T. (1992). The psychodynamic formulation: An aid in assessing suicidal risk. In R. W. Maris, A. L. Berman, J. T. Maltsberger, & R. T. Yufit (Eds.) *Assessment and prediction of suicide* (pp. 362–380). New York: Guilford Press.

Maris, R. W. (1992). The relationship of nonfatal suicide attempts to completed suicides. In R. W. Maris, A. L. Berman, J. T. Maltsberger, & R. T. Yufit (Eds.) *Assessment and prediction of suicide* (pp. 362–380). New York: Guilford Press.

Marzuk, P. M., Tardiff, K., & Hirsch, C. S. (1992). The epidemiology of murder-suicide. *Journal of the American Medical Association, 267,* 3179–3183.

Maxmen, J. S. & Ward, N. G. (1995). *Essential psychopathology and its treatment* (2nd ed.). New York: W. W. Norton & Co.

McNeil, D., & Binder, R. (1991). Clinical assessment of risk of violence among psychiatric inpatients. *American Journal of Psychiatry, 148,* 1317–1321.

Meloy, J. (1987). The prediction of violence in outpatient psychotherapy. *The American Journal of Psychotherapy, 41,* 38–45.

Monahan, J. (1995). *The clinical prediction of violent behavior.* Northvale, NJ: Jason Aronson.

Mulvey, E., & Lidz, C. (1995). Conditional prediction: A model for research on dangerousness to others in a new era. *International Journal of Law & Psychiatry, 18,* 129–143.

National Institute of Mental Health. (2009). The numbers count: Mental Disorders in America. Retrieved from: www.nimh.gov/health/publications/the-numbers-count-disorders-america.htm.

National Center for Health Statistics. (1998). *Vital statistics in the United States 47*(9). Washington, D.C.: U.S. Government Printing Office.

National Center for Health Statistics. (2001, Oct. 11). Suicide as a leading cause of death by Age, Race and Sex: 1999. *National Vital Statistics Report, 49*(11). Retrieved from: www.cdc.gov/nchs/fastats/suicide.htm.

National Institute of Mental Health. (2002). Suicide facts. Retrieved from: www.nimh.gov/research/suifact.htm. April 8, 2002.

Nock, M. K., & Marzuk, P. M. (1999). Murder-suicide: Phenomenology and clinical implications. In D. G. Jacobs (Ed.) *The Harvard Medical School guide to suicide assessment and intervention.* San Francisco: Jossey Bass.

Palmer, S., & Humphrey, J. A. (1980). Offender-victim relationships in criminal homicide followed by offender's suicide, North Carolina, 1972–1977. *Suicide & Life Threatening Behavior, 10,* 106–118.

Pope, H. G., & Katz, D. L. (1990). Homicide and near-homicide by anabolic steroid users. *Journal of Clinical Psychiatry, 51,* 28–31.

Pope, H. G., & Katz, D. L. (1994). Psychiatric and medical effects of anabolic-androgenic steroid use: A controlled study of 160 athletes. *Archives of General Psychiatry, 51,* 375–382.

Reed, B. J., & May, P. A. (1984). Inhalant abuse and juvenile delinquency: A control study in Albuquerque, New Mexico. *International Journal of Addictions, 19,* 789–803.

Schneidman, E. (1985). *Definition of suicide.* New York: Wiley.

Schneidman, F. (1999). Perturbation and lethality: A psychological approach to assessment and intervention. In D. G. Jacobs (Ed.) *The Harvard Medical School guide to suicide assessment and intervention.* San Francisco: Jossey Bass.

Shaffer, D. A., Gould, M. S., & Hicks, R. C. (1994). Worsening suicide rates in black teenagers. *American Journal of Psychiatry, 151,* 1810–1812.

Slovic, P., & Monahan, J. (1995). Probability, danger and coercion: A study of risk perception and decision making in mental health law. *Professional Psychology: Research & Practice, 26,* 499–506.

Sontag, D. (2002, April 28). A suicide at M.I.T.: *In loco parentis* is dead. Is that why Elizabeth Shin is, too? *New York Times,* Section 6, 57–61.

Tarasoff v. Board of Regents of the University of California, 551 P2d 334(1976).

Truscott, D., Evens, J., & Mansell, S. (1995). Outpatient psychotherapy with dangerous clients: A model for decision making. *Professional Psychology: Research & Practice, 26,* 484–490.

Tsuang, M. T., Fleming, J. A., & Simpson, J. C. (1999). Suicide and schizophrenia. In D.G.Jacobs (Ed.) *The Harvard Medical School guide to suicide assessment and intervention.* San Francisco: Jossey Bass.

Warner, E. A. (1993). Cocaine abuse. *Annals of Internal Medicine, 119,* 226–235.

Weiss, R. D. & Hufford, M. R. (1999). Substance abuse and suicide. In D. G.

Jacob (Ed.) *The Harvard Medical School guide to suicide assessment and intervention.* San Francisco: Jossey Bass.

Chapter 12 School Crisis: Prevention and Intervention

American Psychological Association Zero Tolerance Task Force (2008). Are zero tolerance policies effective in the schools? An evidentiary review and recommendations. *American Psychologist, 63,* 852–862.

Athey, J., & Moody-Williams, J. (2003). *Developing cultural competence in disaster mental health problems: Guiding principles and recommendations.* Washington, D.C.: U.S. Department of Health and Human Services.

Brock, S. (2003). Crisis theory: A foundation for the comprehensive crisis prevention and intervention team. In S. Brock, P. Lazarus, & S. Jimerson (Eds.), *Best Practices in School Crisis Prevention and Intervention* (pp. 5–17). Bethesda, MD: National Association of School Psychologists.

Brock, S. E. (2006). *Crisis intervention and recovery: The roles of school-based mental health professionals.* (Available from National Association of School Psychologists, 4340 East West Highway, Suite 402, Bethesda, MD 20814).

Brock, S. E., Nickerson, A. B., Reeves, M. A., Jimerson, S. R., Lieberman, R. A., & Feinberg, T. A. (2009). *School crisis prevention and intervention: The PREPaRE model.* Bethesda, MD: National Association of School Psychologists.

Brock, S., Sandoval, J., & Lewis, S. (2001). *Preparing for crises in schools: A manual For building school crisis response teams.* New York: John Wiley.

Brooks, K., Schiraldi, V., & Ziedenberg, J. (2000). School house hype: Two years later. Washington, D.C.: Justice Policy Institute/Children's Law Center.

Cavaiola, A., & Colford, J. (2006). *A practical guide to crisis intervention.* Boston: Houghton Mifflin Company.

Cornell, D.G. (2006). *School violence: Fears versus Facts.* Mahwah, NJ: Lawrence Erlbaum Associates.

DeVoe, J. F., Peter, K., Noonan, M., Snyder, T. D., & Baum, K. (2005). *Indicators of school crime and safety: 2005.* U.S. Departments of Education and Justice. Washington, D.C.: U.S. Government Printing Office.

Jimerson, S. R., & Huff, L. C. (2002). Responding to a sudden, unexpected death at School: Chance favors the prepared professional. In S. E. Brock, P. J. Lazarus, & S. R. Jimerson (Eds.), *Best practices in school crisis prevention and intervention* (pp. 449–487). Bethesda, MD: National Association of School Psychologists.

Moscicki, E. K. (1995). Epidemiology of suicidal behavior. *Suicide and Life-Threatening Behavior, 25,* 22–35.

National Institute of Mental Health. (2004). *Suicide in the U.S.: Statistics and prevention.* Washington, D.C.: Author.

Pagliocca, P. M., Nickerson, A. B., & Williams, S. (2002). Research and evaluation directions in crisis intervention. In S. E. Brock, P. J. Lazarus, & S. R. Jimerson (Eds.), *Best practices in school crisis prevention and intervention* (pp. 771–791). Bethesda, MD: National Association of School Psychologists.

Paine, C. (1998, November). Tragedy response and healing: Springfield unites. *NASP Communique, 27*(3), 16–17.

Pitcher, G., & Poland, S. (1992). *Crisis intervention in the schools.* New York: The Guilford Press.

Poland, S., & Gorin, S. (2002). In S. Brock, P. Lazarus, & S. Jimerson (Eds.) *Best Practices in School Crisis Prevention and Intervention* (pp. 5–17).

Bethesda, MD: National Association of School Psychologists.

Poland, S., & McCormick, J. (1999). *Coping with crisis: Lessons learned.* Longmont, CO: Sopris West.

Reddy, M., Boram R., Berglund J., Vossekuil B., Fein R., & Modzeleski, W. (2001). Evaluating risk for targeted violence in schools: Comparing risk assessment, threat assessment, and other approaches. *Psychology in the Schools, 38,* 157–172.

Sandoval, J., & Lewis, S. (2002). Cultural considerations in crisis intervention. In S. Brock, P. Lazarus, & S. Jimerson (Eds.) *Best Practices in School Crisis Prevention and Intervention* (pp. 5–17). Bethesda, MD: National Association of School Psychologists.

Underwood, M., & Dunne-Maxim, K. (1997). *Managing sudden traumatic loss in the schools.* Piscataway, NJ: University of Medicine and Dentistry of New Jersey.

U.S. Department of Education. (2006). *Indicators of school crime and safety: 2006.* Washington, D.C.: Author.

U.S. Secret Service and the U.S. Department of Education. (2002). *The final report and findings of the safe school initiative: Implications for the prevention of school attacks in the United States.* Washington, D.C.: Author.

Young, M. (2002). The community crisis response team: The national organization for victim assistance protocol. In S. Brock, P. Lazarus, & S. Jimerson (Eds.), *Best Practices in School Crisis Prevention and Intervention* (pp. 5–17). Bethesda, MD: National Association of School Psychologists.

Chapter 13 Crises in the Workplace

Andrews, E. (2008, March 8th). Sharp drop in jobs adds to grim economic picture. *New York Times.*

Armstrong-Stassen, M. (1993). "Survivors" reactions to a workforce reduction: A comparison of blue-collar workers and their supervisors. *Canadian Journal of Administrative Sciences, 10*, 334–343.

Bohen, S. (2002). *Psychiatric emergencies*. Eau Claire, WI: PESI Healthcare LLC.

Bureau of Justice Statistics. (2009). Workplace violence. U.S. Dept. of Justice Press Release. Retrieved from: www.ojp.usdoj.gov/bjs/pub.

Cavaiola, A., & Lavender, N. (1999, March). Personality disorders in the workplaces: Arc we driving each other crazy. Paper presented at Work, Stress and Health APA-NIOSH Conference, Baltimore, MD.

Cavaiola, A. A., & Lavender, N. J. (2000). *Toxic Co-Workers: How to deal with dysfunctional people in the workplace.* Oakland, CA: New Harbinger Publications.

Eggen, D. & Ferdinand, P. (2000, Dec. 26). 7 die in Massachusetts office shooting. *Washington Post*, Washington, D.C.

Eggen, D. & Ferdinand, P. (2000, Dec. 27). Major shootings in the workplace since 1995. *Washington Post*, Washington, D.C.

Eisenberg, P. & Lazarsfeld, P. E. (1938). The psychological effects of unemployment. *Psychological Bulletin, 39*, 358–390.

Ellis, A. (1952). *Reason and emotion in psychotherapy.*

Gilbert, B. (Producer), & Higgins, C. (Director). (1980). *Nine to Five*, (Motion picture), United States: 20th Century Fox.

Hickok, T. A. (2000, Nov.). Downsizing and organizational culture. Retrieved from: www.pamij.com/hickok.html

Johnson, K. (2004, July 4). Death toll rises to six in workplace shooting. New York Times, pp. Section 1, Page 10.

Kaufman, H. G. (1982). *Professionals in search of work.* New York: John Wiley & Sons.

Leana, C. & Feldman, D. C. (1992). *Coping with job loss: How individuals, organizations and communities respond to layoffs.* New York: Lexington Books.

Levinson, H. (1994). Why the behemoths fell: Psychological roots of corporate failure. *American Psychologist, 49*, 428–436.

Lewis, G. W. & Zare, N. C. (1999). Workplace hostility: Myth and Reality. Philadelphia, PA: Taylor & Francis Co.

Maiuro, R. D. (1998, Oct. 4). Murder becoming a real job hazard. *Newsday*, Long Island, NY.

Mohrman, S. A., & Mohrman, A. M. Jr. (1983). Employee involvement in declining organizations. *Human Resources Management, 22*, 445–465.

New York Times (1996). *The downsizing of America.* New York: Time Books.

Noer, D. (1993). *Healing the wounds: Overcoming the trauma of layoffs and revitalizing downsized organizations.* San Francisco, CA: Jossey-Bass.

Rayner, C. (2000) Bullying research: Global Allies Bullying At Work, Survey Report – UNISON (UK union), Campaign Against Workplace Bullying, P.O. Box 1886, Benicia, CA 94510.

Rotenberg, M. (Producer), & Judge, M. (1999). *Office Space*, (Motion picture). United States: 20th Century Fox.

Sexual Harassment: Fact v. Myth. (1994). Retrieved from: www.wsu.edu/~ twl/horizon/rights/sexual/ harassfact.html.

Talbot, M. (2002, Oct. 13). Men behaving badly. *New York Times.*

Toufexis, A. (1994, April 25). Workers who fight firing with fire. *Time*, pp. 337.

Suggested Readings:

Cavaiola, A. A., & Lavender, N. J. (2000). *Toxic Co-Workers: How to deal with Dysfunctional People in the Workplace.*

Oakland, CA: New Harbinger Publications.

Levinson, H. (1994). Why the behemoths fell: Psychological roots of corporate failure. *American Psychologist, 49,* 428–436.

Lewis, G. W., & Zare, N. C. (1999). *Workplace hostility: Myth and reality.* Philadelphia, PA: Taylor & Francis Co.

Noer, D. (1993). *Healing the wounds: Overcoming the trauma of layoffs and re-vitalizing downsized organizations.* San Francisco, CA: Jossey-Bass.

Woodward, H. & Buchholz, S. (1987). *Aftershock: Helping people through corporate change.* New York: John Wiley & Sons (Wilson Learning Corp.).

Chapter 14 Community Response to Crisis

Bureau of Labor Statistics (2006). *Volunteering in the United States, 2006.* Washington, D.C.: Author.

Cavaiola, A., & Colford, J. (2006). *A practical guide to crisis intervention.* Boston: Houghton Mifflin Company.

Clary, E., Snyder, M., Ridge, R., Copeland, J., Stukas, A., Haugen, J., & Miene, P. (1998). Understanding and assessing the motives of volunteers: A functional approach. *Journal of Personality and Social Psychology, 74,* 1516–1530.

Dluhi, J., Gilbert, A., Wilton, L., Rogers, T., & Ruane, E. (2001). *Middletown's FAVOR: Our mission.* Middletown, NJ: Authors.

Finkelstein, M. (2007). Correlates in satisfaction in older volunteers: A motivational perspective. *The International Journal of Volunteer administration, 24,* 6–12.

Independent Sector. (2001). *A survey of charitable giving after September 11, 2001.* Washington, D.C.: Author.

National Volunteer Organizations Active in Disaster. (2002). *Preventing a disaster within the disaster: The effective use and management of unaffiliated volunteers.* Arlington, VA: Author.

Sheehy, G. (2005). *Middletown, America: One town's passage from trauma to hope.* New York: Random House.

Index

362.1968
C376

123873

LINCOLN CHRISTIAN UNIVERSITY

3 4711 00202 5619